Encyclopedia of Health and Aging

The Complete Guide to Well-Being in Your Later Years

Evelyne Michaels

438

health and hygiene

PRIMA PUBLISHING

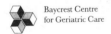
Baycrest Centre
for Geriatric Care

Originally published in Canada as *Look to This
Day—A Complete Guide to Health and Well-
Being in Your Later Years* by Key Porter Books
Limited.

Illustrations © Angela Vaculik

Photographs: © Barros and Barros (p. 91, large
photo); © Gary Beechey p. 58, 59, 122, 123, 190,
191); © David W. Hamilton (p. 16, small photo);
© Ken Huang (p. 256, small photo); © HMS Images
(p. 90, small photo); © Janeart Ltd. (p. 232, small
photo); © Pat Lacroix (p. 233, large photo);
© Margaret W. Peterson (p. 17, large photo); © Jay
Silverman (p. 176, small photo); © Bill Varie (p. 176,
large photo); © Weinberg Clark (p. 257, large photo)

**Library of Congress Cataloging-in-
Publication Data**

Michaels, Evelyne.
   [Look to this day]
   Encyclopedia of health and aging: com-
plete guide to well-being in your later years /
Evelyne Michaels.
           p.   cm.
   Originally published in 1995 under the
title: Look to this day: a complete guide to
health and well-being in your later years.

   Includes index.

   ISBN 0-7615-0856-2

   1. Aged—Health and hygiene. 2.

Aged—Diseases. 3. Aged—Life skills guides.

4. Aging. I. Title.
RA777.6.M53 1997
613 '.0438—dc21   96-37274
                                        CIP

97 98 99 00 01 DD 10 9 8 7 6 5 4 3 2 1

Printed in the United States of America

Permissions: Salaried Live-in Helper Agreement and
The Demographics of Caregiving reprinted with per-
mission of The Free Press, a Division of Simon &
Schuster Inc., *Taking Care of Aging Family
Members: A Practical Guide, Revised and
Expanded Edition* by Wendy Lustbader and Nancy
R. Hooyman. Copyright © 1994 by Wendy
Lustbader and Nancy Hooyman. Copyright
© 1986 by The Free Prees.
   The Stress Test reprinted from *The Book of
Tests* by Dr. Michael Nathenson. Copyright
© 1984, 1985 by Dr. Michael Nathenson. Published
by Viking Penguin Inc.
   Selection by Dr. Seuss from *You're Only Old
Once* by Dr. Seuss. Trademark™ and Copyright © by
Dr. Seuss Enterprises, L.P. Reprinted by permission
of Random House, Inc.

How to Order

Single copies may be ordered from Prima Publishing, P.O. Box 1260BK, Rocklin, CA 95677; telephone
(916) 632-4400. Quantity discounts are also available. On your letterhead, include information concerning the
intended use of the books and the number of books you wish to purchase.

Visit us online at http://www.primapublishing.com

Contents

For my remarkable mother, Edith Michaels

And in loving memory of my father, Sam Michaels

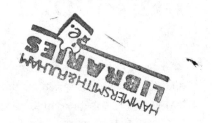

Look to this day!

For it is life, the very life of life.

In its brief course lie all the varieties and
realities of your existence.

The bliss of growth;

The glory of action;

The splendor of beauty:

For yesterday is already a dream
and tomorrow is only a vision;

But today, well-lived, makes every yesterday

A dream of happiness, and every tomorrow
a vision of hope.

FROM THE SANSKRIT

Foreword

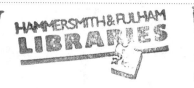

As a geriatrician, I am used to answering many questions every day, questions brought to me by my elderly patients and their families: "Dr. Gordon, will I get better?" "Dr. Gordon, why is this happening to my mother?"

These questions are often challenging, and there may not be any satisfactory answers – a reality that is sometimes difficult to accept, for doctors and patients alike.

When the publisher of this book asked me to provide some answers, I was relieved that the questions were so straightforward: "Why should there be a special book on health and well-being in life's later years?" and "Why should people be confident about information that comes from Baycrest Centre for Geriatric Care?"

Until recently, relatively little attention was paid to the unique needs and wishes of those in later life. But during the past decade, all this has changed. Those over age 65 – whether they are called "seniors" or "elders" or simply "older people" – have become a force to be reckoned with.

While they have always been an integral and important part of our social fabric, their growing presence has finally convinced those who provide care and service that they deserve equal – even special – consideration and treatment.

Over the past 75 years, Baycrest Centre has developed a unique expertise in helping older adults and their families. Besides providing care to elders, we have also learned a great deal about the strength, tenacity and wisdom of this population.

Baycrest Centre has always drawn on the knowledge and skill of its professional staff: the nurses, doctors, social workers, therapists, psychologists, nutritionists and countless others who interact with more than 2,000 older people each day, both within our facilities and out in the community. But we have also made a special effort to listen to the older people whom we serve, since they have always been the best teachers.

Unlike many other books directed to the public, this one doesn't focus on medical care in the traditional meaning of the term. While the importance of medical concerns is not denied here, an attempt has been made to present the information in a much fuller context.

The *Encyclopedia of Health and Aging* assumes that older people are, by and large, as vigorous and concerned about maintaining their health as the younger population. It also assumes that older people can take control of their health and well-being, rather than waiting passively to be "cared for" by others. In harmony with the Baycrest Centre philosophy, it recognizes that, even when the years take their toll and we are assaulted by illness or frailty, we can still find strength and purpose in our lives.

We hope that the information presented here will prompt enquiry, understanding and security. Our ultimate goal is to give you confidence and courage, and thus allow you to make the best health and health care decisions for yourself and older members of your family.

Michael Gordon, M.D. FRCP(C)
Head of Geriatric and Internal Medicine,
Baycrest Centre for Geriatric Care
Professor of Medicine, University of Toronto

Preface

When my grandmother was born nearly 100 years ago, I'm sure she never expected to reach age 97 with most of her physical and mental faculties intact. After all, she lived much of her life in a world where antibiotics, multivitamins and low-fat diets didn't exist.

What seems especially remarkable is that my grandmother survived to the end of her tenth decade without taking major responsibility for her own health. She never exercised, she ate what she pleased (including plenty of butter!) and she had no real hobbies or outside interests. She rarely went for a physical checkup, never had a mammogram, and was never seriously ill, except for the time when she had her gallbladder removed at age 70. She finally died in hospital, several months after falling out of bed and fracturing her hip.

By now you must be wondering why this story appears in a book aimed at helping you take a more active role in maintaining your health as you grow older. After all, if my grandmother lived until age 97 without making much of an effort to preserve her health, why should you bother?

My grandmother's longevity could be explained in several ways. She was a very strong woman, who never allowed life's misfortunes to get her down – she survived the rigors of immigration from Russia, the Depression, a chronically ill husband and the tragic death of her only son at an early age. Two other factors probably contributed to her long life: good luck and good genes.

By good luck, I mean that she escaped

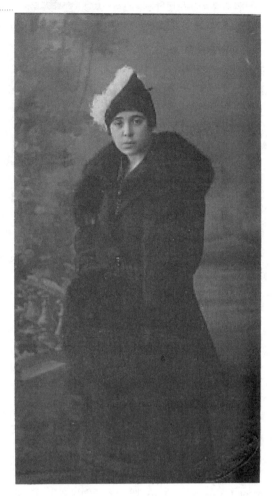

The author's grandmother, Sarah Lena Cantor, age 18, circa 1914

being struck by a streetcar and wasn't exposed to a serious infection before the advent of antibiotics. As for good genes, it's known that some diseases – for example, certain types of Alzheimer's disease and cancer – tend to run in families. If you don't inherit the gene for such ailments, you are likely to live longer than someone who does. But besides inheriting a tendency toward illness, you may also inherit a tendency toward longevity. Scientists who study the biology of aging now believe that the rate at which our cells age and our bodies decline is an astonishingly complex process involving hundreds or even thousands of genes.

Experts estimate that we have a maximum lifespan of between 100 and 120 years, but until recently, very few of us could even dream of reaching those outer limits. Now, thanks to social and medical progress, more of us are living longer. There are now about 3,700 Canadians aged 100 years or more – three times as many as there were 20 years ago – and statisticians predict that the number of centenarians will double in the next two decades.

Ask yourself this question: If you could live to be 100 years old, would you want to? Most of us would probably say, "Of course – as long as my quality of life was good."

If my grandmother didn't actively preserve her own health, it was partly because she expected that someone else – her husband, her adult children or a professional caregiver – would look after her when she finally became sick. But this attitude is changing. If you have adult children, they may certainly care *about* you, but they may not be able to care *for* you. Today many families are split by geography, divorce or the demands of two-career marriages. Because of this, and because they're more educated about health than most people in my grandmother's generation, many older adults have decided they must take up the challenge of self-care.

What is self-care?

It means that you must assume a great deal of responsibility for your life and well-being, even if you're already suffering from acute or chronic health problems. Others – a spouse or adult child, your doctor or pharmacist – can certainly help, but you shouldn't depend on them completely.

It means not taking your health for granted and refusing to accept such symptoms as pain, depression, fatigue and memory loss simply as "part of getting old." Very few illnesses or conditions are caused solely by advancing years, and while not every ache, pain or problem can be cured, many can be diagnosed and significantly improved.

It means honestly evaluating your current situation and educating yourself about certain risk factors for disease. You can do this by talking to your doctor and other health care professionals, by taking an interest in health-related news stories and television programs, and by reading this book.

The elegant dancer and actor Fred Astaire once said: "Old age is like everything else. To make a success of it, you've got to start young."

In fact, it's never too late to start.

Acknowledgments

"Always write about things you know," one of my teachers used to say.

I thought about her advice when I first sat down to write this book on health and well-being for older adults. Considering that I'm not a doctor and am barely in my forties, it seemed a bit presumptuous at the time. With help, I think I've managed to overcome these initial disadvantages and hope that older readers, their families, and caregivers will approve.

Support and encouragement have come from many people and places.

My sincere thanks to the professional staff at Baycrest Centre for Geriatric Care in Toronto, Ontario. Over its remarkable 75-year history, Baycrest has done more than simply serve those who need it. It has provided service in a particular context, where aging is not seen as an enemy, and where older women and men are treated with the respect and dignity each of us deserves.

In particular I would like to thank Jennifer Schipper, Moshe Greengarten, and Stephen W. Herbert for their trust in me and their commitment to this project. I am also grateful to the dedicated medical and professional staff whose names and credentials appear at the end of the book. Special thanks to Dr. Paula Rochon, Dr. Michael Gordon, Dr. Morris Freedman, Dr. David Conn, Carol Robertson, Shayna Alpern, Etta Ginsberg-McEwan, Sorele Urman, Margaret Mac-Adam, Rabbi Norman Berlat, Blossom Wigdor, Dr. Victor Marshall, Dr. Rory Fisher, Judy Chu and members of the Wellness Education Group at the Joseph E. and Minnie Wagman Centre.

I would also like to thank Sylvia Teaves and Dr. Donald Stuss for generously providing me with a home at the Rotman Research Institute of Baycrest Centre during the writing of this book.

Thanks to my editor Laurie Coulter for her thoughtful pruning of the material and her many excellent suggestions. My gratitude and admiration also extend to Anna Porter, whose excellent instincts told her that as the population ages, her readers are growing older and they will demand reliable, accurate information about aging well.

I must also thank some personal sources for their support and encouragement: Pat Dickinson, Cindy Weiner, Diana Thomson, Daniela Teti, Dr. Harvey Kaplovitch, Rhonda Katz, and my brother, Dr. George Michaels.

Special thanks to David Nayman, who entered my life 24 years ago as my very first editor. He now plays the dual role of husband and editor, a challenging job that he performs superbly.

Finally, to my sons, Adam and Matthew Nayman – I hope that by the time you are both "old enough" to need this book or one like it, many of the problems that faced your parents and grandparents in their later years will no longer exist.

Introduction

Age wins and one must learn to grow old.

LADY DIANA COOPER

Why a special book on health care for people over 65?

Even before Dr. Benjamin Spock wrote his complete guide to baby and child care more than 50 years ago, it was widely accepted that the health problems and concerns of young children differ vastly from those of adults.

Parents take their children to family doctors and pediatricians who have been specially educated about healthy physical and emotional development during childhood, and who have detailed knowledge about diagnosing and treating illnesses in infants and children. For example, they know that certain drugs aren't recommended for children and that dosages must be tailored to a child's specific needs. Good child-oriented family doctors and pediatricians also have a special understanding of and appreciation for their young clients, and years of hands-on experience with tearful toddlers and anxious parents have equipped them with vital communication skills.

In many ways an 80-year-old requires the same kind of sensitive, knowledgable and, at times, specialized health care as an eight-year-old. This is true for many reasons. As you age, your body changes internally as well as externally. You become more prone to certain diseases and conditions. Your symptoms may be quite different from those of a younger person with the same illness. You respond differently to various medications and treatments.

You may also be more vulnerable to negative physical and psychological effects from the change and loss that tend to occur later in life. The chronic illness or death of a spouse may cause depression and loneliness. A new living situation – for example, moving from a house into an apartment or seniors' residence – may create stress. Retirement may lead to feelings of boredom or loss of self-esteem.

Today most older people continue to rely on their family physicians and other health professionals who may have gaps in their training when it comes to age-related issues. While the level of care they receive can be quite satisfactory, older people can still slip through the cracks in a system that isn't geared to recognize and meet their particular needs.

But as people live longer and the ranks of those over 65 continue to swell, this situation is bound to change.

What do we mean by "old"?
Some people believe they're old the moment they turn 65, or when they become grandparents or when they finally retire from their jobs.

Our idea of old age has changed radically

as advances in medical science and improved social conditions (at least in some parts of the world) have extended our average life expectancy. Just a few centuries ago, when infant mortality was common and infectious disease was rampant, people were elderly at 40. Today we consider those who are 40, 50, 60 and even 70 to be relatively young.

"Old" can have many meanings. Is it the number of birthdays you've had (your chronological age) or is it how well your body and mind are holding up? A healthy 75-year-old may be biologically similar to someone 20 years younger. In the same way, a 55-year-old whose body has deteriorated due to illness or neglect may be much older than his or her chronological age.

However, being "old" may have less to do with your body than with your attitudes toward life.

For example, most people would probably consider Eleanor Mills old. The 82-year-old Toronto woman has a severe spinal deformity due to osteoporosis and needs the support of a walker to get around. This amazing lady wanted to increase public awareness of osteoporosis and raise funds for research, so she decided to walk across Canada over a two-year period. Not long ago she reached her goal. If we define old age as a time when we no longer welcome new experiences and challenges, then Eleanor Mills isn't old, despite the fact that she's 82 and suffers from a serious illness.

It's important to keep a balanced view of aging that recognizes that there are potential negative and positive aspects to growing older.

How do people in general feel about aging? See how many of these statements you honestly agree with:

Some negative aspects of aging

◆ You lose your feeling of physical attractiveness (still more of an issue for women than for men, but this is changing);

◆ You lose some of your physical strength;

◆ You become isolated as children grow up and leave home, as a partner dies and as treasured friends pass away;

◆ You become more dependent on family, friends or other helpers;

◆ You feel less productive because of retirement from work;

◆ You may have financial problems because you're on a fixed income;

◆ You feel undervalued by society, which highlights the achievements and culture of the young;

◆ You have a sense that life has passed you by;

◆ You must confront issues around illness and your own death, which gets closer with each passing birthday;

◆ You worry about how your last years will be spent.

Some positive aspects of aging

◆ There are fewer pressures to look young and fit in with society's idea of what is attractive;

◆ If you raised children, you can now begin to focus on your own needs because no one is dependent on you any longer;

◆ You have the chance to give up full-time employment and begin some other work which you've always wanted to do;

◆ You have more free time to pursue interests, hobbies and personal commitments;

◆ You have more time to spend with your partner and/or friends;

◆ You are able to deal with problems by applying the wisdom of lessons learned over many decades of living.

If your perceptions of aging have been formed largely by media images, it's likely that you identify more with the negative aspects of aging. But if you are an older person who has managed to retain a fair degree of physical and emotional health, chances are that you appreciate the positive aspects of growing older.

In fact, these two lists aren't mutually exclusive. Growth, creativity and wisdom can and do exist along with feelings of loneliness and anxiety. To partially quote Forrest Gump, aging – like life – "is a box of chocolates: You never know what you're going to get!"

What do we mean by "healthy"?

Health – which derives from the Anglo-Saxon word "haelth," meaning "safe, sound or whole" – means different things to different people.

In the past you could count yourself healthy if you were free from disease. But more recently we have moved toward a much broader definition of health or wellness: a combination of physical, mental and

The four keys to good health

◆ *Biology*: You haven't inherited genes that make you susceptible to illnesses such as certain cancers, heart disease, Alzheimer's disease and Huntington's disease.

◆ *Lifestyle factors*: A nutritious, well-balanced diet; sufficient exercise and sleep; avoiding the abuse of alcohol, tobacco and other drugs; stress reduction; safer sexual practices; accident prevention.

◆ *Emotional well-being*: Having sound, supportive relationships with other people; feeling good about yourself; feeling that you have some control over your life, that you can deal with important psychological challenges and changes.

◆ *Social and environmental well-being*: Having enough money for adequate food, shelter and health care; having access to clean air and water; being able to socialize adequately for your personality and your needs.

social well-being that allows us to achieve our full potential and leaves us energy to deal with unforeseen crises.

What's the link between aging and health?

There's a perception, especially among younger people, that growing old inevitably leads to sickness, poor functioning, dependency and institutionalization. Unfortunately, this belief causes many of us to dread growing older, and it even affects how some doctors and other health care providers respond to older adults who come to them with specific complaints, for example: "Of course your memory isn't what it used to be," or "Back pain is just part of growing old."

While these situations can and do occur later in life, especially among the very old (those past age 85), they are not synonymous with older age.

A recent survey of more than 10,000 people over 65 disputes the notion that getting older means getting sick:

◆ More than 82 percent of the men and 80 percent of the women rated their health as either "very good" or "pretty good";

◆ 45 percent of the total group said that health problems didn't stop them from doing what they want to do;

◆ Only 12 percent were currently living in institutions.

Your expectations and your ability to cope with changes can also play an important role in whether you perceive yourself to be healthy. Many people with chronic or serious disease such as cancer, osteoporosis and diabetes still say they feel well and continue to enjoy their lives to the fullest.

While it's true that many older people remain relatively healthy for most of their lives, it's also a fact that chronic illnesses such as arthritis, heart disease, and vision and hearing problems are more likely to occur later in life.

In the following chapters you will be given clear, concise information and practical advice that can help you maximize your own chances for health and well-being. These include:

◆ strategies for healthier aging such as making good food and fitness choices;

◆ ways you can participate in your own health care, including how to choose and communicate with your doctors; how to make positive lifestyle changes; how to use medications safely and effectively; how to cope with change and stress; how to make the most of your retirement years; how to stay safe both inside and outside your home;

◆ information and advice about common age-related complaints such as constipation, fatigue, heartburn, palpitations, dizziness and memory problems;

◆ an in-depth look at special health problems that affect older adults, including heart disease, stroke, cancer, arthritis, incontinence, Alzheimer's disease and depression;

◆ special sections "for older women only" and "for older men only" answering common questions and concerns;

◆ common-sense advice on important family matters, such as coping with the illness and death of a partner, grandparenting and getting along with your adult children, and information on issues such as competency and elder abuse;

◆ and finally, vital information about getting help if and when you need it, including how to choose community services; a checklist for selecting a retirement facility or nursing home; advice on how to cope with the anxiety, fear and guilt that often arise during this time; and finally, a section on how to face terminal illness.

The information that follows is presented in a way that assumes that good health is – or certainly should be – the norm for people of any age. Does this mean that you shouldn't expect any sickness and trouble in your later years? Of course not. But as you will learn here, these trials are not an inevitable part of growing older, and you can do a great deal to prepare yourself for what might come.

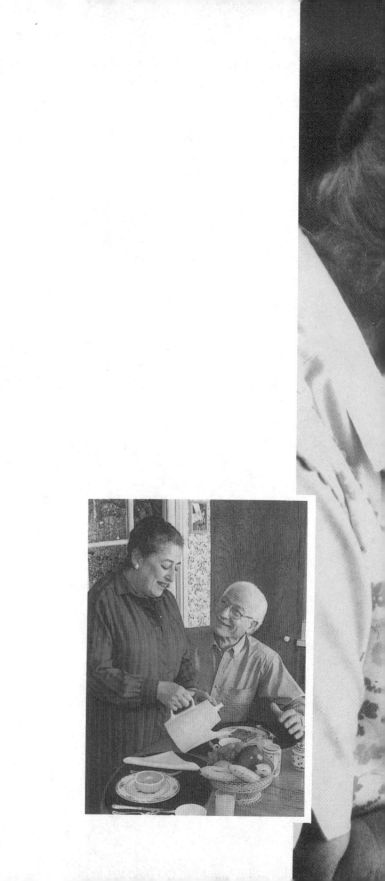

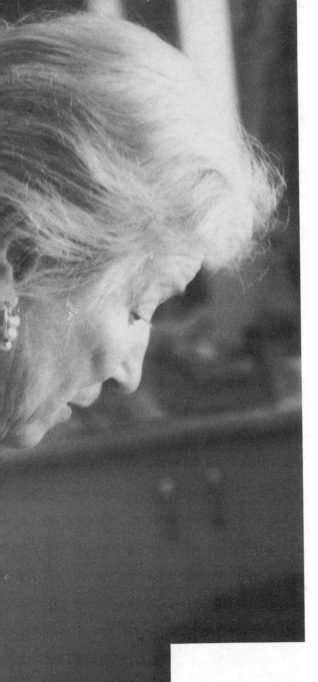

1

A sound mind in a sound body, is a short, but full description of a happy state in this World: he that has these two, has little more to wish for and he that wants either of them, will be little the better for anything else.

JOHN LOCKE

Healthier Aging

IT MAKES SENSE THAT THE BODY OF a healthy 15-year-old is quite different from the body of a healthy 40-year-old. They vary in many ways – nutritional needs, physical and mental stamina, sexual and emotional development. In the same way, your body is quite different today at age 65, 75 or 85 than it was when you were younger.

It's important that you understand how your body is likely to change with normal aging. Such knowledge can be reassuring because it explains how you feel and may prevent you from becoming unduly anxious about certain aspects of your physical and emotional state. You are also better equipped to recognize when you aren't functioning properly for a person of your age and can then seek help from your doctor.

Eating well to live better

He that takes medicine and neglects diet, wastes the skill of the physician.

CHINESE PROVERB

Like most people, you probably feel overwhelmed by the sheer volume of news and advice related to diet and nutrition that appears every day in newspapers and magazines and on television.

Unfortunately, much of this information is still geared to the needs and interests of younger people – for example, advice about how to lose weight. While shedding unwanted and unhealthy pounds is an important health issue for many older people, the fact remains that some of you, especially those over age 75, may have quite the opposite problem: You need to gain weight. When was the last time you saw a magazine article titled "How to Put on 15 Pounds This Summer"?

When it comes to concern about nutrition, most people fall into three basic groups. Where do you belong?

◆ *Those who eat to live:* You've always been interested in healthy eating and have taken an active role in eating the right combination of nutritious foods and maintaining an ideal body weight.

◆ *Those who live to eat:* You haven't paid much attention to your diet and have always eaten pretty much what you please. You have a fatalistic attitude about diet and believe that changing your diet won't have much of an impact on your quality of life.

◆ *The vast majority:* You've tried to eat well but haven't always followed the healthiest possible diet. You may have been a "yo-yo" dieter for most of your life, losing weight by severely limiting your calorie intake, then gaining it back and beginning the whole dismal cycle again. Now that you're older and more concerned about your health, you may feel ready to make changes that could improve your quality of life.

There's no doubt that sensible nutrition is the foundation for better health in your later years. Food is important, not just as a source of sensual and social pleasure, but also as a source of fuel for your body's continued activity and well-being. This body fuel is composed of nutrients that are used to produce energy and other vital substances such as enzymes, immune agents, blood cells and hormones. The main nutrients you get from your diet are carbohydrates (starches and sugars), proteins, fats, water, vitamins and minerals. If you don't get enough of them, your body can't function properly. You may become fatigued, your physical and mental functions may be affected, and you may develop deficiency diseases such as anemia, the result of too little iron in the diet.

It's important to understand that your diet – what kinds of food you eat, how much and how often – is affected by many physical, psychological and social changes that take place as you grow older.

Physical changes

Ways to make eating easier

You may find it harder to chew and swallow because of a natural decrease in saliva flow, which can also make food seem less tasty. Keep fresh water handy for sipping, or try a non-prescription, mouth-moistening spray if your mouth is especially dry. Swallowing may become more difficult because of weakness or reduced coordination in your throat and neck muscles. Make sure you eat sitting in an upright position with your chin slightly forward. If you notice that food is getting stuck often or you cough frequently while eating or drinking, speak to your doctor. Good dental habits are important, too, since chewing and swallowing problems can be caused by missing or diseased teeth, inflamed gums or poorly fitting dentures (see page 114).

Normally food passes directly through your esophagus into your stomach. But a weakening of the sphincter between your esophagus and stomach may allow food to back up, causing that sour-tasting, painful experience known as heartburn. Staying in an upright position for at least an hour or two after meals helps the food move down through your digestive tract.

As you age, your body may become less efficient at absorbing nutrients from food. That's why it's important to eat foods that provide you with high-quality nutrition.

Tickling your taste buds

Those little bumps on your tongue, your taste buds or papillae, may become less effective with age, and this can make your sense of taste less acute. So can decreased saliva flow. You may find it easier to detect sour or bitter tastes, while you need some foods to be a little sweeter in order to enjoy them. Your sense of smell, which plays a major role in how you perceive flavors, may also diminish, and this dulling of senses can make food seem less appetizing.

One way to increase the appeal of food is to use flavor-boosting seasonings such as herbs, spices, tangy lemon juice and vinegar. Adding a modest amount of sugar or honey is also fine, unless your doctor or dietitian has advised you to avoid them.

Finding new ways to manage meals

Your fine coordination can decline with age, and this, combined with arthritis or vision problems, can make it more difficult for you to cook or prepare foods and to handle eating utensils. There are many adaptive devices – special jar openers, plates and utensils designed for easier use, cutting boards that hold foods in place – that can make meal preparation and eating easier for you. These may be available at medical supply houses listed in your telephone directory, or through the rehabilitation department at your local hospital.

If mobility is a problem and you have trouble getting around to shop, try to find a grocery store that takes orders by phone and delivers them free. Or try to arrange a "buddy" system with a more mobile friend or neighbor. Perhaps the friend could shop for you once a week, and in return you could prepare and serve a special dish or meal.

If you find cooking difficult, try out some of the prepackaged frozen "meals" now available at many supermarkets. Be sure to check the labels and choose only those meals that are low in saturated fat and sodium. You can make the meal more nourishing and satisfying by adding a salad, bread and fruit for dessert. You might also consider taking advantage of a community meals program, such as Meals-on-Wheels, which can deliver ready-made nutritious meals right to your door for a fee arranged to fit your budget.

Psychological and social changes

If you are a woman and had growing children to consider when you were younger, you probably spent more time then shopping for a variety of foods and cooking well-balanced meals than you do now. With children grown and gone, there may be less of an incentive for you to think about good nutrition. But it's important to understand that better nutrition is more important to you now than ever before, and by making it a priority, you can minimize health problems and maximize your enjoyment of life.

The loss of a spouse can also have a profound impact on diet and nutrition. Loneliness and grief may cause you to use food as a source of solace, and you may begin to overeat. If this happens, you should consider talking to someone about your feelings and try to replace food with some other kind of comfort or reward – a pot of fresh flowers or some scented bath salts. If you can afford and care for one, a pet can be a wonderful source of companionship and distraction.

The loss of companionship can also have the opposite effect, reducing your desire to shop, cook and eat balanced meals. This can be a special problem for older widowers who relied on their wives to prepare meals, and they may face a serious risk of becoming malnourished. Again, a buddy system – sharing shopping and meal preparation chores with someone else – is worth trying, or you might investigate a basic cooking course where you can learn new skills and meet new friends. If this isn't an option, then a community meal service such as Meals-on-Wheels may be needed.

Your finances can also affect your diet. Some older women who have been widowed or divorced find it difficult to shop for food on a reduced income. You can stretch your food budget by avoiding expensive processed foods, and, if possible, by buying items on sale and in bulk. Many communities have food co-ops or discount stores that can also help you save money.

Your individual needs count

It's good to learn all you can about healthy eating. You can start by reading books and articles about nutrition, by speaking to your doctor or by consulting a registered dietician through your local public health department. However, be aware that nutrition guidelines are extremely general and may not address the following factors:

Healthy weight ranges for older adults

Height		Healthy Weight Range	
Imperial (ft. in.)	Metric (cm)	Pounds	Kilograms
4'9"	145	92–125	42–57
4'10"	147	95–128	43–58
4'11"	150	99–134	45–61
5'0"	152	101–136	46–62
5'1"	155	106–143	48–65
5'2"	157	108–147	49–67
5'3"	160	112–152	51–69
5'4"	163	117–158	53–72
5'5"	165	119–163	54–74
5'6"	168	123–167	56–76
5'7"	170	128–172	58–78
5'8"	173	132–178	60–81
5'9"	175	134–183	61–83
5'10"	178	139–187	63–85
5'11"	180	143–191	65–87
6'0"	183	147–198	67–90
6'1"	185	150–202	68–92
6'2"	188	156–209	71–95
6'3"	190	158–213	72–97
6'4"	193	163–220	74–100
6'5"	196	170–229	77–104
6'6"	198	172–233	78–106

Source: Baycrest Centre for Geriatric Care

◆ *Your individual body size and build*, which are largely genetic, determine your need for calories. A slender, fine-boned person may need fewer calories than someone of equal height with a heavier frame. The best way to determine the healthiest possible weight for you is to figure out your "Body Mass Index." Your doctor may be able to calculate it for you, or you can use an easy-to-read chart (see opposite).

◆ *Certain health problems*, such as diabetes or hypertension, may require you to make changes in your diet, for example, limiting your intake of calories, sugar, fat or salt. (Making these changes is a good idea even if you're still healthy!)

◆ *Your current activity level* is also important. If you're physically active, you can afford to take in more total calories than someone who lives a more sedentary life. Ask yourself why you're less active. One factor could be poor nutrition – if you don't eat properly, you might feel less energetic and less enthusiastic about getting out and about.

? **How can you make positive changes in your diet now?**
If you have any concerns about your own way of eating and nutrition in general, it's best to ask your family doctor to refer you to a qualified dietitian, particularly someone who is familiar with the different nutritional needs of older adults. (Even if you live in a small community, you can probably get access to a dietitian through your nearest hospital.)

This person will take a detailed look at how, what and why you're eating and can tailor-make a meal plan to suit your unique needs

and current lifestyle. Remember: The changes don't have to be drastic to be effective.

The building blocks of a healthy diet

Protein
◆ found in meat, poultry, fish, eggs, dairy products, nuts, and combinations of legumes and whole grains;

◆ should make up about 15 percent of your total calories.

Although dietary protein is vital for good health, most adults eat far too much of it. You certainly don't need to eat meat or poultry every day to get enough; instead, eat adequate amounts of fresh or canned fish, eggs (prepared with little or no fat), and reduced-fat or nonfat dairy products. Combinations of whole grains, such as rice, and legumes, such as peas or lentils, are a tasty and nutritious source of protein.

Fat
◆ found in meat, poultry, fish, whole dairy products, butter and margarine, plant-based oils, and hidden in many packaged foods such as chips, crackers, and commercially baked cakes, cookies and crackers;

◆ should make up no more than 30 percent of your total calories.

Most people eat way too much fat, especially the fat that is often found in baked goods, snack foods and processed meats. Experts agree it's important to keep your total fat intake down because research has linked high-fat diets to many health problems, including heart disease and some types of cancer.

Getting rid of hidden fat in your diet

◆ Steam, poach, bake or broil instead of frying.

◆ Read product labels carefully. Some foods labeled "low cholesterol" may still contain high levels of saturated fat. Products that list "hydrogenated" or "partly hydrogenated" oils are not as good as foods without any hydrogenated oils. (Hydrogenation is a process that changes the structure of the fat – for example, it allows vegetable oils to take on a hardened form as margarine – and also renders the oil less healthy for consumption.)

◆ If you choose to use margarine, select products with the greatest amount of nonhydrogenated fat according to the label. The rule here is the softer the margarine stays in your refrigerator, the less saturated fat it contains.

◆ Make soups or stocks in advance, refrigerate and then skim off hardened fat.

◆ In recipes, substitute low-fat yogurt for sour cream, nonfat or 1 percent for whole milk, and fat-reduced products for regular cottage and hard cheeses. If a recipe calls for half a cup of saturated fat, such as butter, substitute vegetable oil: For every cup of solid fat, use about three-quarters of a cup of liquid fat. (This method works well for cakes, cookies and muffins, and once you get used to an oilier-feeling dough, it can also be used in making pastry and pie crusts.)

All the talk in the media about fat and different types of fat can be extremely confusing. Here's a basic primer on fats.

Reducing your total fat intake is the best strategy, but the worst culprit is *saturated fat*, found in animal products such as meat, butter and cream, and in palm and coconut oils used to make cookies, potato chips, crackers, granola cereals and other packaged foods. These fats raise your body's levels of harmful low-density lipoprotein (LDL) cholesterol, triglycerides and trans fatty acids, which may be associated with disease in some people.

Moderate amounts of *polyunsaturated fat*, found mainly in fish and vegetable oils such as corn, walnut, safflower or sunflower oil, are considered to be better for you, and may even help lower overall cholesterol levels.

Monounsaturated fats, found in olive, canola and peanut oils, can help to improve your body's balance of harmful LDL cholesterol and helpful high-density lipoprotein (HDL) cholesterol.

Fiber

◆ soluble fiber is found mainly in fruits, vegetables, barley, oats and oat bran, and legumes such as peas and lentils;

◆ insoluble fiber is found mainly in whole grains and the chewy peels of fruits;

◆ you should be eating both types of high-fiber foods daily.

Research suggests that a diet containing enough dietary fiber and fluid can prevent certain health problems such as constipation, which is especially common in older people (see page 98). The insoluble fiber combines with water to soften and expand stool, making elimination easier and more regular. If you have diabetes or high levels of cholesterol and other fats in your blood, increasing your fiber intake may also be helpful. Some research even suggests that a high-fiber diet reduces your risk for certain types of bowel cancer.

If you have chronic digestive problems such as ulcerative colitis or diverticulitis, let your doctor know if you are planning to boost your fiber intake. Caution may be needed.

It's best to increase your fiber consumption gradually, otherwise you may experience bloating. If gas and bloating occur after you eat certain vegetables and grains, you may benefit from a product called Beano, which comes in tablet or liquid form and is available without prescription in many drugstores. Beano contains an enzyme that breaks down the complex sugars contained in beans, peas, lentils, soy, broccoli, cauliflower, corn and oats. This can make these foods easier to digest and less likely to cause gas. However, if you have a penicillin allergy,

Some ideas for cutting down on fat

Cutting down on the amount of fat in your diet doesn't have to be difficult or interfere with your enjoyment of food. Here are some common situations and suggestions from a registered dietitian on how to make healthier food choices:

Meeting your friend at the doughnut shop

◆ *Your usual menu*: a doughnut or muffin, coffee with cream;

◆ *A better menu*: a bagel with jam or butter on the side, coffee with low-fat milk.

Lunch at the chicken restaurant

◆ *Your usual menu*: salad with dressing, half chicken dinner (including skin) with french fries, roll and butter, pie and ice cream, coffee and cream;

◆ *A better menu*: salad with dressing on the side, quarter chicken dinner (skinless) with baked potato and sour cream or yogurt (on the side), roll dipped in sauce, pie *or* ice cream, coffee with low-fat milk.

The idea is to choose the lower-fat items more often: a bagel has much less fat than either a doughnut or a muffin, and a skinless quarter chicken has less fat than a half chicken with skin. You can still indulge in higher fat items, such as butter, salad dressing and sour cream, but ask for them "on the side," so you can control how much you use. You'll find that a touch of butter or sour cream is often enough to make food taste good. Many people don't want to give up dessert, so try splitting dessert with your companion or have a sweet treat every second time you go out instead of every time. Most restaurants will be happy to substitute 1 or 2 percent milk for cream.

diabetes or a condition called galactosemia, don't use Beano without consulting your doctor or a dietitian.

Water

◆ found in fruits, vegetables, juices, milk and other beverages, as well as tap or bottled water;

◆ most older people don't drink enough. The need for fluids varies, but at least 8 to 10 cups per day are recommended for the average older adult to stay healthy. In hot weather or if you have a fever, you may need more to make up for water lost in perspiration.

Many people begin to reduce their intake of water and other beverages as they grow older. They worry about having to make extra trips to the bathroom, especially at night, and some are concerned that drinking too much will aggravate a tendency toward urinary incontinence. But if you don't get enough fluids each day, you may be prone to a variety of health problems, including constipation, urinary tract infection and kidney disorders. Water also works to hydrate your skin, helping it stay soft and smooth.

You don't have to drink a lot at one time – keep a glass of water or your favorite beverage handy and take several sips every hour. If you drink tea, coffee, cola drinks or chocolate beverages, remember – the caffeine they contain may act as a diuretic, increasing your output of urine, which can be a problem at night. Four cups of caffeine-containing beverages each day is considered a moderate amount, unless your doctor has recommended otherwise.

Vitamins

◆ found in foods or can be taken in the form of non-prescription vitamin supplements;

◆ vitamins are crucial to good health, enabling your body to perform essential functions.

Some research suggests that certain vitamins (mainly A, C and E, which are known as antioxidants) may reduce your risk of developing some types of cancer and heart disease.

If you eat a balanced diet that includes a variety of foods from the four food groups (dairy, grains, fruits and vegetables, meats and fish), you're probably getting most of the vitamins your body needs. However, as you get older, you should know a little more about two important vitamins: vitamin B_{12} and vitamin D.

Vitamin B_{12} is found in most animal source foods. The incidence of B_{12} deficiency is more common among older adults – but not usually because of low intake. As you age, your gastrointestinal tract becomes less able to absorb this nutrient. Some older people whose bodies don't absorb food properly may become chronically deficient in this vitamin and develop nervous system problems or a disease called pernicious anemia.

Vitamin D is found in fortified milk, fish liver oil, sardines, hard cheeses, navy beans and broccoli, or can be obtained by exposure of your skin to sunlight. Your body needs this vitamin to absorb calcium and maintain strong teeth and bones.

There are two reasons why you may become more prone to vitamin D deficiency as you get older: You may drink less fortified milk because of digestive problems, and you may spend most of your day indoors – either because of poor health or because you live in a region that experiences long winters.

If milk intolerance is a problem, see if drinking lactose-reduced milk lessens symptoms of digestive upset. You don't have to get a lot of sunlight for your body to receive adequate exposure. In the summer, or even on sunny winter days, 5 to 15 minutes of sunlight a day will produce enough vitamin D, but try to avoid exposing skin at midday, when the rays are strongest and may damage your skin.

Minerals

◆ found in most vegetables, legumes, poultry, fish, bran, liver;

◆ these nutrients work in combination to ensure the healthy functioning of your organs, muscles and nervous system.

Although your body contains trace amounts of more than 50 minerals, only 22 seem to be vital. Some, such as iron and calcium, are

Vitamin supplements

Before you decide to take a multivitamin or an individual vitamin in supplement form, you should be aware of certain drawbacks and risks.

◆ Vitamin supplements are expensive. If they aren't really necessary for your health, why not spend the money on something else?

◆ Some research suggests that vitamins consumed in the diet are better absorbed by the body than vitamins taken in supplement form.

◆ In high doses vitamins no longer act as useful nutrients but can become toxic. Although it's easiest to overdose on vitamins such as A, D, E and K, which are stored in body fat, you can also take too much of the water-soluble vitamins; for example, too much vitamin C can cause diarrhea and increase your risk of developing kidney stones.

Is it ever a good idea to take supplements?

◆ If you have a chronically poor appetite due to health or other problems, a daily multivitamin may be useful.

◆ If you take ASA (acetylsalicylic acid, or aspirin) for arthritis or to prevent blood clots, this can interfere with vitamin absorption. Speak to your doctor or dietitian about whether taking a supplement is appropriate for you.

◆ If you smoke, your body may need extra vitamin C.

◆ If you often use medications such as antibiotics or laxatives, this can interfere with the normal absorption of vitamins and minerals. Again, speak to your doctor.

◆ If you do take vitamin supplements, never exceed the daily dose recommended by your doctor or dietitian.

well understood, but recent studies have shown that zinc, copper and other minerals also play an important role in health and disease.

If you eat a well-balanced diet, it's likely that you're getting enough minerals. But certain diseases are known to be partly related to mineral deficiencies; for example, osteoporosis is linked to inadequate calcium, and anemia is sometimes associ-ated with inadequate iron intake. Extra minerals can be obtained through adding mineral-rich foods to your diet, or if your doctor advises it, you can take mineral supplements.

 Why should you be concerned about nutrition in your later years?

Even if you weren't vigilant about healthy

Shake your excess salt habit

Sodium, found in table salt and other compounds, helps to regulate the amount of water in your tissues. It's one of your body's most essential components, and either too much or too little can cause a variety of health problems.

If you're like most people, you probably use too much added salt – sodium chloride – and as your taste buds become less sensitive with age, you may feel like adding even more salt to your recipes and at the table.

Most healthy adults can tolerate fairly high levels of salt, but there's some evidence linking dietary salt intake with high blood pressure – a condition known as hypertension – in some individuals (see page 172). Even if you aren't affected by this condition, it's probably a good idea to try cutting back on your salt intake:

◆ Eliminate regular intake of high-salt items such as cured meats, sausage, hot dogs, luncheon meats, pickles, canned soups and vegetables (unless they are labeled "reduced in salt"), potato chips and other salted snack foods. But unless your doctor has ordered absolutely "no salt," you can still indulge in them occasionally.

◆ You may enjoy switching from salted butter or margarine to an unsalted variety.

◆ Many people use salt by habit alone. Always taste your food at the table before reaching for the salt shaker – you may be surprised to find that you like how it tastes.

◆ Gradually decrease the amount of salt you use in cooking by two-thirds, and at the same time decrease and finally eliminate adding salt at the table.

◆ To boost food's flavor, try using spices, herbs, lemon, vinegar and wine. Many people find that once they stop using so much salt, they begin to enjoy the real taste of food!

eating when you were younger, it's still not too late to start eating right. Many studies have shown that changing your diet in certain ways – for instance, reducing saturated fats, eating more fiber, getting enough vitamins and minerals – can improve the quality of your life and decrease the risk or delay the onset of some diseases. Recent evidence suggests that a well-balanced diet can actually boost your body's ability to fight infection.

Eating well can also give you more energy, which will have a positive effect on your ability to stay active and to socialize with others. This, in turn, may help you avoid feeling isolated or unhappy.

Do you need fewer or more calories as you get older?

A common mistake many older people make is that they consume the same amount and kinds of food they did when they were in their 20s. As you age, your metabolism changes, and your calorie needs may decrease. Unless you adjust your calorie intake, it's easy to gain unnecessary weight. But although you may need fewer calories now, your body may require extra nutrients that are vital to healthier aging.

Is it bad to be 10 or 15 pounds overweight?

In fact, carrying around some extra weight may be an advantage when you're older. If you develop an infection or other serious illness, a little extra weight may help you bounce back faster. Heavier people, particularly women, are also less prone to osteoporosis, a disease characterized by pro-

gressive thinning of bone and risk of multiple fractures. The extra weight stimulates bone formation by providing you with a bit of a workout.

However, if you have health problems such as arthritis in your knees or hips, or if you suffer from hypertension or diabetes, your doctor may suggest that you try to lose those extra pounds.

Should you be worried about a small appetite?

It's not uncommon for people to lose interest in food as they grow older because of physical, psychological and social changes. This loss of appetite can have serious health repercussions. Your energy level dwindles, you lose vital bone and muscle mass, and you may experience health problems related to deficiencies of essential vitamins, minerals and other nutrients.

What kind of foods should you be eating?

Eating right doesn't have to be a complicated affair. The secret is to consume a variety of foods, with an emphasis on complex carbohydrates, which come from fresh fruits and vegetables, legumes, whole grains, fresh fruits and rice. Starchy foods like bread, pasta and potatoes, once the dieter's taboo, are actually good for you – as long as you don't slather them with high-fat sauces and butter.

Try to eat fresh or frozen foods, depending on the season, rather than highly processed foods. And avoid trendy diets that rely on single foods or food groups.

❓ Should you still eat three meals a day?

The number of meals you eat per day is less important than what foods you eat and the size of your portions. Because eating a big meal is more likely to upset your digestion now, you may prefer smaller, more frequent meals throughout the day. If gaining weight is a problem, be careful about portion size – those five or six meals or snacks a day should be small ones – high in good taste and nutritional value, but low enough in total calories so that you don't begin to put on weight.

Try not to skip breakfast – it gets your day off to a good start and may reduce your desire to snack, especially on less nutritious foods, later in the day. If you prefer to have snacks and just one big meal each day, some experts suggest you have it at midday rather than evening. Eating later in the day, when you're less likely to be active, can sometimes cause digestive discomfort.

The dietary changes that you make now should be ones you can live with for the rest of your life. There's no point in establishing a diet that's so restrictive you give up on it after a few weeks or months. Don't be so strict with your diet that you stop enjoying life. Food is an important source of pleasure. That occasional slice of pie or piece of fried chicken probably won't shorten your days. Remember – it's what you do most of the time that counts, not what you do just once in a while.

Staying active:
The importance of exercise

Vitality shows in not only the ability to persist but in the ability to start over.

F. SCOTT FITZGERALD

Imagine your life as a magnificent building that is going to be under construction for 70, 80 or even 100 years. If good nutrition is the foundation of your life, then regular physical activity is the superstructure holding everything firmly in place.

Older adults, though, are less likely than those in their middle years to keep up a healthy level of physical activity – perhaps because many accept society's negative, rocking-chair image of older age. Each of us, however – even those with physical limitations due to health problems – has the responsibility to define and strive for our own healthy level of activity.

It's not hard to understand why your level of physical activity is more likely to decline after age 65, especially if you haven't been accustomed to regular exercise:

◆ You may be starting to feel some of the aches and pains that come with increasing age and think you shouldn't exercise because of them.

◆ If you're retired from work and active parenting, you may simply have less to do each day.

◆ If you've lost your spouse or friends who used to share in enjoyable activities, you may not be interested in exercising alone.

◆ If you've gained extra pounds during your middle or later years, you may feel physically uncomfortable when you move around, or you may be embarrassed about appearing in shorts or a bathing suit.

This slowing down can trigger a negative cycle that some experts have dubbed "the inactivity-stress syndrome." The less you do, the worse you feel, and the less you get out of life.

If your doctor told you that taking a certain drug could make you feel better physically and mentally without any harmful side effects, you'd probably ask for a prescription. Well, according to one expert, there's no drug in current or prospective use that holds as much promise for sustained health and well-being as a lifetime program of physical exercise!

An important goal of exercise at any age should be physical fitness: a combination of strength and flexibility and cardiovascular fitness. Assuming you don't have any significant illness or other physical limitation, how can you tell if you're physically fit? You probably *aren't* fit if you:

◆ feel tired most of the time;

◆ are unable to keep up with other people who are your own age;

◆ avoid physical activity because you know you'll tire quickly;

◆ become short of breath or tired after walking a short distance.

You probably *are* fit if you can:

◆ carry out your daily tasks without feeling tired and have some energy left over to enjoy leisure activities;

◆ walk a block or two or climb a flight of stairs without feeling out of breath or experiencing heaviness or fatigue in your legs;

◆ carry on a conversation during light to moderate exercise such as brisk walking.

What kind of exercise is best?
The best way to develop a realistic fitness program for yourself is to consult an exercise specialist, especially one who is familiar with the needs of older adults or people with disabilities. Such specialists, who work at many community and seniors' centers, can design a sensible exercise program for you to use at home.

Most programs will contain the following types of exercise:

◆ *Aerobic exercise,* which is designed to promote cardiovascular fitness, improves your body's ability to supply itself with life-sustaining oxygen ("aerobic" means "with

Sensible exercise tips for older adults

Before you exercise

◆ A prominent Swedish physiologist, Per Olaf Ostrand, has written that people should seek their doctor's permission *not* to exercise! Even so, it's probably a good idea to check with your family physician before you start an exercise program or new fitness activity.

◆ Wait two to three hours after a large meal before exercising. Digestion directs blood to your digestive system and away from your heart. Drink something (preferably water or juice rather than coffee or beer) about an hour before you begin exercising to make sure you don't become dehydrated.

◆ If you're exercising outdoors, pay attention to the weather. It's best not to exercise during extremes of heat, cold, rain or wind, especially if you have respiratory or heart problems. Make sure the location is safe, away from the hazards of heavy traffic. Another reason to avoid traffic is the emission of carbon dioxide, which can be a problem for older people who are sensitive to less oxygen in the air.

◆ During the summer and even on sunny winter days, don't forget to wear sunscreen on all exposed skin areas. In summer you should wear a broad-brimmed hat to shade your neck, face, scalp and ears, and sunglasses to protect your eyes and reduce glare; in winter a warm hat that covers your ears will prevent you from losing vital body heat.

◆ Make sure you have the proper equipment for your activity – the right tennis racket, an approved bicycle helmet, or properly fitted walking shoes.

◆ Always begin with a five-minute warm-up of stretching and slow walking. This raises your body temperature, which increases muscle flexibility, reducing the chance of harmful muscle strain.

While you exercise

◆ It's natural to breathe in during exertion – but many people don't exhale fully, which can make them tire more easily. Concentrate on breathing out in a regular and controlled fashion.

◆ It's especially important for older people to listen to their bodies during exertion. If you have a cold or aren't feeling well, it may be advisable to skip exercising for a day or two. If you feel tired, slow down your pace a

oxygen"). The best kinds of aerobic activities for older adults include brisk walking, swimming, dancing, bicycling, rowing and other low impact exercises. When sustained over time (i.e., regular periods of exercise each week), these activities place a heavier-than-normal demand on your cardiovascular system – your heart, lungs and blood vessels. This allows them to work more efficiently, both during exercise and at rest.

◆ *Strength exercise* increases your muscle strength (the amount of weight you can lift without injury in one try) and also your

bit. If you develop any of the following symptoms, stop immediately (see cool-down advice below): dizziness, fainting, nausea, excessive shortness of breath, severe fatigue or distress, any pain in your chest or lungs, wheezing during breathing, irregular heartbeat. If these symptoms persist, seek medical attention or advice.

◆ If you feel thirsty, stop for a drink of water or diluted fruit juice.

◆ Avoid sudden or extreme movements of the neck and head. These could cause muscle strain or circulatory problems resulting in dizziness.

After you exercise

◆ A cool-down period of at least five minutes will allow your pulse and respiration to slow down gradually to resting levels. To avoid dizziness during this period, don't lower your head below your heart.

◆ Your muscles may feel sore after exercise, but the pain should go away within a few hours. If it lasts longer, you may be overdoing it and should slow down. After a day's rest, exercise again, though a bit more gently. If you think you've injured a joint or muscle, apply a cold pack and rest. (Never use a heating pad or hot water bottle – while the warmth may initially relieve the pain, it will actually increase inflammation and prolong the recovery time.) An injury that seems severe should be seen by your doctor.

◆ Avoid hot showers, steam rooms and/or saunas after exercise, at least until your body has cooled down. The heat can make tiny surface blood vessels dilate, keeping blood away from the heart and causing faintness.

◆ One final and important word: Don't be disappointed if you don't see or feel instant results from exercise. The key to success is to be realistic, consistent and patient – with yourself as well as your body.

endurance (the ability to lift a certain percentage of that weight many times) through regular, repeated motions against resistance. One way to accomplish this is by using specialized gym equipment designed to work various muscles and joints in your arms, knees, ankles and back through a system of weights and pulleys. If you don't have access to such equipment, an exercise specialist can design strength exercises that you can do at home using homemade weights. New research suggests that even frail elderly people can benefit significantly from this type of strength training.

◆ *Flexibility exercise* encourages easier movement of your body's joints. This usually involves a series of exercises where your arms, legs, waist, neck and spine are repeatedly and gradually stretched, held and released.

◆ *Relaxation exercise,* often combined with stretching and breathing techniques, encourages you to be more aware of unhealthy tension in your mind and body that can contribute to muscle spasms, headaches and shallow breathing.

? Why should you exercise?

Many studies, including those of people in their 60s, 70s, 80s and even 90s, have shown that regular physical exercise can help lower the risk for certain diseases and conditions, not to mention improving the quality of your later years.

People who are fit feel better, look better and are better able to cope with the stress created by negative events such as physical illness and bereavement. Here are the major

Walk your way to better health

Most of us walk just to get around, but walking is also one of the best ways to improve your overall fitness. It's easy, and inexpensive, and can be varied to suit your individual needs and preferences.

While any kind of walking – strolling in the park, walking the dog, making your way to the store on foot instead of driving – is good for you, walking for fitness requires a bit more effort and planning. If you are overweight, if you have a heart condition, or if you haven't walked or jogged to keep fit before, check with your doctor first.

◆ Fitness walking must be done regularly, three or four times a week for at least 20 minutes each time. Walking should be brisk enough to increase your heart rate and respiration, giving your cardiovascular system a good workout.

One way to chart your progress is to check your pulse and respiration rates while resting (this means while sitting in a chair before exercise). Find your pulse either on the inside of your wrist or the side of your neck. Then, using a clock or watch with a second hand, count the number of beats in 60 seconds while resting. Next, count the number of breaths you take in 60 seconds while resting. You might want to jot down these numbers in a notebook. You should then check your pulse and respiration rates during or just after walking. The goal is to increase them. A fitness specialist or your doctor can tell you how much of an increase is safe for you, according to your age and level of fitness.

◆ Always start with a warm-up period. This should include flexibility exercises, which stretch the muscles in your lower legs, preventing injury to joints and muscles. Walk slowly for a few minutes to give your body time to adjust to the increased demand.

◆ To start, walk on level ground and avoid hills. If possible, never walk against the wind since this will increase your workload.

benefits of a sensible program of regular physical exercise:

♦ *Your heart and lungs:* Cardiovascular fitness can reduce your risk of heart attack and stroke in a number of ways. Regular aerobic exercise enables your heart to withstand any sudden exertion – for example, running for a bus – that demands extra oxygen for your muscles. If your heart is fit, it pumps blood more efficiently, which means it can pump less frequently. As your fitness level increases, you may notice that your resting pulse rate (the number of times your heart beats per minute while you're at rest) actually drops. Exercise can also improve your lung capacity, allowing you to stay active for a longer time without becoming tired or breathless.

Exercise burns calories, so if you're overweight (a known cardiovascular risk factor), this is an excellent way to shed extra pounds, so long as you don't increase your intake of food. Many people worry that physical exertion will make them hungrier

♦ Start out slowly and increase speed and distance (see the Three-Month Walking Program on page 37).

♦ Don't strain yourself to the point of physical discomfort or compete with other walkers. It's fun to walk with a companion, but never push yourself to keep up with someone who walks more quickly.

♦ Wear well-fitted, appropriate walking shoes with good arch support and cushioning for your feet. To avoid blisters, always "break in" new shoes by wearing them for a few weeks before you begin a walking program.

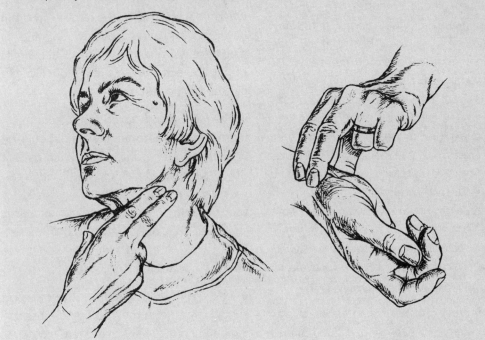

and more likely to overeat, but many people swear that exercise actually curbs their appetites.

Exercise is known to reduce blood pressure, to increase levels of good cholesterol and to decrease levels of bad cholesterol and blood fats known as triglycerides. In addition, it can reduce your level of blood sugar, which may help prevent or delay the onset of some types of diabetes.

◆ *Your bones, muscles and joints*: As you age you tend to start losing bone tissue, which makes you more prone to fractures. Some older people lose so much bone mass that they develop a potentially serious condition called osteoporosis (see page 163). Weight-bearing exercise such as walking, dancing and bicycling can prevent and even reverse some of this bone loss. Recent studies have found that swimming, although not traditionally considered weight-bearing, may also improve bone strength.

The health of your bones and joints depends on the support of strong muscles, ligaments and tendons, and these are also improved by exercise. Exercising your back muscles can improve posture, which may suffer as you get older, leading to problems with your spine. Not only does keeping your spine erect make you look better, but it also allows you to breathe more deeply and digest your food properly.

Exercise can also improve your sense of balance. When done regularly, even a very simple activity – standing on your toes while steadying yourself by holding onto the back of a chair – can sharpen your balance and prevent falls.

◆ *Your sleep*: Exercise is an excellent way to improve your chances for a good night's sleep. Physical activity during the day or early evening releases stress and relaxes your body.

◆ *Your mental health*: Some studies have found that when you exercise, your pituitary gland releases beneficial hormones called "endorphins." In fact, some researchers think that regular physical activity may be as effective as medication or psychotherapy in relieving mild depression and anxiety. Other potential benefits include improved body image and self-esteem, a greater feeling of control and the opportunity to socialize.

How much exercise is enough at your age?

Many people make the mistake of thinking that a bit of exercise is better than no exercise at all. In fact, irregular attempts at extreme exertion can have negative effects. If you don't exercise regularly, those "day-after" sore muscles that are common when you first start an exercise program never really go away. You never experience the real physical and psychological benefits of physical activity, so you're more likely to give up on the attempt.

◆ *Frequency and duration*: For the maximum benefit, aerobic exercise should be done three or four times a week, for at least 20 to 30 minutes per session. If this is too much, begin more gradually and build up toward your goal. Stretching exercises should be done daily, before and after exercises, while strength exercises should be done two or three times a week.

◆ *Intensity*: When you first start out, you should exercise to the point where breathing and heart rate are increased, but never to the point where you are gasping, over-

A three-month walking program

You should walk three times per week. Each session begins with a slow, five-minute warm-up walk and ends with a slow five-minute cool-down walk. The target exercise period, which involves brisk walking, increases gradually each week from five minutes the first week to thirty minutes the last week:

Week 1
Warm-up: walk slowly for 5 minutes
Target exercise: walk briskly for 5 minutes
Cool-down: walk slowly for 5 minutes
Total: 15 minutes

Week 2
Warm-up/cool-down: 5 minutes each
Target exercise: 7 minutes
Total: 17 minutes

Week 3
Warm-up/cool-down: 5 minutes each
Target exercise: 9 minutes
Total: 19 minutes

Week 4
Warm-up/cool-down: 5 minutes each
Target exercise: 11 minutes
Total: 21 minutes

Week 5
Warm-up/cool-down: 5 minutes each
Target exercise: 13 minutes
Total: 23 minutes

Week 6
Warm-up/cool-down: 5 minutes each
Target exercise: 15 minutes
Total: 25 minutes

Week 7
Warm-up/cool-down: 5 minutes each
Target exercise: 18 minutes
Total: 28 minutes

Week 8
Warm-up/cool-down: 5 minutes each
Target exercise: 20 minutes
Total: 30 minutes

Week 9
Warm-up/cool-down: 5 minutes each
Target exercise: 23 minutes
Total: 33 minutes

Week 10
Warm-up/cool-down: 5 minutes each
Target exercise: 26 minutes
Total: 36 minutes

Week 11
Warm-up/cool-down: 5 minutes each
Target exercise: 28 minutes
Total: 38 minutes

Week 12
Warm-up/cool-down: 5 minutes each
Target exercise: 30 minutes
Total: 40 minutes

Adapted from "A Three-Month Walking Program" by the American Heart Association

heated or unable to carry on a normal conversation.

Once you've passed the beginner stage, however, you may decide to expand your fitness horizon. Vary the intensity of your workouts, allowing yourself to move into the "discomfort zone" more often. (Note: This means mild muscular discomfort, not pain or dizziness!) Only by working more intensely can your body adapt and improve.

? What's the best way to get started?

If you never enjoyed the benefits of physical exercise when you were younger, you probably aren't convinced about starting now. You may have developed one or more ways to rationalize your choice to avoid or postpone regular physical exercise. How many of the following excuses have you used? Be honest!

◆ *"I'm too old to start exercising."* You're quite right – it's certainly better to begin fitness habits early in life. But many studies show that older people, including those who already suffer from heart disease, arthritis, cancer, hypertension and other chronic ailments, can still derive important health benefits from a supervised program of regular exercise.

◆ *"I'm just too tired."* Fatigue can certainly be caused by physical illness and conditions such as anemia, depression and thyroid problems. But you might be surprised to learn that a major cause of fatigue in older adults is lack of activity. Sitting in a chair all day saps your physical and mental energy, which further reduces your motivation to move around. Lack of exercise can also cause poor sleep, which makes you even more tired and less motivated the next day.

◆ *"I don't have time."* Many older people continue to lead busy, productive lives, and sometimes it's a challenge to find time for regular exercise. Convince yourself that it's worth it, and you'll have no trouble finding 20 to 30 minutes three or four times a week for fitness activities. One sure way to succeed is to choose an activity you enjoy that fits into your current lifestyle. If you hate jouncing around and feeling overheated, don't sign up for an aerobics class – try swimming or aquabics instead. If you like socializing, then an organized fitness class will be more fun than walking alone.

You can also incorporate physical activity into your day. Walk to the mall instead of driving or taking the bus, or at least get off a few stops earlier and walk the rest of the way. If you live in an apartment building, try walking up one or two flights before taking the elevator. If you have a garden, spend 15 minutes each morning pulling weeds or raking the grass.

◆ *"It's too complicated and expensive."* Too many people believe that starting an exercise program requires a lot of planning and money for classes or equipment. In fact, the path to fitness doesn't have to be complicated or expensive.

Check out your local community center, YMCA-YWCA, and municipal swimming pool – you'll find that they provide excellent facilities that are, in some cases, free of charge. Many shopping malls now offer indoor walking programs. These are free and have the advantage of being protected from the weather. Walking for fitness costs virtually nothing, except the price of some well-fitting, supportive shoes. If you have trouble with your feet, pay a visit to a foot specialist to see if you might need special inserts for your shoes, called "orthotics," to protect your feet from damage and allow you to walk more comfortably.

◆ *"I don't look good exercising."* As we get older, it's natural for our bodies to change their shape and appearance. Many people may hesitate to exercise outdoors because they feel that they no longer look good in shorts or a bathing suit.

If this is a problem for you, it's one that's well worth resolving. Start by honestly examining whether your attitudes toward appearance and aging are having a negative effect on your self-esteem and are keeping you out of the game. Very few people over age 65 can live up to the impossible ideals of slenderness, smoothness and rippling muscles portrayed in our youth-obsessed culture. If you cheerfully accept who you are and how you look at any age, then others will accept you too. In fact, they'll probably admire your energy and applaud your zest for life!

◆ *"I'm not well. It's not safe for me to exercise."* Even if you have a health condition or chronic illness, it may still be perfectly safe and even beneficial for you to engage in physical activity. Studies show that even older adults recovering from heart attacks or

Stengthening exercise for the lower legs

Here's a simple strengthening exercise for lower legs: Fill a sock with sugar or flour, fasten the end securely, and then balance the sock on your ankle. While sitting in a chair, raise and lower the weighted ankle 10 times, then switch to the other ankle. Try to increase the number of lifts each day.

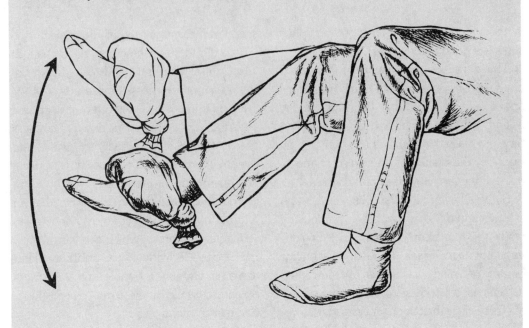

coronary bypass surgery benefit from a supervised program of cardiovascular exercise and strength training.

If you are physically frail and feel you can barely walk around your own home, you can still take part in activities to improve your body's strength and endurance.

If you normally get up from your chair once every hour, try doing it twice per hour for a few days, then increase the frequency and duration of these standing periods. You'll soon find that your legs feel much stronger and moving around seems to tire you less.

Try to increase the amount of walking you do in your home or apartment. You can start with "living room laps" – walking around the edge of your living room – and then move into other areas of your home. Begin with just a few minutes of slow walking with a cane or walker, if necessary, and if you feel all right, continue. Soon you may find yourself feeling strong and energetic enough to begin walking around the block!

All about sleep

That we are not much sicker and much madder than we are is due exclusively to that most blessed and blessing of all natural graces, sleep.

ALDOUS HUXLEY

Without a doubt, one of life's greatest pleasures is a good night's sleep.

The duration and quality of our sleep changes over our lifespan. Newborn infants spend between 16 and 18 hours a day asleep, but as we grow older, our sleeping time gradually diminishes. For some people over 65, the quality of sleep also changes, and these changes cause great distress.

Surveys have found that between 25 and 40 percent of older people – particularly women – report sleep problems, including disturbed or "light" sleep, frequent awakenings or early morning awakenings, and unwanted daytime naps. For these reasons, older people are more likely than younger ones to use prescription medications to help them sleep.

In order to understand how sleep changes later in life, you first need to know something about the process of sleep.

At one time it was believed that sleep was a period of inactivity. But now researchers tell us that sleep is really an active and dynamic process with physical, chemical and hormonal components.

Your own sleep pattern is governed by an internal body clock, a set of rhythms called "circadian rhythms," which can vary slightly from one individual to another. That explains why some people are early risers or "larks," while others – the "owls" – function best at night.

? **How much sleep do you need when you're older?**

You probably think you need a certain amount of sleep each night in order to function properly. In fact, studies show that healthy people can be deprived of sleep for two days or longer without showing much deterioration in how well they perform tasks. However, while occasional sleeplessness isn't generally harmful, it can leave you feeling fatigued and out of sorts.

Your need for sleep remains fairly constant from early adulthood into your later years. Most people need between six and eight hours of sleep per night in order to stay physically and mentally healthy.

When asked to rate the quantity of their sleep, many older women and men complain that they sleep fewer hours now than when they were younger. Actually, most older people continue to sleep between six and eight hours, but they may not sleep for long hours at a stretch – for example, they may sleep four or five hours at night, an hour in the early morning, and then take two half-hour naps during the day.

The quality of sleep does seem to change with normal aging. Older adults don't sleep as deeply or soundly as younger ones and are more easily awakened.

? **Why is it sometimes so hard to fall asleep or stay asleep?**

All of us have experienced insomnia – trouble falling or staying asleep or early morning awakening – at one time or another. Researchers found that one-third of older people in a test group reported problems

The anatomy of sleep

You can expect to spend about one-third of your adult life asleep. By the time you're 75, that means you've spent a total of 25 years sleeping! But what really happens when your head hits the pillow?

◆ *Relaxed wakefulness:* This is the period of drowsiness that occurs before you fall asleep, and in healthy sleep it can last from a few minutes to half an hour.

◆ *Non-REM sleep:* "Rapid eye movement," or REM, is a stage of sleep associated with dreaming. If you are awakened suddenly during REM sleep, you're far more likely to recall dreams than if you sleep through until morning. After you first fall asleep, you enter a phase of non-dreaming known as non-rapid eye movement or non-REM sleep.

◆ *REM-sleep:* About 70 to 90 minutes after you fall asleep, you experience your first REM sleep, which lasts about five minutes. Your body changes quite dramatically during REM sleep – for example, blood pressure and respiration increase, your body temperature drops slightly, your muscles become extremely relaxed, and men experience penile erections. For the rest of the night, you alternate between non-REM and REM sleep, with the periods of REM sleep growing longer as morning approaches. Researchers believe that in order to awaken feeling rested and refreshed, you must get adequate, uninterrupted REM sleep.

How to get a better night's sleep

Here are some do's and don'ts that may help increase your chances of getting a good night's sleep:

DO's

◆ DO get some physical exercise during the day – it relaxes you and makes you tired and ready to sleep. But avoid a brisk workout right before bed.

◆ DO indulge in some relaxing activity (a warm bath, soothing music, light reading, television) before going to bed. Some people – but not all! – find that sexual activity is an excellent tranquilizer.

◆ DO make sure that your sleeping environment encourages sleep. Although individual preferences vary, it should probably be quiet, dark and not too warm or cold. The bed should be comfortable and no bedside clock should be visible, so you don't lie awake watching the clock and worrying. If a partner's sleep habits are keeping you awake, you might sleep better in another room until the problem is solved, or you might consider sleeping in separate beds.

◆ DO keep to a regular sleeping schedule if possible, including a set time for going to bed and waking up.

DON'Ts

◆ DON'T eat a heavy meal or snack at the end of the day. If you're hungry, try something light – crackers or cereal with milk (milk is high in a natural substance called "tryptophan," which encourages drowsiness).

◆ DON'T consume too much caffeine, a stimulant found in cola drinks, regular coffee, tea, cocoa and also in some over-the-counter cold and pain remedies.

◆ DON'T use tobacco, which is also a stimulant, or alcohol – a glass of wine or a hot toddy may make you feel sleepy initially, but alcohol interferes with normal, refreshing sleep.

◆ DON'T drink too many liquids right before bed, especially if the need to urinate wakes you often during the night.

◆ DON'T spend your waking hours lying in bed reading or resting. Bed should be for sleeping only.

◆ DON'T take long or frequent daytime naps. They will interfere with your need for sleep later. A one-hour nap each day isn't harmful, however, and it may actually relax you so you sleep better at night.

◆ DON'T use tranquilizers, sedatives or other medication unless your doctor has prescribed them.

◆ DON'T become obsessed with your inability to sleep. If after a reasonable time in bed you're still awake, get up, go into another room and read, knit or watch TV until you start to feel sleepy.

falling asleep; nearly half had trouble with nighttime awakening; and one-fifth complained about waking up too early in the morning.

There are many reasons why older adults are more likely to complain about or experience insomnia:

◆ Your sleeping habits and behavior tend to change as you grow older, especially if you don't have a schedule of activities that keeps you active. For instance, you may go to bed very early – around 8 or 9 P.M. – and awaken at 3 or 4 A.M. This feels like insomnia or a sleep problem, but in fact, you've already slept a full seven hours.

◆ Because the quality of sleep changes with age, it may take longer for you to fall asleep. You may also sleep less soundly and may awaken during the night, which interferes with restful sleep.

◆ You're more likely to have worries about your own health or that of others, or about other troubling issues.

◆ You may be suffering from an illness or other condition such as arthritis that causes pain or discomfort and prevents you from sleeping well.

◆ You may be taking medications for health problems – for example, propranolol hydrochloride used to treat high blood pressure – that interfere with normal sleep.

◆ You may be suffering from an undiagnosed depression or other illness that is upsetting your normal sleep patterns.

◆ Finally, you may be upset about your inability to sleep. This can cause a vicious cycle of sleeplessness, worry and more sleeplessness.

If you feel sleepy during the day, is it all right to nap?

Some people can incorporate daytime napping into their regular schedule without any problem at all. They may be accustomed to sleeping for an hour before dinner, or they may take several quick catnaps throughout the day.

If you find yourself feeling sleepy during the day, it could be because you aren't sleeping well at night. In some cases this situation may be solved by doing whatever you can to avoid daytime sleeping. But it's also possible that your daytime sleepiness is due to an undiagnosed sleep disorder (see page 44).

Daytime sleepiness can also occur if you aren't physically active or don't have enough to do to keep you feeling alert and occupied during the day. You may be limited because of illness or other physical problems. Or perhaps you haven't replaced those activities that used to fill your days when you were younger – going to work, caring for the family, socializing with friends – with new pursuits.

If you think that boredom is a factor in making you sleepy during the day, it's important to do something about it: Get involved in a new hobby or pursuit, make an effort to see friends and neighbors, look around your community and see if there's a task or role you'd like to take on. Consider talking to your family, your doctor or a spiritual counselor who may have some constructive ideas for you.

Should you take medication to help you sleep?

Because sleep problems become more common later in life, older adults are more likely than younger ones to resort to sedating medication to help them sleep. But you should be aware of the many hazards associated with sleeping pills.

You are more likely than a younger person to experience side effects such as sedation, anxiety and lightheadedness because barbiturates and tranquilizers are metabolized differently in older age. This can sometimes lead to problems with balance, resulting in falls. You and your doctor should know that, because of these age-related changes in metabolism, older people may need a much lower dose of certain sleeping medications to achieve the desired effects.

If you're taking other kinds of medication for certain diseases or conditions, these drugs can interact with sleeping medication. This is a real problem if you are getting prescriptions from more than one physician and having them filled at different pharmacies.

You can develop a tolerance for sleeping medication, which means you need to take more to obtain the desired result. This can lead to unpleasant side effects, including rebound sleeplessness where the drug itself makes you feel restless and wakeful instead of relaxed and sleepy.

Before you resort to over-the-counter sleep aids or seek a prescription from your doctor, make sure you're practicing good sleep habits (see page 42). If your sleeping problems persist, consult your doctor. (In the past most doctors were male, but today you're likely to encounter many female doctors, so throughout this book you'll see doctors referred to as both "he" and "she.") She should take a detailed medical history, evaluate any other medications you are currently taking, and perform a thorough physical examination to rule out any underlying phys-

ical or mental problem that could be interfering with your sleep.

If your doctor does prescribe a sleeping medication, be sure to use it *according to her directions only*. That means taking it in the prescribed dose and only for a limited period of time. Your pharmacist can answer any questions you may have about specific prescription or non-prescription sleep aids.

How do you know if you have a sleep disorder?

You should consider the possibility that you have a sleep disorder if:

◆ you have chronic trouble falling or staying asleep;

◆ you never wake up feeling rested;

◆ you feel excessively sleepy during the day and need to nap;

◆ your bed partner complains that you're always restless or that you snore loudly;

◆ any of these problems persist for longer than three to four weeks, causing you significant distress.

If you think you might have a sleep disorder, consult your family doctor who may refer you to a sleep specialist. You may be suffering from one of the following disorders:

◆ *Sleep apnea* occurs when an irregular breathing pattern prevents you from enjoying deep, refreshing sleep, and you awaken feeling exhausted. In most cases, the sleeper isn't aware of the problem, although your bed partner may notice that you take a deep breath (often accompanied by a loud noise), stop breathing for a brief period of time, and then start breathing again. Sleep apnea can be treated by wearing a mask-like device called a CPAP (Continuous Positive Airway Pressure), which delivers a flow of air into your mouth to keep your throat open and prevent interruptions in breathing.

◆ *Nocturnal myoclonus* involves regular, repeated kicking or jerking of the legs during sleep. You may be completely unaware that this is happening (although chances are your bed partner isn't), but the kicking prevents you from sleeping deeply enough to feel refreshed. Nocturnal myoclonus often responds to treatment with the drug clonazepam.

◆ *Narcolepsy* is a fairly rare, inherited sleep disorder that causes the sufferer to fall asleep suddenly and frequently during the day.

Sexuality in later life

Old age has its pleasures, which, though different, are not less than the pleasures of youth.

W. SOMERSET MAUGHAM

Sex appeal is fifty percent what you've got and fifty percent what people think you've got.

SOPHIA LOREN

If you enjoyed a healthy, fulfilling sex life when you were younger, chances are you don't plan to give it up after your 65th birthday. Yet many of us, young as well as old, find it hard to envision active, lusty sex between people old enough to be grandparents or even great-grandparents. There is no problem accepting that a couple in their 80s might still enjoy holding hands or sharing a tender hug and kiss, but what about their having a sexy romp in the shower?

Sexuality and the ability to express that basic human urge are vital to your well-being at any age. Not only does sexual activity – including intercourse, masturbation, kissing, caressing and other types of pleasuring – relieve physical stress, it also reinforces many positive emotions. You are able to express your deepest feelings to another person, you may feel less alone, and the fact that you are loved and/or desired by someone else is a wonderful way to increase self-esteem.

Of course, some older people are relieved and happy to finally put sexual activity on the shelf. Your previous sexual experiences may have been less than satisfying and, in some cases, traumatic. Or it's possible that you never really had a strong sex drive to begin with. Regardless of your age, you should have the same freedom to abstain from sex as to revel in it, as long as the choice isn't a problem for your partner, if you have one. ("Partner" in this book refers

Myths and facts about love and sex after age 65

There are many myths about sex and age that can interfere with sexual satisfaction later in life. These ideas are rooted in personal beliefs.

We form our attitudes toward physical and emotional intimacy early in life by listening to what our parents say (or don't say) about the subject and by observing what they do. Were your parents openly affectionate with each other? Were they comfortable answering questions about sex? Did they make negative comments about other people's sexual preferences or activities?

Your attitudes toward sexuality are also influenced by cultural and religious beliefs. Judeo-Christian religions, for example, are strictly opposed to sex outside of traditional marriage, and they forbid a variety of practices which many now accept as part of normal, healthy sexuality.

Some myths about late-life sex are based on certain prejudices and misconceptions about older age. All older people were once considered frail and ill, or at the very least, past their prime. As we grow older, we may believe that advanced age demands a certain amount of dignity and self-control that is at odds with sexual passion and abandon.

The psychiatrist Sigmund Freud believed that children have a powerful need to see their own parents as sexless. Some experts have suggested that we find it difficult to accept the idea of older people as sexual beings because it presents the (unthinkable!) possibility that our own parents and even our grandparents are engaging in sex.

◆ *Myth:* Older people don't have sexual urges anymore.

◆ *Fact:* It's true that sexual activity does decline with age, but this may have less to do with an age-related decline in sexual interest and function and more to do with the availability of a sexual partner. When researchers surveyed older women and men about whether they still enjoyed sex, the majority replied that they did.

◆ *Myth:* Older people are so fragile that sexual activity might hurt them.

◆ *Fact:* Loss of strength and vigor are not synonymous with older age. Unless you were devoted to gymnastically exotic sexual positions when you were younger, chances are you aren't too frail to indulge in sex.

◆ *Myth:* Older people are physically unattractive and undesirable so no one would want to have sex with them.

◆ *Fact:* This is clearly not the case, since many older people continue to enjoy the look, feel, smell and taste of a beloved partner. Women and men of any age can still be attractive to (and attracted to) others – including people close to their own age, and even those who are younger. This myth of undesirability has been encouraged by our youth-oriented culture, where only slim, taut bodies and smooth, unlined faces are portrayed in a sexual context. It also reflects a belief that sexual desire is purely physical and based on how a person looks, excluding the reality that desire for a partner can be based on familiarity, emotional compatibility, trust and deep affection.

to a spouse or lover of the opposite sex or, in the case of older gay men and lesbian women, a lover of the same sex.)

? Do sexual desire and function change as you get older?

In general, sexual desire and function do change with age, but not as much as you might think.

◆ *Older women:* The loss of hormones after menopause may mean that you take longer to respond to sexual stimulation. Vaginal lubrication becomes less effective and may take longer to achieve than it once did, and your vagina may become less elastic. Some of these problems can be overcome by taking small doses of female hormones after menopause, or applying the hormones as a cream (see page 183) or using a non-petroleum based lubricant jelly, such as K-Y jelly or Astroglide, before intercourse. The good news is that a woman's ability to experience orgasm doesn't seem to decline with age.

◆ *Older men:* You may notice a change in your erections. It may take you longer to achieve one, and you may require more stimulation than you did when you were younger. Your erections may be less sturdy than they used to be, you probably need more time between erections, and ejaculation may be less forceful. But the enjoyment

---

Sexually transmitted diseases after age 65

If you're past menopause or having sexual intercourse with someone who is, then age will protect you against unwanted pregnancy. Age won't protect you, though, from sexually transmitted diseases such as herpes, gonorrhea, and Acquired Immune Deficiency Syndrome (AIDS), which is linked to infection with the human immunodeficiency virus, or HIV.

Talking about safer sex practices is difficult at any age, and it may be especially difficult for you if you were raised in an era when sex wasn't discussed openly. But if you are sexually active at any age, you must assume responsibility for your own health and the health of your partner.

If you're thinking about becoming sexually involved with someone new, you should discuss practicing safer sex well before you end up in the bedroom. There are many ways to protect yourself: You may agree to avoid certain high-risk activities such as vaginal or anal intercourse and oral sex, and focus instead on other kinds of pleasuring such as hugging, kissing and mutual masturbation. Or you can reduce the risk of infection during high-risk activities by using a latex condom *every time you have intercourse*. If you need a lubricant, ask your pharmacist to recommend one. Don't use Vaseline or other petroleum-based products because they can cause the latex to break down (see above for suggested lubricants).

If you're in a committed relationship – a marriage or long-term arrangement – you may feel confident that your partner has been and continues to be monogamous. In such a situation, you may not need to use condoms or practice safer sex.

of sexual activity – yours and your partner's – doesn't depend on the rigidity of your erection as much as it does on your physical and emotional contact with your partner.

Although the male hormone testosterone does decline very slightly with age, most older men continue to produce it in sufficient quantities throughout their lifetime. Even so, some researchers believe that the age-related drop-off in testosterone causes a subtle type of male menopause that reduces some older men's interest in sex and affects sexual function (see page 187).

The sexual organ that causes the most trouble for older women and men is the brain, which is much less vulnerable to the aging process than other parts of the body! There may be a gap between your own self-image (you continue to see yourself as being sexually interested and interesting) and how society regards older women and men (they are seen as no longer attractive or desirable).

In some parts of the world this attitude is beginning to change and the next generation of elders may begin to demand that society's images and institutions reflect a new reality – where the experience and expression of human sexuality aren't limited to the young.

What other factors can cause sexual problems?

Certain illnesses and conditions that are more likely to occur when you're older can affect your ability and desire to have sex:

◆ If you or your partner have had a heart attack, you may worry about resuming sex because you fear it could trigger another one. But studies show that heart attacks that occur during sex are extremely rare. Based on your doctor's advice, most people can and should resume sexual activity within a few months of a heart attack.

◆ Older men suffering from diabetes or prostate disease may experience impotence. If you have this problem, don't be embarrassed to consult your family doctor. Many types of impotence can be successfully treated with medication, or by using external or implanted devices that assist in achieving and maintaining an erection (see page 187).

◆ Other conditions, such as depression and anxiety, can impair sexual interest and arousal, but these, too, can be successfully treated (see page 211).

◆ If you have undergone a hysterectomy (removal of the uterus) or a mastectomy because of breast cancer, you may avoid sex because you now feel less feminine and attractive. If you have a strong relationship, your partner should be able to reassure you that you are still desirable. If you are entering a new relationship, this is an issue that you might wish to discuss with your partner once you feel comfortable together.

◆ If you or your partner suffers from arthritis that causes pain, or if you have been left with some type of paralysis following a stroke, this can interfere with enjoyable sex. Your doctor or a physiotherapist may be able to recommend alternative sexual positions that will be more comfortable for you.

◆ Some medications, including drugs to control high blood pressure, diuretics (water pills), barbiturates, tranquilizers, narcotics and some antidepressants, can interfere with normal sexual response. If you think a certain drug is affecting you in this way, mention it to your doctor, who may be able to switch you to one with fewer side effects.

◆ You may find that using tobacco or drinking too much alcohol dulls your sexual responses.

What's the major obstacle to a good sex life in older age?

Alex Comfort, a renowned geriatric psychiatrist, once said: "Old folks stop having sex for the same reasons they stop riding a bicycle – general infirmity, thinking it looks ridiculous, or they don't have a bicycle."

In fact, not having a bicycle – the lack of a suitable partner – is the main obstacle to sex later in life. This is a particular problem for older married women, who tend to outlive their husbands and find there are fewer older men available.

If you've been widowed or divorced, you may want to find a new partner to love and enjoy. But you may be held back from acting on this healthy impulse by your own attitudes and those of others:

◆ It can be daunting to consider romance and sex with someone new if you've been married to one person for most of your life.

◆ If you aren't planning to remarry, you may hesitate because you believe that sex outside of marriage is wrong.

◆ Although an older man may not hesitate to become involved with a younger woman, older women may reject the less traditional option of seeking a younger man.

◆ If you do find a suitable partner for love or remarriage, your adult children may attempt to discourage the relationship because it upsets them to think of you with someone new, or because they want to protect you from making a mistake.

◆ Lack of privacy can hinder your sex life – for example, if you live with an adult child or other relative, or if an adult child lives with you, if you share living space with a roommate, or if you live in a nursing home or other long-term care institution.

One alternative to enjoying sex with someone else is to enjoy it alone. Studies show that nearly all men and many women – even those who have satisfactory partners – create their own physical pleasure through masturbation. If you indulged when you were younger, there's certainly no reason to abandon this normal human pleasure now.

What can you do when your partner is chronically ill?

Loss of a sexual partner through bereavement isn't the only problem that tends to occur later in life. You might find yourself coping with a chronic illness – your own or your partner's – and in some cases, this leads to long-term institutionalization in a hospital or nursing home.

While some people find that serious illness robs them of the energy and desire for sex, others still want to maintain some type of physical intimacy. Unfortunately, few chronic care facilities are equipped in terms of space and policy to provide you with the necessary privacy. But while intercourse and other activities may no longer be possible, there's still great satisfaction to be gained from touching, stroking and kissing your partner.

If your partner is extremely debilitated with chronic neurological or dementing illness, you may be faced with the difficult decision about whether to seek sexual gratification outside your relationship. Some people never see this as an option and find other ways to cope without a sexual partner. This is a deeply personal and private choice that you may want to discuss with a trusted friend or counselor.

Mental and emotional well-being

The best tunes are played on the oldest fiddles.

SIGMUND Z. ENGEL

The connection between mind and body may never be more important than it is now, when your physical health can have a major impact on your state of mind and vice versa.

Aches and pains, acute or chronic illness, age-related declines in vision or hearing – any of these can rob you of pleasure in living. At the same time, negative emotions can contribute to or worsen many physical ailments and may even affect your immune system, making you more prone to infection.

While people continue to change and grow throughout their entire lives, certain personality traits tend to remain fixed. If you were relaxed and easygoing when you were younger, you'll probably stay that way in older age. If you started out stubborn and hard to please, that probably won't change either. Some experts believe that personality traits, particularly negative ones, become even more fixed and exaggerated later in life.

But while you may not be able to change your basic nature, you can do a great deal to encourage mental and emotional well-being.

How can age affect your mental capacities?

Certain physical changes that occur with aging – for example, gradual shrinkage of the brain and the loss of neurons – can affect how well you function mentally. The decline in mental abilities such as reasoning, language fluency and spatial comprehension begins in the mid- to late 60s and accelerates in the 70s. Men are less likely than women to lose some of their spatial abilities – for instance, how to read a map – while women are less likely than men to suffer a decline in inductive reasoning skills – for example, how to assess complex information.

The most obvious change in healthy older women and men occurs in how well they remember certain things. Knowledge that you've accumulated over the years –

history and geography (experts call this "crystalized memory") – is least affected by aging. But so-called fluid memory – the ability to store and retrieve new information or to recall something that happened recently – does decline with aging (see page 197).

? How can age affect your psychological well-being?

Your psychological well-being includes whether or not you feel generally satisfied with your life. Illnesses such as depression and anxiety disorders threaten psychological well-being (see page 210). But many other factors, including a loss of purpose, lack of self-esteem and feelings of isolation, can also threaten your sense of well-being. While the biological process of aging doesn't cause these feelings, how you feel about yourself as you age (including how others make you feel) can have a major impact on contentment later in life.

? What personal traits are important in successful aging?

As we grow older, our attitudes and feelings are continuously reshaped. This can happen as a direct result of some profound life experience, or as part of a conscious effort to change – for example, many people have found that psychotherapy can help them break free from certain negative patterns of thought or behavior.

Researchers who study how people age have identified several key traits that seem to be important in what they call "successful aging."

◆ *Resilience:* the ability to adapt to various expected and unexpected stresses, including physical, psychological and social stress.

Resilience comes from having maintained good physical health – if you've never smoked and kept your weight at a healthy level, you'll probably withstand a bout of pneumonia better than someone who has smoked and is underweight. If you've developed a variety of interests and social connections, chances are you'll adapt better to the death of a spouse or close friend than someone who has been totally dependent on one person.

◆ *Autonomy:* the feeling that you retain some control over your life. When you feel that you no longer have any choices in where you live and what you do every day, you're more likely to suffer from physical and psychological problems.

◆ *Social integration:* an awareness that, even at the end of your life, you are valued by others and there's a place for you in the larger society.

◆ *Integrity:* the sense that when you reflect upon the past, reviewing your experiences and accomplishments, you feel that your life was meaningful. Failure to achieve this sense of integrity at the end of your life can lead to despair, experts say, while doing so can lead you toward a sense of peace.

◆ *Wisdom:* the feeling that you have reached a certain level of experience and insight that is valued by others who have not yet reached that stage.

These last two traits – integrity and wisdom – may be the most difficult to attain because we don't grow older in isolation. Aging is part of a dynamic process in which your self-image and self-esteem are profoundly influenced by how society in general values aging and the aged.

? What can you do to keep mentally and psychologically fit?

The old saying about "a healthy mind in a healthy body" is especially true later in life, and it's one more reason to work at maintaining your physical health through sensible lifestyle habits such as proper diet and adequate exercise.

There are also steps you can take to keep your mind in the best possible condition:

◆ *Exercise your brain.* There's evidence that if you have keen interests later in life, you're more likely to retain your mental abilities. Research has found that even those who have already experienced some age-related mental decline can be helped by courses in problem solving. Read or listen to books, take some adult education or even university courses, do puzzles or join a reading club (if there isn't one in your neighborhood, start one).

◆ *Don't stop having new experiences.* If you're well and can afford to travel, do so. If you don't want to travel alone, ask your travel agent about seniors' tours, and if money is limited, explore the Elderhostel program, which offers older adults inexpensive accommodation away from home. New experiences aren't limited to travel – why not go out to a restaurant that serves a type of food you've never tried before, or attend a jazz concert if you've always chosen the symphony?

◆ *Don't keep company only with people your own age.* Of course it's great to be with those who share your experiences, but don't avoid the younger generation – grandchildren, great-grandchildren and their friends. Although it's sometimes easier for older people to look backwards, where the landscape is familiar, you should also stay in touch with the present and the future. Take a look at some of the books and movies that younger people are talking about and listen to their music. Ask them about their interests, and chances are they'll start asking you about your own. If you don't have grandchildren or if they live far away, get involved at a seniors' center that offers intergenerational programs. These bring older adults and kids together to sing, take photographs or go on outings.

◆ *Keep a daily journal or taped diary, or write your autobiography.* Such activities encourage you to review your life and accomplishments, and may help you identify what you would still like to achieve.

◆ *Seek out stimulating companions.* Studies have shown that just having an intelligent, stimulating person around – whether it's a spouse, a partner, a roommate or a close friend – can have positive effects on your own mental sharpness.

◆ *Practice preventive mental health.* If you start to feel lonely, bored or unhappy, don't wait for these feelings to take hold and make you sick. Just as you would seek medical help for a persistent ache, talk to your doctor or a trusted friend about how you feel and try to take some constructive action.

Looking in the mirror: Changes in appearance

So much has been said and sung of beautiful young girls, why doesn't somebody wake up to the beauty of old women?

HARRIET BEECHER STOWE

Bald as the bare mountain tops are bald, with a baldness full of grandeur.

MATTHEW ARNOLD

How you look is probably the most obvious sign to you and to others that you're growing older. But it can be difficult to age gracefully in a society that prizes slender, well-muscled bodies, a healthy smile, a full head of hair and smooth, unlined skin.

Our attitudes about the importance of physical appearance can vary greatly. If you took special pride in being beautiful or handsome in your youth, you may feel especially upset by the changes that accompany older age. However, if your identity and self-esteem were linked to factors other than appearance – for example, your sense of humor or your intellectual ability – you may have no trouble accepting what you see in the mirror.

In general, women have always felt that their attractiveness, including a more youthful appearance, matters more than it does for men, and they have been the ones to use cosmetics, hair dye and plastic surgery. Now as some women rebel against social pressures to stay young-looking, some men are starting to take a greater interest in their appearance.

It's easy to say that how we look on the outside should matter less than who we are on the inside. But for many people, keeping up a fine appearance remains important later in life because it boosts their self-esteem and encourages a sense of well-being.

What then should your ultimate goal be? Is it to look as well-groomed and wonderful as you can at your age? Or is it to look wonderful by trying to look younger? This is an extremely personal decision that no one else can or should make for you.

? How does growing older affect your skin?

As your skin ages, it becomes thinner and drier. It loses its supporting layer of fat, and there's a deterioration in the blood vessels that nourish it. There is also a decrease in sweating and the production of sebum. This moist, oily substance is secreted by glands in the skin and protects it from drying out.

The wrinkling of facial skin, which actually began when you were in your 20s, probably became noticeable by the time you were 40, and will continue for the rest of your life. How soon your skin begins to wrinkle and the extent of wrinkling are based on factors such as heredity, sun exposure during early and middle life, and smoking.

Aging skin is more prone to *brown spots or patches* caused by exposure to sunlight. These tend to appear on your face, upper arms or the backs of your hands. Some older adults also develop *rosacea*, a long-term condition that causes redness in the nose, forehead and cheeks due to widened blood vessels.

Also more common in older age is *intertrigo*. The skin becomes red with itching and raw patches, usually occurring in body folds and creases – for example, in the groin, between the legs, under the arms, and, in women, under the breasts. Friction and lack of ventilation cause the skin to become raw and, if a fungal infection develops, it can produce an odor.

? What can you do to keep older skin looking great?

Here are some ways you can protect and care for your skin now:

◆ Wash your face less often, avoiding harsh soaps and astringent cleansers. Pat skin dry (but not too dry) with a soft towel and use a daily moisturizer. Expensive "anti-aging" creams and exotic extracts that promise amazing skin renewal work no better than less pricey creams and lotions available at your grocery store or pharmacy. Men should also moisturize their skin after shaving.

◆ Drink plenty of water to moisturize skin from the inside, and if dryness is a persistent problem, especially in the winter, a portable humidifier can help. If dry skin becomes itchy, or if a rash or broken areas develop, consult your doctor.

◆ Wear a sunscreen with a sun protection factor (SPF) of 15 or higher whenever you go outdoors, even on bright winter days. Shade your face and the back of your neck with a broad-brimmed hat, protect the eye area with sunglasses, and wear light, loose, long-sleeved clothes.

◆ Like darker moles, brown age spots should be watched carefully – most are harmless, but any change in their shape or appearance should be reported to your doctor. Some people try to conceal or fade these spots by using lemon juice or commercial "fading" products. Check with your doctor first.

◆ If you are prone to intertrigo, keep body creases dry and cool. After bathing, apply a dusting of cornstarch. If the skin becomes red and sore, see your doctor, who can prescribe medications to dry the area and control fungus infection. If extra weight is a factor, try to lose a few pounds.

? What effect does aging have on your hair?

You grow and shed hair in cycles throughout your life. Each hair cell or follicle (you had about 100,000 of them when your hair was at its fullest) alternates between a resting stage and a growing stage. Both men and women begin to lose their hair – that is, hairs are shed but don't grow back – by about age 50, and this loss becomes more rapid in the 70s and 80s.

Thinning and loss of hair are just one sign of aging. As you get older, hair begins to appear gray or white because the new hairs growing in no longer contain the pigment that gave your hair its natural black, brown, blonde or red color.

Body hair, including eyebrows and eyelashes, pubic and underarm hair, and chest and facial hair in men, also becomes thinner and loses its color.

Significant hair loss in men is usually caused by an inherited tendency known as "male pattern baldness": Hair begins to recede at the forehead and/or the crown, leaving a fringe of hair around the back and sides of the head. Serious age-related hair loss in women is less common, although women's hair does tend to become thinner and more difficult to manage with age.

In addition to hair loss, you may also develop areas of new or excess hair growth. In men this can occur in or on the ears, in the nostrils, and on the upper back and arms. Women may develop hair growth on the upper lip, the chin, and the lower abdomen. Such hair growth could be a sign of some hormonal problem and should be reported to your doctor.

? How should you care for your hair?

Here are some suggestions about hair care later in life:

◆ Men who are bothered by baldness can try several things. A few – about 10 percent of those who try it – have been able to grow new scalp hair by regular applications of a cream containing the drug *minoxidil*. The drawbacks are that hair grown by using minoxidil is usually sparse and short, hair may stop growing when the drug is stopped, the drug is costly and it can have side effects such as headaches.

Other options include *hair transplants* (plugs of healthy, growing hair are removed from one part of the head and transplanted elsewhere); *scalp reduction surgery* (the bald area is removed and skin covered with hair pulled over to replace it); or a *hairpiece* (designed to blend into the color and texture of your remaining hair). Finally, you could choose to glory in your baldness and identify with the virile, balding look sported by the late Yul Brynner (the King in *The King and I*), Sean Connery (the former James Bond), and the British actor Patrick Stewart (Captain Picard on the television show "Star Trek: The Next Generation"), who was recently named one of the world's sexiest men of any age!

◆ Excess hair can be left alone, although women with this problem often want to hide or get rid of it. You can do the former temporarily by *bleaching* or the latter by hair removal methods, including *plucking, waxing* or *chemical depilatories*. A more permanent solution is *electrolysis*. A technician uses a needle to deliver a tiny burst of electricity to each unwanted hair follicle, which may prevent it from growing back. This procedure is expensive and time consuming, and it should be done only by a skilled technician who either uses disposable needles or provides you with your own personal needle (preventing the transmission of bloodborne infections such as hepatitis and human immunodeficiency virus, or HIV). If you have heart trouble or wear a pacemaker, never have electrolysis without consulting your doctor first.

◆ To avoid pulling out or breaking hair, don't brush or comb it too often or when it's wet. Avoid pulling hair back too tightly and using brush rollers.

Cosmetic surgery

Society's obsession with youth has caused many people to seek out cosmetic surgery in the hope that it will make them look younger. Again, this is a very personal choice, but one which should be carefully considered.

It's important for you and your doctor to discuss why you want cosmetic surgery. Even though these procedures are widely available, they aren't risk-free, they can be painful, and the cost – often thousands of dollars – is probably not covered by your health insurance.

You shouldn't have cosmetic surgery to please your spouse or partner, or to raise your spirits if you are feeling low. You should also be realistic about what can be achieved. While some of these procedures may make you look younger, the change is temporary and you may need to repeat surgery periodically to maintain the desired effect.

One type of cosmetic surgery may actually be recommended for older women. Large, pendulous breasts often cause back and shoulder pain, as well as irritation of the skin where the breasts rub against the chest and abdomen. Breast reduction can be used to reduce their size.

The most common cosmetic procedures that doctors consider to be fairly safe are:

◆ *eye tucks*, where the surgeon removes sagging skin and puffiness above the eyelid and below the eyelid;

◆ *face lifts*, where facial skin is peeled away from underlying structures, then trimmed, draped and sutured to give a tighter, smoother appearance to the face. Liposuction may be done to remove pockets of unwanted fat. New procedures also involve surgery to facial muscles and underlying tissue;

◆ *chemical peels*, where a type of acid is used to remove the top layer of dead skin. This softens fine lines and wrinkles, but heavy lines can't be erased with this procedure.

Procedures that are commonly done but are *definitely not recommended* include:

◆ *injections of silicone or body fat* to plump up wrinkles and lines in the face. Silicone is not considered safe for injection, and fat injections may cause hardened calcium deposits;

◆ *liposuction*, where fat is suctioned out of areas such as the thighs, buttocks, abdomen and face. This can cause torn blood vessels and blood clots in older patients.

If you've thought it all through and still want to go ahead, ask your family doctor to recommend a reputable cosmetic surgeon. A good surgeon will want to know about your motives, your expectations and your general health.

◆ If you don't like your gray hair, you can color it, but nothing will ever restore it to its original color. One way to liven up your appearance and show that you're proud of your age is to color dull gray or partially gray hair a beautiful white or silver.

? **What effect does aging have on your teeth?**

If you're over 65, it's likely that you grew up expecting to lose many, if not most, of your teeth later in life. In fact, many older people alive today *are* missing teeth and must rely on full or partial dentures to help them eat and talk properly.

But older age itself doesn't cause diseases that lead to tooth loss. Other factors are involved:

◆ When you were younger, the quality of dental care and the understanding of dental hygiene were much poorer than they are today.

◆ Dental techniques were less advanced, so many dental procedures were painful, which caused people to avoid seeking treatment.

◆ Techniques such as orthodontia (the use of braces) to straighten crowded teeth and make them easier to clean were not widespread two generations ago. Dentists were more likely to treat problems by extracting teeth rather than trying to preserve them.

◆ Most communities didn't have fluoridated water, which is known to reduce the prevalence of dental caries, or tooth decay.

Fortunately, the situation has changed in recent decades, and thanks to improvements in dental treatment, your adult children and their children have an excellent chance of keeping all their teeth for life.

How should you care for your teeth?

Taking care of your mouth and your remaining teeth is extremely important.

◆ Decayed or broken teeth can cause infections in the bone, which may put your overall health at risk.

◆ If your teeth are causing you pain, or if they're missing, this can affect your ability to chew food properly. This in turn can lead to problems with swallowing and indigestion. Both can cause you to lose interest in food, increasing your risk for malnutrition and serious health problems.

◆ Missing teeth can affect your ability to form words properly. This may make conversation difficult, which can cause you to become isolated from other people.

◆ Diseased and unattractive teeth can affect your self-esteem, and you may stop smiling or avoid talking to other people.

If you've been seeing a dentist regularly until now, don't stop! If you've avoided having regular dental checkups and haven't been caring for your teeth, it's not too late to start:

◆ If you don't have a regular dentist, ask friends and family to recommend one who is accessible and affordable. The high cost of dental care can be a problem for older people on a fixed income, but some dentists may be willing to discuss a reduced fee.

◆ It's a good idea to look for a dentist who has experience in treating older clients. Call your local dental association for advice.

◆ You should see your dentist at least once or twice a year for a full examination, and possibly X-rays, of your teeth, gums and facial structures. You should also have your teeth professionally cleaned at least once or twice a year, or more frequently if your dentist advises it.

You are responsible for taking care of your teeth and gums in between visits to your dentist. The dental hygienist who cleans your teeth can instruct you on how to brush and floss your teeth, paying special attention to your gums.

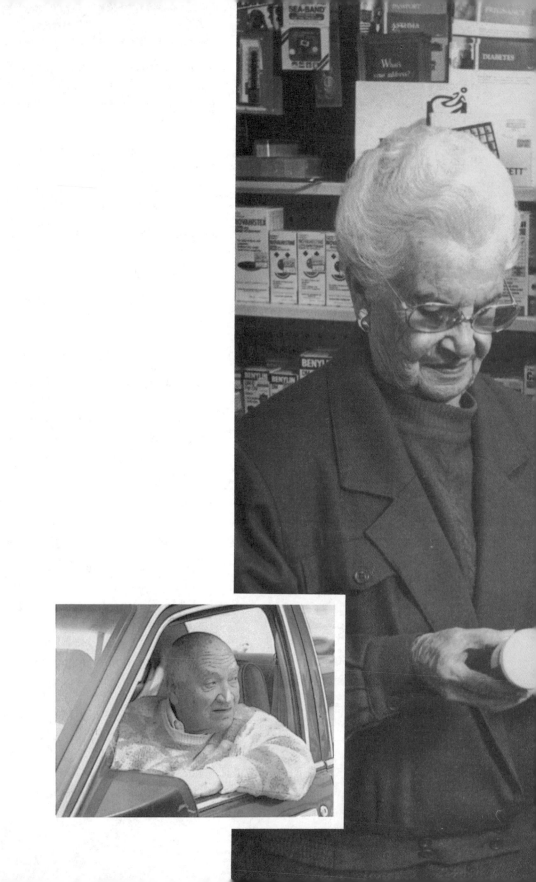

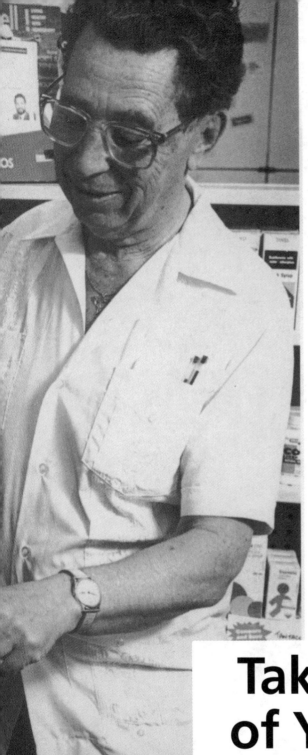

2

To be (human) is to be responsible ... . It is to feel, when setting one's stone, that one is contributing to the building of the world.

ANTOINE DE SAINT-EXUPERY

Taking Charge of Your Health

UNDERSTANDING HOW YOUR BODY changes with the years is just the first step toward health and well-being later in life. You must also consider whether you're doing everything you can to help yourself achieve a healthier, happier lifestyle.

In this chapter we'll look at some important issues and areas of concern – how to deal effectively with your doctors, how to avoid problems with medication, how to cope with change and stress, and finally, how to take charge of your personal safety.

Dealing with your doctors

What I call a good patient is one who, having found a good physician, sticks to him till he dies.

OLIVER WENDELL HOLMES, SR.

The patient-doctor relationship is probably quite different today from what it was years ago, when you were much younger. Back then doctors expected patients to accept what they were told without question, and patients followed medical advice passively, often keeping important information, questions and concerns to themselves.

These days patients are better informed about health matters, and are more likely to take an active role in their health care. Good doctors have always welcomed this attitude, saying it relieves them of pressure to be omnipotent, and also returns some control and responsibility for health back where it belongs – with the patient.

In some surveys of attitudes toward doctors, people say they don't like doctors in general, but they do like their own doctor in particular. How you feel about doctors has

an important effect on your health. For example, you may have had some negative experiences that make you reluctant to have periodic checkups or seek medical help when you're sick. If you feel that doctors have a great deal of power, you may feel intimidated or fearful – or you may see them as gods, unable to do any wrong.

It's important to have a realistic view of your own doctors. Physicians are highly trained, sometimes overworked professionals who must deal with stressful situations on a daily basis. But they're also people who have their own families, problems and illnesses. We expect a lot from our doctors: We want them to protect us from illness, relieve our pain, heal our diseases and listen to our troubles. While some physicians fall short, it's a wonder that so many are able to deliver.

? ## How do you choose the best doctor for you?

It's amazing how many people don't have a regular doctor – sometimes called a family physician or "primary care doctor." If you do, chances are he has cared for you for many years and knows your medical history and health status.

You may wonder whether to seek the services of a geriatrician, a doctor who specializes in the care of older adults. If you're relatively healthy and already have a good relationship with your family doctor or internist, this isn't necessary. However, if you're over 75 and have a number of health problems, your doctor may want to refer you to a geriatrician or to another primary care doctor who has experience and interest in treating older patients.

Here are some tips to keep in mind if you're choosing a new primary care doctor:

◆ His office should be fairly close to your home and accessible by public transit if you don't drive. Having the doctor nearby makes it easier for you to visit, and if your physician makes house calls this is also convenient.

◆ It's a good idea to find a doctor who is located in a clinic or medical complex that has an on-site laboratory, X-ray, and pharmacy. You should also look for someone in a group practice – that means the doctors cover for each other 24 hours, seven days a week. The office should have an answering service that can reach the doctor, rather than an answering machine that takes messages only.

◆ The doctor should be associated with a hospital in your community. Ask friends and family if they can recommend their own doctors, or call your local medical association, the family practice unit in any large hospital or the public health department. Decide whether you feel more comfortable seeing a male or female doctor.

◆ When you call or visit, check to see if the staff, including receptionists, nurses and technicians, are pleasant and well organized, and if the waiting room looks comfortable.

◆ It's best to choose a new doctor when you're feeling reasonably well and not during a crisis. That way you won't feel under any pressure to stay with the doctor if you don't seem to get along.

? ## How often should you see your primary care doctor?

How often you see the doctor depends on your current age and health. Although many younger people have stopped having yearly checkups, if you're over age 65, an annual exam is probably a good idea. Your doctor may pick up an early sign of illness, and it's a good opportunity to let the doctor know if there are any problems or stresses in your life that could affect your health.

While some doctors will have their office staff call and remind you to come for a checkup, in most cases, it's your responsibility. Pick a date – your birthday is a good cue – and make an appointment. If the doctor wants to see you more often, she'll tell you.

? ## When should you see a specialist?

Many problems can be diagnosed and treated by a good primary care doctor. But if symptoms persist or your doctor feels it's necessary, he will refer you to a specialist. People don't normally choose what specialist they will see – doctors tend to refer their patients to other doctors whom they know and trust. Specialists work in cooperation with your primary care doctor, if you have one.

Specialists are usually very busy and they may not get to know you as well as your own doctor. Even so, a good specialist should take the time to talk to you and answer questions.

Here's a list of specialists you're most likely to see if you're over 65:

◆ *Anesthesiologists* choose and administer anesthesia during surgery and monitor you during the operation.

◆ *Cardiologists* diagnose and treat disorders of the heart and blood vessels.

◆ *Dermatologists* diagnose and treat skin diseases and conditions.

◆ *Endocrinologists* specialize in diseases of the hormone-producing glands such as diabetes mellitus, and also treat disorders of the thyroid and adrenal glands.

◆ *Gastroenterologists* diagnose and treat disorders of the digestive system (esophagus, stomach, intestines, gallbladder, pancreas).

◆ *Geriatricians* are usually internists who specialize in treating people over age 65.

◆ *Gynecologists* diagnose and treat disorders of the female reproductive system.

◆ *Hematologists* diagnose and treat disorders of the blood.

◆ *Internists* diagnose and treat (although not surgically) internal disorders.

◆ *Nephrologists* diagnose and treat disorders of the kidneys.

◆ *Neurologists* diagnose and treat disorders of the brain and nervous system, including the spine and nerves.

◆ *Oncologists* diagnose cancer and recommend appropriate treatment. Radiation oncologists specialize in the use of radiation to control cancer.

◆ *Ophthalmologists* diagnose and treat disorders of the eyes.

◆ *Otorhinolaryngologists* (also known as ear, nose and throat, or ENT, doctors) deal with these areas.

◆ *Physiatrists* coordinate many aspects of physical rehabilitation after illness or injury.

◆ *Psychiatrists* diagnose and manage most mental, behavioral and emotional illnesses. Geriatric psychiatrists specialize in treating these illnesses in people over age 65.

◆ *Radiologists* order and interpret X-rays and ultrasound scans to diagnose medical problems.

◆ *Respirologists* or chest doctors specialize in diseases of the trachea, bronchi and lungs.

◆ *Surgeons* diagnose and operate on many parts of the body and usually specialize in one area – for example, neurosurgery, eye surgery or gastrointestinal surgery.

◆ *Urologists* diagnose and treat urinary tract diseases and, in men, problems of the reproductive organs. *Urogynecologists* specialize in urinary problems affecting women.

While medical doctors are a vital part of

Making the most of your office visit

Setting up the appointment

If possible, schedule appointments when they're most convenient for you – you're more likely to keep them. Write down the date and time on your calendar, and if you want an extra reminder, ask the doctor's secretary to call you the day before.

Before the appointment

Write down any questions you have for the doctor and take them with you. Get your medications together and take them along, too. Take a bath – you'll feel less self-conscious about your body during the physical examination, and your doctor will appreciate it.

The day of the appointment

Call in the morning and ask if the doctor is on schedule. If she's running late, at least you'll be ready for a wait. Bring along something to do while you wait – a book, some magazines, a knitting project.

What to expect

A good doctor is like a detective. She will look for important clues about your health – for example, she may watch how well you move, whether your hearing is clear, whether your breathing seems too fast, too slow or labored. She may also listen "between the lines" of your answers for any emotional or social problems affecting your health.

Here's what the doctor will do during an office appointment that includes a thorough history-taking and a physical examination:

◆ Take a complete medical history, including any previous illnesses and treatments; any previous surgery; what medications you've taken or are taking now; your family history to see if you're prone to any diseases; where you used to work, to see whether you were exposed to any toxic substances that could have damaged your lungs or other parts of your body; whether you've traveled anywhere in the past five years, to see if you might have been exposed to a parasite or infection.

◆ Check to see if your immunizations are up to date. He may recommend that you have an annual influenza shot and a vaccine to protect you against pneumococcal pneumonia (a common type of pneumonia in older adults).

◆ Check your height and compare it with your records – if you lose a certain amount of height, this can be a symptom of osteoporosis (see page 163).

◆ Check your weight to make sure you haven't gained or lost too much.

◆ Examine your eyes for abnormalities that could be a sign of nervous system disease, eye disease or thyroid disorder.

◆ Examine your ears to look for signs of infection, tumors, damaged eardrums, and a buildup of ear wax, which can impede hearing.

◆ Check the mucous membranes of your mouth and throat for abnormalities, and also examine your teeth, gums and tongue.

◆ Feel your neck to check your lymph nodes, thyroid gland and the major arteries that nourish the head and brain.

◆ Listen to your chest and back with a stethoscope to check for abnormal sounds that could mean heart or lung disease. You may be asked to cough or do simple exercises, and it's not unusual for the doctor to order a chest X-ray and an electrocardiogram if she wants to check your heart and lung function more thoroughly.

◆ Take your blood pressure to see whether it's too high or too low. This may be done several times while you're standing, sitting or lying down, and it may be done by checking pressure in both arms. If you feel nervous about having your blood pressure taken, tell the doctor – many people suffer from "white coat hypertension," which means their blood pressure rises at the sight of the doctor or blood pressure cuff.

◆ Feel the tops of your feet or behind your ankles for pulses. If they're not strong enough, this could signal a narrowing of arteries due to a buildup of fatty deposits.

◆ Examine your abdomen and pelvic area to check the size and shape of your internal organs and to probe for abnormalities such as hernias. The doctor should also do a digital rectal exam (DRE) with a gloved finger to check your lower bowel for polyps or cancer, and, in men, to check for signs of prostate disease.

◆ Check your body's range of motion, including how flexible your joints are, how well you bend and move, how strong your muscles are and whether you have normal balance.

◆ Examine your legs for signs of swelling that could mean you're retaining fluid, and for varicose veins or other abnormalities.

◆ Examine your feet for problems that may need treatment – for example, bunions, corns or hammer toes.

◆ Check your skin for rashes, dryness or excessive perspiration. The doctor will also examine parts of your body that you can't see, such as your back, for suspicious looking moles or other growths that could be an early sign of skin cancer.

For women only
◆ Examine your breasts while you're sitting up and lying down, including probing the nipple areas and armpits for lumps or thickenings. This is very important for women over 65 who are at greater risk for breast cancer than younger women.

◆ Do an internal examination to feel your ovaries and uterus. The doctor will also check the vagina for any signs of cancer or sexually transmitted diseases and may take an internal smear to check for cancer of the cervix.

For men only
◆ Check your prostate gland for changes, which could mean infection or cancer, by inserting a gloved finger into the rectum. This is a very important test for older men, who are at increased risk for prostate disease.

◆ Examine your penis and testicles for signs of infection or other abnormalities.

◆ Check your breasts – while breast cancer in men is rare, it's not unheard of.

The health care partnership

Each time you visit a doctor, it's a good idea to keep in mind that you are a consumer as well as a patient. You're paying for the services you receive, either directly if you don't have a health plan, or indirectly through taxes and fees paid to government or group health-insurance plans. While it's not quite the same as paying plumbers or mechanics for their services, you do have the right to expect certain things from your doctor, and your doctor has the right to expect certain things from you.

What you have the right to expect from your doctor

◆ She should listen and respond to you appropriately. This means she avoids medical jargon, takes time to explain things to you and answer questions, and doesn't make you feel rushed unless there's a good reason.

◆ He should show concern for your dignity. This means you should be allowed to undress in private, unless you ask for assistance. When he examines your body, the parts not being looked at should be covered with a sheet. A doctor should never make flippant, complimentary or off-color remarks about your body, and should never touch you in any inappropriate way. Many patients don't mind and even welcome appropriate touching, such as a gentle pat on the shoulder or a warm handclasp. A hug or embrace is fine if you've known your doctor for many years and consider him a friend. But it's a good idea for both of you to keep some professional distance during an office visit.

◆ She shouldn't treat you differently because of your age, gender, sexual orientation, race, religion, ethnic background or economic status.

◆ He is required by law to respect patient confidentiality. What you tell him should not be reported to other family members without your permission, and your records should be kept secure and confidential. Rules governing access to medical records are set by state and federal law. In general, while the records themselves belong to the doctor (who must keep the original copy for legal reasons), as the patient, you own the information in the record as it relates to you.

the health care team, they aren't the only component. Older adults are more likely than younger ones to encounter other health professionals.

◆ *Dentists* treat problems of the teeth and gums and recommend procedures to keep your teeth and gums healthy.

◆ *Denturists* design and create full or partial dentures to replace missing teeth.

◆ *Dietitians that* advise people about healthy eating and recommend foods that can help in the prevention and control of various diseases and conditions. They also provide information about all matters related to healthy nutrition.

◆ *Nurses* assist doctors in taking certain tests such as blood pressure measurement, and may also take medical histories. In hos-

You can request that a copy of your records be sent to another doctor, and in some cases, you can refuse to have them sent.

◆ She should fully explain everything she's doing. This includes examinations and tests that she may order. You should be told how long it will take to get test results and whether the office will call you (most doctors only call if the tests uncover a problem).

◆ He should never try to explain away a symptom as "just a normal part of getting older."

What your doctor has the right to expect from you

◆ If you're a new patient, you should make sure she has access to your previous medical records.

◆ You should provide a complete list of your medications, or better still, bring them along in their original containers so he can see the dosage, the type (brand name or generic drug), and any instructions. Also show him any unfilled prescriptions you may have been given by another doctor.

◆ Be honest about how you're feeling. Your doctor can't help you if you hide physical or personal problems out of shame or embarrassment.

◆ Follow the doctor's advice – it's part of the partnership. For example, if you continue to smoke after being advised to quit, you have no right to complain when you're diagnosed with lung disease. If the doctor gave you advice that you didn't follow, let him know about it and tell him why. Perhaps you found it too hard to stick to a certain diet, or a medication he prescribed upset your stomach. He may be able to tailor the advice so it's easier for you to comply.

◆ Keep socializing to a minimum. A good doctor won't mind spending some time talking to you – you may reveal something important during a social conversation. If you feel lonely, by all means tell your doctor – this can have a major impact on your physical and mental well-being. But too much chatting may make it hard for her to accomplish everything she'd like to in the time available.

pital, they dispense medications and treatments and play a vital role in assisting surgeons during operations. Public health nurses visit older adults at home to change dressings, carry out certain treatments and discuss health concerns. In some communities, nurse practitioners diagnose common ailments and recommend treatments.

◆ *Nursing assistants and health care aides*

provide care and assistance to people in hospitals and nursing homes.

◆ *Physiotherapists* specialize in mobility and movement disorders, using various exercises and other treatments to help people with conditions such as arthritis and paralysis achieve their maximum level of physical functioning.

◆ *Podiatrists* specialize in problems of the feet.

Common medical tests for older adults

Your doctor may order one or all of these tests, depending on what he's checking for. Most are done as part of your periodic health examination, while others are usually used to diagnose or rule out specific health problems.

If you have any questions or concerns about a medical test, always ask your doctor. He should tell you why the test is being done, when you can expect results, and what could happen if results are positive. (In medical language, a "positive" test means an abnormality has been found, while a "negative" result means everything looks normal.)

Laboratory tests

You may be requested to avoid eating before giving samples of blood or urine. Don't cheat, because if you do, it can distort the results.

◆ *Blood analysis*: Your blood is normally tested to see whether you're producing the right type and proportion of blood cells, and to pick up signs of disease or deficiencies – for example, too much or too little glucose, or abnormal levels of cholesterol and other blood fats.

◆ *Pap test:* A sample of cells taken from your cervix is analyzed for changes that could be a sign of infection or cancer.

◆ *PSA (prostate-specific-antigen) test*: This test can pick up a substance in your blood that is a marker for prostate cancer, but its use in mass screening is still controversial, and not all doctors recommend or offer it (see page 138).

◆ *Stool analysis*: A stool sample is checked for the presence of blood, which could be a sign of gastrointestinal disease, including cancer of the colon or rectum.

◆ *Urinalysis*: A sample of your urine is tested to make sure your kidneys are working properly, to check for signs of infection, and to look for sugar, which could be a sign of diabetes, or for protein, which may be a sign of kidney disease.

Specialized tests

◆ *Electrocardiogram* (ECG or EKG): Electrodes attached externally to your chest record patterns that help your doctor detect any heart abnormalities. (Painless, non-

◆ *Occupational therapists* help people with physical injury, illness or mental disorder to work and live by themselves despite their health problems.

◆ *Optometrists and opticians* are involved in non-medical aspects of eye care, such as vision testing and making glasses and contact lenses.

◆ *Social workers* help people and their families cope with stresses and decision-making associated with illness and other problems.

◆ *Speech-language pathologists* diagnose and treat defects of speech due to neurological illness or diseases affecting the throat and larynx; they may also diagnose and help people with swallowing disorders.

invasive, can be done in doctor's office.)

◆ *Endoscopy:* The doctor uses special equipment that allows him to see into your stomach (gastroscopy) or colon (colonoscopy) for evidence of abnormalities. This test is usually done if you have symptoms or a family history of gastrointestinal disease. (Invasive, some discomfort, usually done in hospital or clinic.)

◆ *Pulmonary function:* You will be asked to breathe into a device which measures lung function and may reveal signs of emphysema, bronchitis and asthma. (Painless, noninvasive, usually done in hospital or specialist's office.)

Diagnostic imaging
◆ *Chest X-ray:* This X-ray can show infections, emphysema, tumors, heart enlargement and damage caused by smoking or exposure to hazardous substances. (Noninvasive, usually done in doctor's office or clinic.)

◆ *CT (Computerized Tomography) and MRI (Magnetic Resonance Imaging) Scans:* These use specialized X-ray equipment to give doctors a detailed and highly accurate look at structures inside your body. They are used to diagnose or rule out disease. (Non-invasive, may require you to remain motionless for up to an hour, usually done in hospital.)

◆ *Mammogram:* You'll be asked to place your breasts in a special device that compresses the tissue and exposes them to small doses of radiation. Screening mammograms pick up very early tumors and other abnormalities, while diagnostic mammograms are done to check out a suspicious growth. (Non-invasive, some discomfort, usually done in clinic or hospital.)

◆ *Ultrasound:* This test uses high-frequency sound waves to make a picture of various organs and structures, which your doctor can then check for signs of disease. External ultrasound involves moving a special wand across your skin (a special gel is applied first to reduce friction); internal ultrasound uses a smaller wand. (Can be invasive, little discomfort, usually done in clinic or hospital.)

? Should you go to your doctor's office alone?

Having someone else – your spouse, an adult child or friend – accompany you to the doctor's office may be helpful in some cases – for example, if you feel extremely anxious or physically shaky, or if you have trouble communicating because of language problems. Some women may feel more comfortable having a third person, such as a female nurse, in the examining room when they're being examined by a male doctor. But having someone else join you in the examining room or office may cause certain problems. A recent study found that when people had companions, the following occurred:

◆ The patient and doctor were less likely to make joint decisions.

◆ The companion answered for the patient, even when she was quite capable of answering for herself.

◆ The companion and doctor tended to talk *about* the patient rather than *with* the patient.

However, when patients saw the doctors alone, the following happened:

◆ The doctor and patient laughed together more.

◆ The patient was more likely to bring up topics important to her. (Although the companion also brought up topics, they were different from the ones mentioned by the patient.)

If you feel you need moral or physical support, or if you want someone with you when you receive test results or follow-up instructions, then it's a good idea to bring someone along. But you should spend part of your office visit alone with your doctor.

When should you get a second opinion?

You rely on your doctor to give you her best medical advice. But if your primary care physician makes a certain diagnosis or recommends a course of action such as surgery or chemotherapy, or concludes that a particular symptom is harmless, you may want to get another doctor's opinion before deciding what to do.

If you don't have complete trust in your doctor, and if a few weeks' delay won't jeopardize your health or prognosis, then there's no harm in getting a second opinion. Your doctor should be willing to arrange it for you. However, if she won't, then it's up to you to seek out another doctor.

If your primary care doctor has sent you to a surgeon who recommends surgery, you may feel the issue isn't clear. However, you have already received two opinions – your doctor's and the surgeon's. In this case, you may still want to return to your primary care doctor and discuss what the surgeon told you. If you still aren't sure, you could ask to be referred to another surgeon.

You have to weigh several factors here. While it's good to educate yourself about your alternatives, it can also be confusing to hear too many opinions. As one geriatrician says: "I often tell patients that if they keep looking, they will probably eventually find an opinion that they like, but one that is not necessarily sound."

Should you consult a chiropractor or other non-medical healer?

There's ample evidence that medical science still has a lot to learn about many factors that affect our health. You may already believe in the possibility of non-medical healing and health maintenance – for example, through the use of traditional remedies, herbs and foods, and techniques such as spinal manipulation used by chiropractors. Perhaps you feel that, since your doctors haven't been able to help you, it's worth trying something else.

Some alternative healers are physicians who practice a more "holistic" type of medicine – treating the whole person rather than various body parts. Other healers, such as naturopaths, homeopaths, herbalists and chiropractors, may have no medical training.

There may be a fine line between practitioners who genuinely believe their methods to be helpful and those whose main objective is to make money by charging for products and questionable services, including analysis of your hair, nails or skin to detect health problems.

When it comes to seeking help outside traditional medicine, the best advice is "caveat emptor – let the buyer beware." Recently some medical doctors have become more open-minded about these alternatives, as long as the methods used aren't harmful and don't replace accepted treatments. If you want to try one of these alternatives, consider discussing the matter with your doctor first.

Using your medicines wisely

This small white pill is what I munch
at breakfast and right after lunch.
I take the pill that's kelly green
before each meal and in between.
These loganberry-colored pills
I take for early morning chills.
I take the pill with zebra stripes
to cure my early evening gripes.
These orange-tinted ones, of course,
I take to cure my charley horse.

FROM "YOU'RE ONLY OLD ONCE" BY DR. SEUSS

Like so many other things in life, drugs are a mixed blessing. When properly prescribed and taken as directed, they can prevent and cure countless diseases, relieve pain and soothe other unpleasant symptoms, and help us cope when life's problems overwhelm us.

But when drugs aren't prescribed or used properly, they can cause problems. As you grow older, you may develop certain illnesses and conditions that will require you to take prescription or over-the-counter med-ication. So it's important that you understand how to use drugs wisely and avoid medication-related risks.

 Why are you more vulnerable to problems with medication now?

When older adults get into trouble with their medications, they may feel that it's somehow their fault. Of course you carry some responsibility, but so do others: your doctors, your pharmacist and the companies that develop and market prescription and non-prescription medicines to older people. Here are some reasons why you may encounter problems:

◆ Age-related changes in your body affect how various drugs are absorbed, used and eliminated. In some cases, absorption may be slowed down, making the drug less effective. Because you may excrete drugs less quickly, they can build up in your body, causing unpleasant side effects.

◆ You're more likely to suffer from diseases and conditions that affect how your body uses drugs – for instance, if you have congestive heart failure, reduced blood flow to your intestines can reduce the absorption of medication. Because you suffer from more than one condition, you may be taking several medications at the same time, both prescription drugs and over-the-counter products. This can lead to unwanted interactions between drugs – or one of your drugs may actually cancel out the benefits of another.

◆ If you have more than one ailment, you may also be seeing several different doctors who are giving you different prescriptions. Unless each doctor knows what other drugs you're taking, again you run the risk of unwanted drug interactions or one drug canceling out the benefits of another.

◆ Many of the drugs now in use were tested on younger people, most of them men. They may have subtly different effects on older adults, with special problems depending on whether they are used on women or men.

◆ Older people may need to take a lower dose of certain drugs because of age-related

changes in body weight and the distribution of body fat.

◆ Some doctors may feel it's more important to relieve the stress of loneliness and anxiety by prescribing tranquilizers and antidepressants than it is to help their older patients solve these problems without medication – for example, by using therapy and stress management techniques.

◆ Studies show that if you think of yourself as "unhealthy" – even if your health is relatively good – you're more likely to take medicines.

❓ What are the most common medication mistakes?

When doctors talk about how well people follow their prescriptions, they say we are either "compliant" (that is, we follow directions well) or "non-compliant" (we don't).

Being a compliant patient is usually a good idea – after all, how can you possibly benefit from your doctor's advice if you don't follow it? But some studies have found that, especially among older adults whose doctors *overprescribe* medication, non-compliance (not taking medication or taking less medication) actually leads to better health.

Your doctor should be reviewing your medications regularly to make certain there are no problems. If he isn't and you have some concerns, it's important to mention them during your office visit. You can also discuss any questions you might have about side effects or unwanted drug interactions with your pharmacist.

Let's assume that your doctor is prescribing wisely. What are the common medication errors you're most likely to make?

◆ *You stop taking the medication or reduce the amount you take without telling your doctor.* Don't assume you can stop taking a certain medication just because you feel better. Antibiotics, for instance, may clear up your symptoms, but you must take the full course of medication to kill bacteria causing the infection.

Many drugs have side effects when used by younger as well as older people. Typical minor side effects include dry mouth, upset stomach, headaches, rashes, blurred vision and drowsiness. It's dangerous to stop taking medication because of side effects without first discussing it with your doctor. You were given the medication for a reason – for example, to lower your blood pressure, to cure an infection or stop it from getting worse. Let your doctor know about the side effects, and he may be able to adjust the dose or switch you to a different drug.

◆ *You take too much of the medication.* You may think that if one pill is good, two pills are better. This is false and can even be harmful. It's also easy to take too much medication if you forgot when you took your last dose. If you forgot or missed a dose, ask your doctor what to do. It may be all right if this happens occasionally, or else your doctor may suggest that you double the next dose. (See page 197 for suggestions on keeping track of your medication.)

◆ *You take the right medicine but at the wrong time.* Some drugs should be taken with food to prevent an upset stomach or to slow down absorption; others need to be taken on an empty stomach or right before bedtime. Some medicines should never be taken with milk or acidic fruit juice, which reduces their effectiveness, and most drugs should never be taken with alcohol. Alcoholic beverages taken with sedating medications such as barbiturates, tranquilizers, antidepressants and antihistamines can cause drowsiness, sleepiness and poor coordination. Very large doses or overdoses of these medicines combined with alcohol can be fatal.

◆ *You "borrow" unused prescription medications from a family member or friend.* This may seem easier and more economical than asking your doctor for a prescription, but it's also dangerous. Your friend's pills weren't prescribed for you – the dose may be wrong or perhaps the drug has expired and is no longer effective.

? **What are some other reasons for medication mistakes?**
Studies have shown that the number of medication mistakes you make is directly related to the number of different drugs you're taking – the more drugs you take every day, the more likely you are to make an error.

You're also more likely to make an error if you don't understand why you're taking each drug. It's not enough to know that you have to take a blue capsule every morning, an orange tablet with meals and two red pills before bed. Be sure your doctor explains why each drug is being prescribed. If you don't understand, ask again.

When taking pills, don't reach for them in the dark or keep them on your bedside table (except in special cases, such as nitroglycerine pills for angina pain). It's too easy to take the wrong pills or too many pills.

Taking stock of your medicine chest

Every few months it's a good idea to weed through your medicine chest and review your stock of prescription drugs and over-the-counter medications.

◆ Get rid of any drugs or products that have passed the expiration date (usually printed on the packaging). They may no longer be effective.

◆ Throw out any products that look dried up or discolored.

◆ Get rid of any drugs that you are no longer using. The best way is to return them to your pharmacist in their original containers for safe disposal. It's not a good idea to flush prescription drugs down the toilet into the water supply or to put them in the garbage where they could be found by a child.

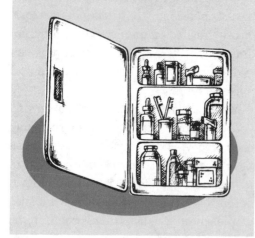

Simple problems can also lead to medication errors or non-compliance. Some older people find they can't manage to open the child-proof caps found on most prescription and non-prescription drugs. There's no rea-son to struggle – ask your pharmacist to give you some regular, easy-to-remove caps, and consider writing a letter to drug manufacturers telling them that they should offer a greater choice in packaging. (If you have young grandchildren or great-grandchildren who visit or stay with you, don't forget to put your medications safely out of their reach!)

? Where can you get help with your medicines?

While your neighborhood pharmacist can't diagnose or treat your problem, he or she can be very helpful when it comes to your medications. Pharmacists are often more accessible than your doctor, their knowledge of drugs and side effects is likely to be more up-to-date, and they are usually happy to answer questions about prescription and over-the-counter drugs. Some drugstore chains now provide drug information sheets, and many keep computerized information on each customer's prescriptions. In addition to helping you keep track of your medication history, this may allow your pharmacist to spot any potential serious drug interactions. Of course, if you are filling prescriptions at different pharmacies, this makes it impossible for each pharmacist to keep track of what you are taking.

Older adults who have been hospitalized sometimes find it daunting to leave the hospital on an unfamiliar medication regimen. Many hospitals now offer self-medication programs as part of their discharge planning. These programs teach you about your personal medications, reducing the chance for mistakes when you go home.

If you take several different medications each day, you can purchase a personal dispensing tray at the drugstore that can help you keep track of your pills.

What's the difference between generic and brand name drugs?

When a drug is first developed it's given a generic or official name. The company that developed it has sole rights to market the drug – usually under a trade name – until the patent runs out. Then other companies can manufacture and market the same drug under its generic name or they can give it a brand name. In either case, the drug must contain the same ingredients in the same form and strength. Because generic drugs are somewhat less expensive than brand name drugs, ask your doctor to prescribe them for you if possible. (In some cases you may find that your drug benefit program automatically pays for the less expensive, generic drug.) Here are some examples:

Generic name	Brand name
propranolol hydrochloride	Inderal
nortriptyline hydrochloride	Aventyl
enalapril maleate	Vasotec
acetaminophen	Tylenol
furosemide	Lasix

Can over-the-counter drugs be harmful?

Many people use over-the-counter (OTC) drugs, but older adults use them the most. Surveys have found that people over age 65 use *four times* as much non-prescription medication as those who are younger.

We tend to think of these products, which include antacids, pain relievers, cold remedies and laxatives, as harmless, but they can cause all sorts of trouble:

◆ They can cause side effects, including drowsiness or nervousness.

◆ They may contain caffeine, alcohol and other extra ingredients that can cause side effects such as nervousness, sleeplessness or sedation.

◆ You can become dependent on products such as sleeping aids, laxatives and nose drops. They may also have a "rebound" effect, causing the very symptoms that led you to take them – for example, pain relievers can cause headaches and nasal sprays can cause chronic nasal stuffiness.

Here are some tips for the safer use of over-the-counter medicines:

◆ Before reaching for any of these products, wait and see if the symptoms pass. If they don't, try a non-drug approach to your problem – a relaxing shower and 20 minutes lying down in a darkened room might relieve your headache; inhaling steam from a warm mist vaporizer may relieve a stuffy nose.

Understanding your prescription

Many people don't understand the terminology on the handwritten prescription that they receive from their doctors. Here's a translation:

BID – take twice a day

TID – take three times a day

QID – take four times a day

PRN – take as needed

Q 4 hours – every four hours

Selecting the best type of painkiller

Painkillers come in a bewildering variety of shapes and forms. You can choose enteric pills, suppositories, or timed-release and extra-strength pills that come in tablets, gelcaps, liquids and even chewing gum.

◆ *Enteric or coated pills* are designed to pass through your stomach before dissolving, which reduces stomach irritation. Use them if you need daily relief for chronic pain.

◆ *Timed-release pills* dissolve slowly, prolonging relief. Use them if you need lasting (overnight) rather than immediate relief.

◆ *Extra-strength pills* contain more pain relievers than regular strength products – 500 milligrams vs. 325 milligrams. Use them if your symptoms aren't relieved by one regular strength dose.

Whether you choose tablets, gelcaps or liquids usually depends on what you find easiest to swallow or what is least expensive.

◆ Always read the product label and follow any directions on how much to take, how often and for how long. The label should also list any non-medicinal ingredients such as caffeine or alcohol.

◆ These products are not meant for long-term use. You may be masking a serious underlying problem by taking painkillers or other drugs – call your doctor if pain or other symptoms persist beyond three days.

A big danger in taking non-prescription medicines is that they can interact with other drugs you're taking, making them less effective or causing unwanted side effects. If your doctor prescribes a certain drug, be sure to tell her if you're taking any over-the-counter medicines.

? Can you abuse laxatives or antacids?

These over-the-counter medicines seem to be favored by older adults who have digestive complaints such as constipation and heartburn. But they must be used carefully to avoid problems.

Laxatives are usually taken to ease the symptoms of constipation. They work by softening stool, making it more fluid, and by adding bulk to the contents of your bowel. Enemas or suppositories also soften stool and stimulate your lower intestine to empty. Problems can occur if you take too many laxatives and take them over a long period of time. They can aggravate your constipation and cause diarrhea, cramping and bloating. You may permanently damage how your bowels function.

It's easy to become "hooked" on laxatives if you have an unrealistic idea of what constitutes normal, healthy bowel movements. You may begin to think that *every* ache or discomfort is due to "irregularity." If you think you may be overusing laxatives, speak to your doctor. You may be able to wean yourself off laxatives by making some basic changes in your diet and behavior (see page 99).

Antacids are usually taken to neutralize stomach acidity, which causes heartburn and indigestion. They interfere with the absorption of many drugs, including digoxin, ranitidine, diazepam, tetracycline, levodopa and corticosteroids, and may interact with other drugs such as warfarin and anticonvulsants. Antacids may also be high in sugar and sodium, which can cause problems if you're on a restricted diet because of diabetes or high blood pressure.

When choosing an antacid, always check the label and ask your doctor or pharmacist about possible drug interactions. You may be able to relieve heartburn and indigestion without taking medication (see page 110). If your symptoms persist for longer than a few days or if they recur, call your doctor.

How do you choose the best painkiller for you?
When you go to the drugstore to buy a non-prescription analgesic (painkiller), you're probably confused by the vast array of choices: acetaminophen (e.g., Tylenol or Panadol), acetylsalicylic acid or ASA (e.g.,

Aspirin or Bufferin), ibuprofen (e.g., Advil or Motrin) and naproxen (e.g., Aleve).

When selecting a product, you should try to match the pill to your problem. Acetaminophen is considered the drug of choice for most minor aches, pains and fever. ASA, ibuprofen and naproxen reduce inflammation as well and are called "nonsteroidal anti-inflammatory drugs," or NSAIDs.

Over-the-counter NSAIDs should be used carefully, especially if you're over age 65. They can cause stomach upset and gastrointestinal bleeding, which may be dangerous. They also interact with blood thinning drugs and shouldn't be taken if you suffer from a bleeding disorder or kidney problems. If you suffer from inflammation due to a disease like arthritis, don't take an NSAID unless it's been recommended by your doctor. In fact, some doctors think that NSAIDs should not be taken by older adults without a prescription.

Coping with changes later in life

*Would that life were like the shadow cast by a wall
or a tree, but it is like the shadow of a bird in flight.*

FROM THE TALMUD

From beginning to end, each stage of life presents its own unique set of challenges. These can be described in a general way, but the details vary from person to person, from generation to generation and from culture to culture.

What can you expect now, during this next stage of your life? Your expectations about growing older are probably colored by some widely held beliefs that may not be completely accurate:

◆ *You become "old" suddenly.* You may start to think of yourself as "old" when you become a grandparent for the first time, perhaps because you recall how elderly your own grandparents seemed to you as a child. Or you may feel old when the mirror reflects certain physical signs of aging. For some, the defining moment occurs on their 65th birthday. But becoming a grandparent, noticing new wrinkles and gray hair, or reaching some chronological marker have much less to do with aging than ever before. After all, if you can expect to live another 10, 20 or even 30 years in relative good health, is it realistic to define this stage as "the beginning of the end"?

◆ *You become physically and mentally incapacitated when you age.* As you've already seen in Chapter 1, certain physical changes often accompany healthy aging. For the most part, though, these can be corrected or compensated for, so it's reasonable for you to expect many more years of good health and well-being. It's also wrong to equate age with mental incapacity, since studies show that fewer than 5 percent of people over age 65 will experience dementia-causing diseases. However, it is true that the likelihood of such problems does increase with very advanced age.

◆ *Growing older somehow changes who you are.* Take a moment and think back to who you were at age 15. While you may have shared certain characteristics with other youngsters of that time and place, you were still an individual. You had your own likes and dislikes, your own personality, your own strengths and weaknesses. Growing older is a process of evolution and change. You won't become someone else in older

age, but will continue to be yourself – a person who is the sum of everything that has gone before.

? What changes are you likely to face when you're older?

One important change that happens later in life is retirement. How you cope with it depends on many factors. If you didn't feel ready to retire, and if work was your main source of identity and self-esteem, chances are you will feel a certain amount of anxiety and sadness at first. About 30 percent of retirees initially report having some negative feelings or difficulties in adjusting to retirement.

If you or your partner is in poor health, if your relationship isn't good or if you aren't financially secure, these factors can also affect your plans for a good retirement.

Still, many older people anticipate retirement with a sense of pleasure and relief. This is your chance to sit back and relax after many years of hard work. But that shouldn't mean you're headed for the rocking chair. You now have more time to enjoy old hobbies and interests or to pursue new ones. You can redesign your garden, go back to school, or take up photography, painting, computers, meditation or golf. You can travel, start an aquarium, get involved in your community, do volunteer work, or even take on some part-time, paid consulting work.

Retiring from work isn't the only change facing older men and women. Even if you are healthy and relatively happy in your later years, you can expect to experience certain losses, and these losses tend to pile up as the years go by.

Personal losses can include the illness or

death of a spouse or companion, the gradual or sudden deterioration of your own health, the loss of good friends and beloved relatives and the loss of your own independence due to disability or financial problems.

Unfortunately, there's no magic formula to help you handle the losses that occur in the later stages of our lives. You can only hope that, by this time, you have achieved a certain level of maturity and insight that will allow you to accept and effectively deal with what comes.

You should also take steps now to prepare and strengthen yourself to deal with loss. This means maintaining some stable relationships in your life besides those with your partner, grown children or one close friend. Many studies have shown that people, especially older adults, who have a sturdy network of social support do far better in times of stress and loss than those who don't.

? What is stress and how does it affect your health?

Imagine yourself coming face to face with an escaped lion. How would you react to this threat? Your body would tense up immediately in a "fight or flight" response. Your adrenal glands would release hormones, causing your heart to beat faster and pump more blood to your muscles, preparing them to respond. Once the stressor (in this case, the lion) was safely removed, your body would relax and return to its normal state.

Fortunately, it's unlikely that you will ever come face to face with an escaped lion. But as you grow older, it's likely that you *will* have to cope with a variety of more mundane and realistic stressors. These may include *acute stressors* (the death of a spouse, a sudden personal illness, divorce) and *ongoing stressors* (loneliness, poverty, lessened mobility, chronic illness or disability).

Unless you can find some way to control your response to these stressors, your body will remain in a constant state of tension, and this can have serious physical and emotional consequences. *Physical problems* related to stress may include: headache, muscle ache, back pain, exhaustion, high blood pressure, heart disease, ulcers, increased or reduced appetite, and a weakened immune system, which leaves you more vulnerable to infection. Some people also say that conditions such as arthritis tend to worsen when they are under stress. *Emotional problems* related to stress include: anxiety, poor concentration, feelings of exhaustion and moodiness.

? What can you do to avoid stress?

It's almost impossible to avoid stress, but some strategies do exist for reducing the toll it can take on your physical and emotional health:

◆ Accept that stress is a normal part of life. Some stress is actually beneficial – it stimulates our creativity and courage and may spur us on to special accomplishments.

◆ Decide which stressful situations and activities you can avoid and then avoid them!

◆ If you feel stressed or upset, try to figure out whether your own perceptions and responses may be fueling the fire. Perhaps you have unrealistic expectations of yourself or others that are setting you up for disappointment.

How to plan for a more satisfying retirement

In previous generations, retirement for most people lasted no longer than five or ten years. But because life expectancy is increasing, *you should expect to spend 20 or 25 years of your life in retirement*. When you look at it that way, it makes good sense to plan for the most satisfying retirement possible.

Experts say the best time to begin planning for retirement is many years before you actually retire. However, even if you and/or your partner have already retired, and especially if it isn't working out as you had hoped, it's still not too late to change the situation.

The secret to a satisfying retirement lies in having a sense of purpose and contact with people outside your family, according to recent studies from expert researchers. While financial planning is important, they say people should pay equal or even greater attention to what they will actually do with themselves during their retirement.

Here's some advice on how to improve your chances for a good retirement:

◆ If the idea of retirement scares you, or if you've retired and feel lonely, bored or unhappy, you need to explore your attitudes about work. Perhaps you miss the positive feelings of identity, status and self-esteem that you got at work and need to choose activities that provide some of those feelings. Perhaps you miss the people you knew at work – your co-workers or customers – and need to re-establish some social contacts. Maybe you don't thrive without a schedule and need to do something more structured with your time.

◆ Continuity is the key to a happier retirement. Unless you have to for health or financial reasons, don't make too many drastic changes in your life right now. For example, if you can afford to remain in your home and it gives you pleasure, why move into an apartment? But don't carry continuity too far! For instance, if you always wanted to travel after you retired, don't keep putting it off.

◆ Change, especially negative change, is a common source of stress. It's easier to deal with change if you have already learned and practiced certain stress management techniques (see opposite).

◆ It's good to feel in control, but feeling that you must have complete control over situations and people is a major cause of stress. Learning when and how to give up control may help reduce stressful feelings.

◆ Set your priorities – after all this time, you've earned that right. This means you shouldn't be afraid to say "no" to other people. If you say "no," don't think less of yourself because you can't meet everybody else's needs.

◆ If you fail at something, don't give yourself a hard time. Think back to other failures in your life and realize that you probably learned more from them than you learned from your successes.

◆ Take care of your emotional needs by

◆ With your partner (if you have one), draw up a budget showing your anticipated income and expenses. You may discover that you don't have enough money to cover everything you'd like to do, and you might need to change your plans. Some experts suggest that you ease yourself into retirement by starting to live on your retirement income about six months to a year before you or your partner retires. If you think you could be managing your money better now, it's worth consulting a professional retirement planner. Your bank manager may be able to refer you to one or, in some cases, may be equipped to advise you.

◆ Men and women tend to cope differently with retirement, especially if they took on traditional roles when they were younger. If you're retired now, you probably grew up in an era when men had careers or jobs outside the home, while women took on the important work of child-rearing and caring for the family, sometimes taking on extra paid employment, too.

Men who spend most of their time and energy on the job often don't establish other interests or activities that could give them a sense of continuity after retirement. Women who are full-time homemakers – and even those who work at jobs – are much more likely to develop lasting social contacts and activities that keep them feeling connected after retirement.

In traditional families, men also tend to be somewhat older than their wives, and this can create a situation where you and your partner are "out of sync" later in life. The man reaches age 65 first and retires, expecting to spend more time with his family. But he finds that his wife is either still working or eagerly planning a second career for herself away from home that doesn't include him.

That's why it's important for you to have two retirement strategies: one for you and your partner as a couple, and one for yourself as an individual.

doing at least one thing that gives you pleasure each day.

What can you do to manage stress?

◆ Being physically healthy is your best ally. That means paying attention to your diet, practicing good sleep habits (see page 42), seeing your doctor (both for regular checkups and to report any health problem), following your doctors' advice and using medications properly.

◆ Physical exercise is an antidote to stress. Try to keep active within any limitations you may have.

◆ Don't be a martyr to your problems. Stress does the most damage when you deny it or keep it bottled up. If something is bothering you, express your feelings by talking to someone you trust. This can be your doctor, a family member, a friend, a counselor or member of the clergy. A good cry can also be very helpful, and if you feel angry, look for a way to release the anger

Check out your stress level

Most people can recognize when a problem or event in their lives produces acute stress. But stress can affect you in more subtle, less obvious ways, and you may not realize the toll it's taking on your physical and emotional strength. Noise, crowding, even a happy event such as a wedding or the birth of a grandchild – these can all act as stressors.

To find out your stress level, answer "yes" or "no" to the following questions. The answers should reflect your emotions and experiences during the past year of your life.

YES NO

☐ ☐ 1. Have you lived or worked in a noisy neighborhood?

☐ ☐ 2. Have you changed your living conditions or moved?

☐ ☐ 3. Have you had problems with your in-laws?

☐ ☐ 4. Have you taken out a large loan?

☐ ☐ 5. Have you fallen behind with everyday tasks?

☐ ☐ 6. Have you had difficulty concentrating?

☐ ☐ 7. Have you had problems falling asleep?

☐ ☐ 8. Have you been eating, drinking or smoking more than usual?

☐ ☐ 9. Have you watched three or more hours of television daily for weeks at a time?

☐ ☐ 10. Have you or your spouse/companion changed responsibilities?

☐ ☐ 11. Have you been dissatisfied or unhappy with your activities or felt excessive responsibility?

☐ ☐ 12. Has a close friend died?

☐ ☐ 13. Have you been unhappy with your sex life?

☐ ☐ 14. Have you been worried about making ends meet?

☐ ☐ 15. Has a family member become ill?

☐ ☐ 16. Have you taken tranquilizers?

☐ ☐ 17. Have you become easily irritated when even little things haven't gone your way?

☐ ☐ 18. Have you had trouble relating to people – even loved ones?

☐ ☐ 19. Have you frequently been edgy with your children or other family members?

☐ ☐ 20. Have you often felt restless or nervous?

☐ ☐ 21. Have you frequently had headaches or digestive upsets?

☐ ☐ 22. Have you felt anxious or worried for days at a time?

☐ ☐ 23. Have you been so preoccupied that you've forgotten where you've put things or whether you've turned off appliances or equipment before leaving home?

☐ ☐ 24. Have you recently married or reconciled with your spouse/companion?

☐ ☐ 25. Have you had a serious illness, surgery or an accident?

☐ ☐ 26. Has anyone in your immediate family died?

☐ ☐ 27. Have you divorced or separated?

How to calculate your score:

Questions 1 through 9: score 3 points for every yes answer.

Questions 10 through 20: score 4 points for every yes answer.

Questions 10 through 25: score 5 points for every yes answer.

Question 26: score 6 points if you answered yes.

Question 27: score 7 points if you answered yes.

Now add up your total score and check your stress level below.

33 to 111 points: HIGH

You're under too much stress for your own good. Try to pinpoint the situations and feelings that pushed your score so high. Then, if possible, try to eliminate these stressful factors from your life. If you can't, at least try not to add any new stressors until your present situation changes.

16 to 32: MILD TO MODERATE

Before your stress level hits the danger zone, analyze the situations that cause stress and develop coping techniques. For example, if a lot of stressful personal situations are coming up right now, eliminate or postpone some lower-priority activities.

0 to 15: LOW

Either you have a placid nature or you have learned to handle your stress. Even if your score was a little over 15, you're still dealing well with stress.

Adapted from The Book of Tests *by Dr. Michael Nathenson (New York: Viking Penguin, 1984).*

without hurting yourself or others. Try writing an angry letter to the person who has upset you, holding nothing back – then throw it away. Just getting it down on paper can be a relief.

◆ When people are under stress, they may turn to alcohol, tobacco, drugs or overeating to help them relax. These substances may give short-term relief, but they can impair physical and mental health and actually end up creating even more stress. If you think stress is causing you to abuse yourself this way, speak to your doctor.

◆ Learn some simple relaxation techniques, including progressive physical relaxation and mental imagery. You can buy or borrow books and audiotapes that explain these techniques, or look for an adult education course in stress management.

◆ In the past, many older people were reluctant to seek professional help from a psychologist, social worker or psychiatrist because they felt it meant they were "mentally ill." Others hesitate to get outside help because they feel embarrassed or don't want a "stranger" knowing about their private lives. But not everyone can work things out alone. Don't be afraid to seek counseling during a period of intense stress – for example, the loss of a loved one or a serious personal problem.

◆ Keep your sense of humor. Even in the most distressing times, there may be something you can still smile about, and a good laugh is a wonderful way to relieve stress.

Paying attention
to your personal safety

To fear the worst oft cures the worse.

WILLIAM SHAKESPEARE

Being careful is important at any age. The fact that you've survived this long probably means you aren't a daredevil who takes unnecessary risks. Nevertheless, you shouldn't rest on your laurels and assume that an accident can't happen to you now. In fact, if you're over 65, your risk for an accident is greater than it used to be. And if you do get hurt, the consequences can have a profound impact on your life, jeopardizing your health, your sense of well-being and your independence. If an injury is serious enough to land you in the hospital now, chances are you'll stay there longer than a younger person with the same injury might, simply because your body needs more time to recover.

 What kinds of accidents are most likely to occur later in life?

Losing your footing or balance and falling down is probably the most common accident that happens to older adults. The tendency to fall is greater for you now because of several factors:

◆ Certain changes that occur with normal aging make you more prone to falling. Impaired eyesight may prevent you from seeing an object in your path. Decreased muscle strength may mean you can't right yourself as quickly as you used to. Your reaction time is impaired – it takes you just a bit longer to recognize and respond to a hazard, and your balance control isn't quite the same as it was.

◆ Certain conditions that lead to falling are more common now – for example, arrhythmia, which causes your heart to beat at an abnormally slow or fast rate, diseases of the inner ear that cause dizziness, and sudden changes in blood pressure. Unexplained episodes of falling can be an early sign of neurological or cardiovascular disease.

◆ Taking too much medication or the wrong combination of drugs can cause you to fall, as can intoxication caused by alcohol or other mood-altering drugs.

◆ An unsafe physical environment can increase your risk of falling down and hurting yourself.

Why is it so important to avoid falling?

All of us have taken a tumble now and then without any ill effects beyond a bruise or slight sprain. As children you and your friends probably made a game out of falling down. But for older adults, the consequences of a fall can be serious and long lasting.

Your bones are more brittle than they used to be. This makes them especially prone to fractures. A broken hip will require major surgery and months of recuperation and physiotherapy to help you walk again. A broken wrist will mean that you need help with daily activities such as cooking, shopping, bathing and dressing.

A fall can also make you more prone to falling again by hindering your self-confidence. Because you worry about repeating the experience, you may start to restrict your activities. Becoming less active can cause your joints to stiffen, and your muscles to become weaker, and can make you more, rather than less, likely to fall again.

What can you do to avoid falling?

◆ Report any non-serious episodes of falling or balance problems to your doctor. He may want to check you out and evaluate any medications you're taking.

◆ Make sure you have your vision checked regularly. If necessary, obtain the proper eyeglasses or contact lenses.

◆ Use your medications wisely (see page 71) and avoid drinking too much alcohol or using mind-altering drugs.

◆ If you can, make regular physical activity a part of each day. Some experts now believe that activities such as walking, dancing and gardening can help you maintain good balance control, which may reduce your chance of falling.

◆ Fall-proof your immediate surroundings and be aware of potential hazards when you travel away from home.

How can you increase your personal security?

Most of us, regardless of age, are reasonably concerned about our personal security. But if your senses and reflexes aren't what they used to be, you may feel particularly vulnerable when you're out on the street or even in your own home.

There's a delicate balance between trying to ensure your personal safety and feeling so afraid that you lock yourself in a room and never come out. Besides observing basic rules for staying safe – always knowing where you're going, avoiding poorly lit and deserted areas, keeping your car doors and windows locked – here are some sensible suggestions for older adults.

If possible, choose an apartment with some kind of controlled entry – either a security guard or an intercom system. If this isn't possible, make sure there's a window or peephole in your front door so you can check a visitor's identity before opening the door.

Don't let repair people or others whom you don't recognize into your home, even if they show an official-looking identification badge. Through the locked door, ask them to give you a phone number for their head office so you can verify their identity. If a stranger comes to your door, saying he's in trouble and needs to use the phone, never let him in – direct him to the superintendent or a nearby public payphone. This applies to female strangers as well as males.

If you live alone, don't advertise the fact by identifying yourself as a single person. If you're a single woman, just use an initial – "E. Baker" rather than "Mrs. E. Baker." Set up a buddy system with a neighbor or friend, agreeing to phone each other once a day to

Safety tips for older adults

Getting around

◆ Make sure your footwear is safe. Many people prefer to wear slippers around their house or apartment, but this may not be a good idea after a certain age (ask yourself why they're called "slip-pers"!). A better choice would be comfortable loafers or walking shoes with non-skid soles and good support for your feet and ankles. When you go out, make sure your shoes or boots offer the same support, and take note of the weather: A rain-slicked sidewalk covered with dead leaves can be just as dangerous as one covered in ice and snow.

◆ If you need a walking aid to get around, make certain it is the correct height for you, it is kept in good repair and you know how to use it properly. Never borrow a cane or walker from someone else. It's important to get the right walking aid for your height with the right amount of support. It's best to be fitted by a physiotherapist or an occupational therapist recommended by your doctor.

◆ Today many older adults who can't walk long distances because of arthritis or heart disease are using motorized scooters to get around their neighborhood. Before you use one, be sure that you understand how to operate it safely. You should also make sure that the batteries have been charged before going out, and that the vehicle is in good repair to prevent mishaps.

Your home

◆ If you haven't done a safety check of your living area, now is the time. You should also make this check before moving into a new house or apartment.

◆ Your furniture layout should be simple, with enough space to maneuver between and around chairs, tables, beds and sofas. Furniture should not be equipped with wheels or casters that make it unstable.

◆ The area should be brightly lit, with nightlights in the bathroom and kitchen to help you avoid falls in the dark.

◆ Floor surfaces should be carefully maintained. Get rid of loose rugs (easy to trip on, even if they're taped down), avoid high-pile or "shag" carpeting, and don't polish wood or tile floors so they are slippery. Stairs should be carpeted, or each stair should be fitted with a non-skid tread. A handrail opposite the banister is also a good idea.

◆ Keep your telephone where it can be easily reached – you shouldn't have to stumble over furniture to get to it. If you can afford it, an extension in each room, a portable phone, or an answering machine can save you from rushing to answer a call. Telephone and electrical cords should be tucked away safely so you won't trip over them.

◆ If you smoke, never do it in bed or if you're feeling sleepy. If you're going to answer the phone, never leave your cigarette burning in an ashtray, and don't empty ashtrays into the wastebasket.

◆ You should have at least one properly installed smoke detector in an apartment, and one per floor in a house. Batteries should be changed at least once every year. (Don't climb up on a ladder or stepstool to do this yourself – ask your landlord, a younger neighbor or a family member.)

◆ If you live in your own home, rather than an apartment, ask the city to clear ice and snow from your walk and driveway in the winter, or else pay someone to do it for you.

◆ If you have special needs because of a hearing impairment, ask your phone company if it can install a light that flashes when the phone rings. You can also purchase a flashing device that is activated when your doorbell rings.

Kitchen

◆ Make sure your stove is in proper working order and always check to see that the burners and oven are off before you go out or go to sleep. If you can afford a microwave oven, this might be a safer alternative for warming and cooking. When you cook, don't wear loose-fitting clothing such as a dressing gown or a blouse with wide sleeves – they can easily catch fire.

◆ Look for kettles and toaster ovens with automatic shutoffs, and keep your electrical appliances in good repair, replacing frayed cords or faulty plugs.

◆ Keep a mop handy in the kitchen so you can clean up spills right away.

◆ Store frequently used items on lower shelves so you don't have to use a stepstool to reach them.

Bathroom

◆ Make sure there is a non-slip mat or decals in the tub and shower enclosure, and tape down the bath rug beside the tub.

◆ Many older people benefit from handrails beside the toilet and in the tub (these should be of the proper type and professionally installed so they don't come loose).

◆ A chair or stool in the shower, fitted with non-slip material on the legs, will allow you to wash sitting down, and a hand-held shower head makes it much easier for you to wash your hair. If possible, turn the thermostat on your water heater down to prevent accidental scalds.

◆ Make sure that medications in your medicine chest are accessible as well as properly labeled and stored.

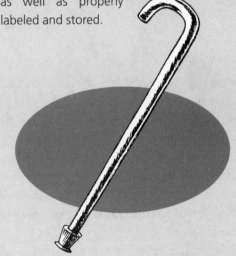

Should you still be driving?

While some older adults continue to drive safely into their 70s, 80s and even 90s, you should regularly review your own situation and decide whether it's still safe for you to drive.

This can be a highly emotional and difficult issue because the car is such a powerful symbol of mobility and independence at any age. It becomes an even greater issue for older drivers, especially if you rely heavily on your car for recreational activities, shopping trips or visits.

Depending on where you live, you may be asked to requalify for your driver's license after a certain age. This may involve taking a written examination, an eye exam and a road test. However, in many areas older drivers aren't required to requalify.

Age itself shouldn't be cause for discrimination against a driver – after all, many younger drivers don't drive as safely as they should. But remember: When you get behind the wheel, you aren't just taking your own life into your hands, you're also responsible for the lives of other drivers and pedestrians.

◆ Consider whether certain ailments or age-related changes have affected your ability to drive safely. These include visual or hearing impairments, problems with joints or muscles, slower reflexes and longer reaction time.

A recent U.S. study of 283 drivers over age 72 noted the following: Older people who walked less than a block a day, who had foot abnormalities such as toe deformities, and who performed poorly when copying

make sure neither of you is in any trouble. You may also be able to sign up for one of many "telcare" programs operated by seniors' groups and health organizations that place daily, friendly phone calls to isolated adults. In some areas, the postal system runs an organized "check-in" program where letter carriers check on older people who live alone.

You can buy or rent a personal alert device. Worn around the neck, it sets off an alarm at the push of a button. Such devices work through the telephone system and, when activated, put you in touch with an outside monitoring service that can dispatch help.

If you have a life-threatening allergy or suffer from diabetes, epilepsy or another illness that might cause you to lose consciousness, wear a medical alert bracelet. You should also consider using the home alert-response system mentioned above.

designs during mental tests were much more likely to be involved in accidents than those with no or fewer risk factors.

◆ Taking certain medications can hamper the alertness and judgment necessary for safe driving.

◆ If you think your driving is still adequate but not as good as it used to be, restrict where and when you drive. Avoid driving at night, during rush hours, on the highway, in bad weather or for too long a stretch.

◆ If you think your driving skills could be upgraded, check with your local transportation authority or a driving school to see if there's a program for mature drivers in your area.

◆ Giving up your car doesn't necessarily mean giving up your independence. With the money you save on gas, insurance and repairs, you can take more taxis or public transportation. Your adult children, grand-children or friends may also be happy to act as occasional chauffeurs.

◆ If you're in the passenger's seat and worry about the driving abilities of your spouse, an older relative or friend, speak to your primary care physician, who can advise you about what to do. For example, if you truly believe your spouse's physical or mental state makes him or her a dangerous driver, your physician can inform the motor vehicle bureau, which may revoke the driver's license. (In some jurisdictions, physicians are legally obliged to make such reports.)

◆ Finally, if you're the driver, don't stubbornly reject the opinion of a spouse or adult child who thinks your driving skills are no longer adequate and expresses fear for your safety. Of course, it's traumatic to be told this, but being killed or injured in an accident or harming someone else would be far more traumatic.

Unfortunately, many scams exist that target older adults. Never sign a contract, send money, give a credit card number or make a down payment for anything before checking out the person or company with your Better Business Bureau or a government consumer affairs department (ask the operator for a phone number in your city or town).

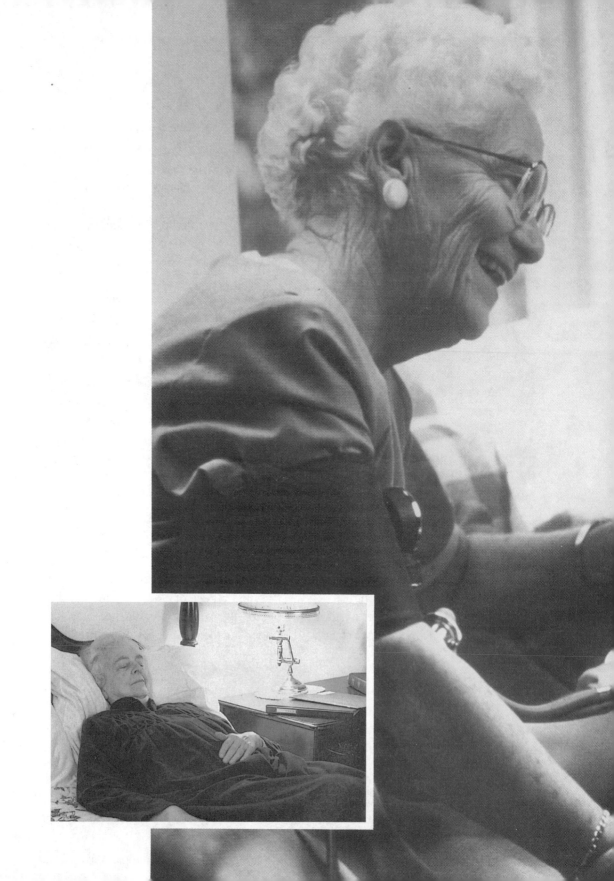

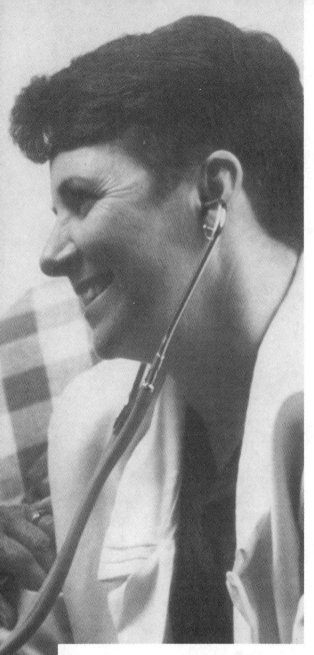

3

*The great secret that all
old people share is that
you really haven't changed
in seventy or eighty years.
Your body changes, but
you don't change at all.
And that, of course,
causes great confusion.*

DORIS LESSING

Aches, Pains and Common Complaints

ONE NEGATIVE IMAGE OF OLDER ADULTS is that they're chronic complainers, always talking about their aches and pains and worrying about their bowels. As your body ages, you do become more prone to certain minor health problems. But all too often older people accept their symptoms – even serious ones – as a normal part of aging, and because they don't believe anything can be done for them, they either suffer in silence or complain constantly. They may also resort to various home remedies or over-the-counter products and medications that don't work and that may actually aggravate the problem or even create new ones.

Fortunately these complaints rarely signal any serious illness or underlying disorder.

But if you suffer from any of them, you know how bothersome they are and how seriously they can interfere with your enjoyment of life.

The following is a guide to aches, pains and complaints commonly experienced in later life. Each section (presented in alphabetical order) will:

◆ describe typical symptoms;

◆ suggest ways that you might be able to prevent or relieve the problem yourself;

◆ give advice about when it's time to call your doctor;

◆ provide information on how your doctor might treat the problem.

Back pain

About 90 percent of us will experience the misery of back pain at some time in our lives. When your back hurts, it's often difficult to know just what's causing the pain. But it's important for you and your doctor to determine why your back is hurting so you can get appropriate treatment.

Symptoms
◆ *Muscle strain:* Your spinal column is supported by various muscles, tendons and ligaments. Any sudden or chronic strain on them can cause pain – for example, a sudden movement (bending over) or injury (from a fall). Poor posture,

tight or weak muscle tone due to lack of exercise, and carrying extra weight, especially around your abdomen, all leave you vulnerable to strained back muscles.

◆ *Osteoarthritis:* As you age, the cartilage covering the surface of your spinal joints tends to deteriorate. The discs between these joints (or vertebrae) become worn, and bony growths, called spurs, may develop. When this happens, the spinal joints rub together, and your back feels stiff and sore, especially when you first get up in the morning or after sitting for long periods.

◆ *Osteoporosis:* The amount of calcium in

your bones decreases with age. This can weaken your spine, making it vulnerable to small fractures. If your bones are very thin and porous, even a simple sneeze or turning over in bed can cause a painful fracture. As these vertebrae or spinal bones collapse, you may become shorter and your posture may become stooped. This problem is more common in women than men.

◆ *Referred back pain:* This can occur when a disease involving another organ – for example, your kidneys, prostate gland or uterus – causes you to feel pain in your back.

◆ *Sciatica:* This condition occurs in about 2 percent of people with back pain. The sciatic nerve, which runs down each leg from hip to heel, may become compressed by a protruding disc or bone spur. When this happens, you may feel pain radiating down from your buttock to your lower leg. There may also be tingling, numbness or muscle weakness, although you don't necessarily feel pain in your back.

◆ *Spinal stenosis:* A narrowing of the spinal canal can occur with aging. The narrowing puts pressure on nerves in your lower back, causing numbness, pain and weakness in your back and legs that grows worse when you walk and eases when you sit or bend forward.

What to try

If you develop sudden back pain related to some activity, such as lifting or bending, you've probably stressed or strained a muscle. Use an over-the-counter painkiller such as acetaminophen, and rest your back for two or three days (no longer, since too much rest can weaken muscles and delay healing). Alternating heat and cold packs applied to your back every 10 to 20 minutes for several hours may also help relieve the pain.

Consult your doctor

Back pain that doesn't improve after a few days, pain caused by a fall or blow to your back, and pain associated with numbness, tingling, or sudden bladder or bowel control problems should always be promptly reported to your doctor.

Treatment

Your doctor may recommend tests to diagnose the source of your pain. This could involve referring you to an arthritis, rehabilitation or orthopedic specialist.

Before resorting to medication, however, you should be aware of certain lifestyle factors that cause, contribute to or aggravate back pain:

◆ Improper bending and lifting can lead to injury. Always bend at the knees, using your leg muscles to lift an object, and avoid twisting your back even slightly when bending or reaching for something. If you have to carry groceries, it's better to push them in a cart.

♦ Try to avoid activities that force you to stay in one position for too long a time – for example, driving or gardening. Interrupt the activity at frequent, short intervals to flex (bend forward) or extend (arch gently backward).

♦ If you spend a long time sitting, you can buy a specially designed cushion to support your lower back, or else try placing a rolled-up towel in the curve of your back.

♦ Avoid sleeping on your stomach, which puts stress on your spine. Instead, sleep lying on your side with the knees bent up toward your chest, or sleep on your back, with one or two pillows under your knees. If

The three sleep positions and placement of pillows

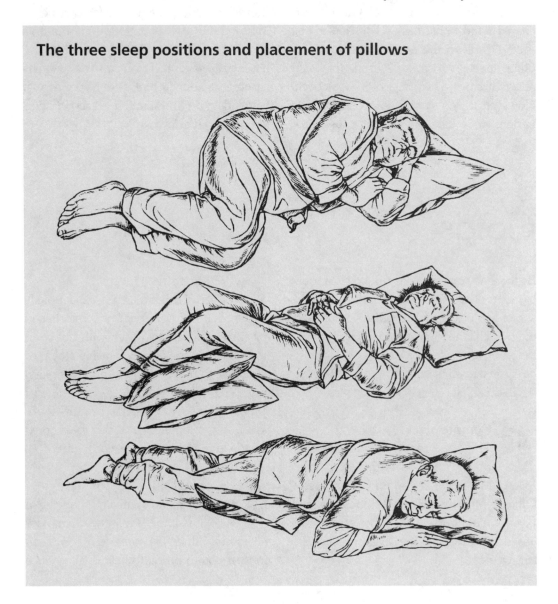

you are devoted to sleeping on your stomach, slide an extra pillow under your hips to reduce the stress on your spine.

◆ Exercise and physical therapy can help avoid and relieve back pain and prevent further injury by improving your flexibility and strengthening your abdominal and back muscles.

◆ Back supports and braces can be purchased at most pharmacies, but shouldn't be used except on the advice of a doctor or other specialist. Properly used, they can relieve strain and help support a weak back. However, they shouldn't be worn for long periods since they can actually cause muscles to weaken and remain "lazy." Your doctor may recommend special back supports to be used only when lifting.

If these strategies don't relieve your pain, your doctor may prescribe medication, including painkillers (analgesics), a short course of anti-inflammatory drugs, muscle relaxants and injections of corticosteroids. Back surgery, usually done when there are complications such as nerve injury, may also be an option, but this should be seen as a last resort unless the damage is severe. If your doctor suggests surgery, listen carefully to her reasons. Depending on the situation, a second opinion may be worthwhile.

Colds

By the time you reach age 65, you've probably had well over 100 colds, based on an average of two colds per year. Colds occur most often in childhood, and fortunately for you, their frequency declines with age. Because colds are caused by viruses rather than bacteria, they can't be cured with antibiotics.

Symptoms
The average, uncomplicated cold usually starts out with a sore throat followed by nasal stuffiness or runniness. Other symptoms include achiness, a mild fever, vocal hoarseness, some chest congestion and a cough that lasts several days to a week.

What to try
Everyone has a favorite cold remedy that's proven useful or comforting in the past: chicken soup, tea with honey, a hot toddy, resting in bed, inhaling steam or cool mist to unclog a stuffy nose, drinking fruit juice, taking vitamin C. The value of some of these remedies may be more emotional than scientific, but if they've worked for you in the past, they're worth a try.

Consult your doctor
If you're fairly healthy, having a cold is simply a nuisance, but older adults are vulnerable to certain complications. If you're prone to bronchial or sinus

Protect yourself against influenza and pneumonia

While a common cold can make you feel miserable, influenza and bacterial pneumonia in people over 65 can be life-threatening. In fact, these illnesses are among the leading causes of death in older adults.

Influenza

Many people who have severe colds believe they're suffering from influenza or "the flu." If you've ever had influenza, though, you know it's much more serious and unpleasant than the average cold. Like colds, influenza is caused by a virus, but the symptoms are more severe. They include chills, a dry cough, high fever, fatigue and loss of appetite. A common complication of influenza in older adults is bacterial pneumonia.

There's no vaccine to protect you against the viruses that cause colds, but you can be vaccinated against many kinds of influenza. It's estimated that vaccines prevent 60 to 70 percent of influenza cases and up to 90 percent of deaths caused by this infection.

If you're over 65, you should have a flu shot every year, preferably in September, before the flu season begins. (It takes about four weeks for the vaccine to become effective in your body.)

Flu shots are also vital if you have a chronic heart or lung condition, kidney disease, severe anemia, diabetes or a weakened immune system.

Your doctor can give you the shot in her office, or you can attend a community clinic. Side effects are usually mild and may involve some soreness at the site of the injection and perhaps a day of low-grade fever.

Pneumonia

This serious infection of the lung or lungs is a major cause of illness and death in older adults. A vaccine now exists that can protect you from pneumococcal pneumonia, a bacterial infection that accounts for about one-third of all adult pneumonias. This is usually a one-time vaccination and is available from your doctor.

infections, or if you suffer from asthma or chronic lung disease, speak to your doctor. You should also let him know if you feel sicker than usual, if your symptoms last longer than a week, if you feel short of breath or notice a wheezing or cracking sound when you breathe, if your temperature, taken orally, goes higher than 102°F (39°C) (which could signal a bacterial infection), and if you cough up thick, greenish-yellow sputum and/or blood.

Treatment

Although over-the-counter cold remedies can ease nasal congestion, cough and other symptoms, these products won't hasten your recovery and may pose certain risks for older people. Many non-prescription remedies take a shotgun approach to treatment. They contain several ingredients such as antihistamines, decongestants, pain relievers and fever reducers, as well as other non-active components such as caffeine or alcohol. These ingredients can interact with other drugs you're taking, causing side effects such as drowsiness or confusion, or they can prevent you from getting a good night's sleep.

The best advice is to avoid any product that contains a combination of ingredients and choose one that uses a single drug. If you have a particular symptom such as nasal stuffiness, ask your doctor or pharmacist to recommend a product specifically targeted to reduce congestion – for example, one containing only pseudoephedrine or phenylephrine. (You should, however, avoid these drugs if you suffer from hypertension, vascular disease or prostate problems.) Nose drops or sprays, which shrink nasal membranes, can help unclog your nose, but don't use them for longer than four days, since they can cause "rebound" or increased stuffiness. Antihistamines, often found in over-the-counter remedies, shouldn't be used for colds – they don't work, can make you feel drowsy and even cause constipation and urinary retention.

To control a dry, hacking cough that keeps you up at night, try a product containing dextromethorphan, which suppresses the cough mechanism in your brain. To make a cough more "productive" – to help loosen and expel mucus – inhaling warm steam is probably more useful than taking non-prescription expectorants containing guaifenesin.

If you feel achy or are running a slight fever, acetaminophen used as directed can be helpful.

Constipation

Constipation is one of the most common complaints voiced by older adults. You may begin to focus on the frequency and quality of your bowel movements, blaming your bowels for any feelings of sluggishness or abdominal discomfort.

❶ Symptoms

Before deciding that you're constipated, you should know a few facts about healthy bowel function. After you eat, the food passes through your stomach and into the small intestine, where vital nutrients and fluids are absorbed. The undigested portion continues to move toward your large intestine or colon, where it can remain for several days until muscular contractions force it out the rectum in the form of feces.

Constipation occurs when the passage of waste (or stool) through the large intestine is delayed or when passage through the rectum is blocked. As you get older, the process of passing stool becomes less efficient, and stool is more likely to remain in the lower bowel or rectum, where it becomes hard and difficult to expel. Besides the unpleasantness of straining, constipation can cause or aggravate hemorrhoids (see page 108), and can lead to irritation and bleeding of the anus.

What to try

You can take certain steps to prevent or control constipation:

◆ Add more fiber to your diet. Fiber, found in fresh or cooked fruits and vegetables, legumes, and whole grain cereals and breads, creates bulkier waste, and this makes moving your bowels easier. But don't overdo fiber consumption – too much fiber may cause you to move your bowels too often. This could impair the absorption of important nutrients and cause excessive gas, or flatus. If you're physically inactive because of an illness or disability, if your intake of fluids is low or if you suffer from intestinal blockages, overdosing on bran can lead to intestinal obstruction.

◆ Drink at least 8 to 10 glasses of water and other liquids each day. Without adequate fluid to lubricate your digestive system, your stool is more likely to become hard.

◆ Reduce your intake of low-fiber, sugar-laden baked goods, and replace them with fruits, vegetables and whole grains.

◆ Become more physically active. Moving your body helps to soften stool in your colon and also keeps your abdominal muscles strong, improving your ability to expel stool during a bowel movement.

◆ Don't take laxative pills, powders, oils and chocolate or use enemas and suppositories without consulting your doctor first. Use natural laxatives such as wheat bran, fruits and vegetables, and fluids. Try prunes, prune juice, figs and unpeeled apples, which have a natural laxative effect. Avoid so-called laxative teas containing senna – they are extremely powerful and may be habit-forming.

◆ You should be aware that a change of environment or stress can sometimes lead to temporary bowel problems.

Consult your doctor

If changing your diet, adding fluids and taking exercise don't seem to help, call your doctor before resorting to laxative medication. It's easy for older people to become "hooked" on laxatives (see page 76).

Constipation can also occur as a side effect of many drugs, including some antidepressants, narcotics, diuretics, antihistamines and antacids (taken for heartburn) containing aluminum or calcium. If you notice a change in bowel habits after starting a new medication, if constipation is accompanied by pain in your abdomen or if you notice any change in your normal bowel habits, speak to your doctor.

Treatment

Your doctor will want to determine whether you are really constipated. She may ask you about your bowel habits, your diet and activity level, and your use of laxatives. If you haven't tried some of the self-help strategies above, she will probably recommend that you do so. She may examine your lower bowel to see if it feels distended with stool and check to make sure there's no obstruction in your rectum. In some cases she may ask you for a stool sample to send to a lab for analysis or order a barium enema. This enema contains barium sulphate, a substance that shows up on X-rays, giving the doctor a clear picture of your digestive tract.

Dizziness

Nearly everyone has felt lightheaded or unsteady after getting up from a sitting or lying position, or from a sudden turn of the head. This is the most common form of dizziness. It usually occurs for no known reason, although it can follow an ear infection or an injury to the ears or head.

In most cases, dizziness doesn't signal a serious health problem. But even so, the sensation can make you feel anxious about your health and reluctant to leave home. Many older people who experience episodes of dizziness also worry that it will lead to fainting.

Your sense of balance is a highly complex and exquisitely sensitive system involving your visual system, vestibular system (located in your inner ear) and perceptual system, which keeps track of where your body is in relation to its surroundings. Problems in the central nervous system, low blood pressure, infections and side effects from medication can interfere with one or more of these systems, resulting in dizziness.

Symptoms

People mean different things when they complain about dizziness. You may feel *lightheaded* (things seem vague or out of focus), or you may feel *unsteady* (things seem to shift around you, making you feel insecure). Or you may experience *vertigo* (things swirl and spin and it's impossible for you to focus or maintain your balance).

What to try

It's difficult to treat yourself if you don't know what's causing your dizziness. Dizziness that lasts for less than a minute or seems to come on after a particular movement (bending over, rising, turning over in bed, raising or lowering your head) can often be avoided by moving more slowly.

A common source of lightheadedness is anxiety. You may be breathing too shallowly and not taking in enough oxygen. Or you may be breathing too rapidly (hyperventilation), which lowers the level of carbon dioxide in your blood and causes blood vessels in your brain to constrict, making you feel dizzy.

If you feel unsteady when standing or walking, this may be due to visual problems, weakened leg muscles or ailments such as arthritis, which make movement difficult. Using a cane or walker with wheels or pushing a shopping cart when you go out may give you an added feeling of stability.

Vertigo can be caused by a variety of illnesses – viral infections that affect cranial nerves (called vestibular neuritis or neuronitis), Ménière's disease (a chronic accumulation of fluid in the inner ear, often accompanied by ringing or buzzing in the ears), and disorders of the central nervous system, particularly transient ischemic attacks (also called TIAs or "mini-strokes" – see page 170).

Consult your doctor

It's important to seek your doctor's advice about persistent, unexplained dizziness. Feeling unsteady can cause you to reduce your activity, making you more prone to falling. Call your doctor right away if dizziness is severe, if it results in a faint or fall, or if it's accompanied by ringing or buzzing in your ears, ear pain, headache, nausea, confusion or problems with speech or swallowing.

✔ Treatment

First your doctor will want to determine the cause of your dizziness. This involves taking a careful history and asking you when the dizziness first occurred and how often and when it tends to happen. He may test your blood and urine to rule out an underlying problem such as anemia or diabetes and will measure your blood pressure to see if it's too low or too high. He will examine your inner ears for signs of infection or another abnormality and will also examine your eyes.

If the doctor suspects your dizziness is related to anxiety or emotional factors, he may ask you to hyperventilate (breathe very quickly) in his office to see if this brings on the dizzy sensation. If it does, he may want to discuss what's making you anxious and look at methods to help you cope better with stress. Sometimes just knowing that there's nothing serious going on is enough to relieve your mind and even your dizziness. In some cases, treatment with a short-term tranquilizer may be helpful.

Certain types of dizziness are relieved by antinausea drugs such as meclizine (Antivert) or dimenhydrinate (Dramamine or Gravol). For severe and very debilitating cases of vertigo, surgery or chemical treatment may be used to destroy the vestibular organs of the inner ear. This procedure generally does not affect your hearing.

If the exact nature of your dizziness isn't clear, your doctor may refer you to a specialist or to a dizziness clinic (if one exists in your area).

Fatigue

Many older people complain that they feel weak and tired all the time and no longer have the "zip" they once did. While fatigue and weakness can be a sign of illness, they occur for other reasons as well.

❗ Symptoms

You may notice that you have to stop what you're doing more often to take a rest. You may feel less alert and sharp than you used to, or you may notice that your arms and legs aren't as strong as they used to be.

Some of these changes can be related to normal aging. As you age you tend to lose muscle mass, and certain changes in sleep patterns may make you feel less alert. But sudden, unusual or persistent fatigue should never be explained away as "part of growing old."

💡 What to try

In many cases, feeling tired all the time may be the result of poor nutrition (including obesity), a sedentary lifestyle, and emotional factors such as loneliness or boredom. Often these factors are related – for example, if you aren't eating properly, you won't have the energy to get out, and because you stay at home, you feel bored and isolated. This can lead to sleep problems that may make you feel even more tired.

Consult your doctor

Unexplained fatigue can be a symptom of many illnesses. The most common ones affecting older adults are major depression, anemia, thyroid disorder, diabetes, and malabsorption (a disorder in how your intestines absorb certain nutrients from food). Sleep disorders can also contribute to a feeling of exhaustion and daytime sleepiness (see page 43).

You should call your doctor if fatigue is persistent, if it is significantly interfering with your normal activities, if it develops suddenly, if it's accompanied by sudden weight loss or if you experience other new symptoms such as shortness of breath, frequent urination, thirst, and changes in appetite or sleep.

Treatment

Your doctor will take a detailed history and may do various tests to rule out an underlying illness. She may also check your medication, since fatigue or weakness can be a side effect of certain drugs, including pain relievers, tranquilizers, antihistamines and medications to manage high blood pressure.

If your tiredness is related to poor nutrition, a sedentary lifestyle or emotional factors, you need to review your diet and physical activity level and make positive changes (see Chapter 1). Finding ways to combat boredom and isolation is important too. Unfortunately, for many older people this is easier said than done. If you're relatively healthy, though, becoming more active and meeting new people should help to increase your energy level.

Foot complaints

Few things can make a relatively healthy person feel more miserable than sore feet. Minor foot problems are a plague for many older adults, resulting in pain and reduced mobility. Some problems affecting the feet are serious, but the majority are merely a nuisance.

Symptoms

Corns and calluses are painful, hardened areas of skin, usually on the toes. They are caused by repeated friction and pressure from shoes. Redness, blisters, peeling and itching between your toes can be caused by *bacterial and fungal infections* such as athlete's foot. Itching can also be a symptom of *dry skin*. *Warts* – hard, raised bumps that often appear on the sole (plantar's wart) – are caused by viruses and can be extremely painful. *Bunions* occur when the joints that connect your big toe to your foot become swollen and painful. *Ingrown toenails* occur when a piece of nail has pierced the skin of the toe and caused an infection.

What to try

Your feet have endured many decades of wear and tear, and you may not be giving them the respect they deserve!

If you're prone to minor foot problems (such as corns), you may be wearing shoes that don't fit properly. Sometimes protective pads can ease the pain of corns, calluses and bunions.

To control bacterial or fungal infections, keep your feet clean and dry, expose them to sun and air whenever possible and dust them daily with fungicidal powder.

Poor circulation in the lower legs and feet, often caused by smoking, diabetes, blood vessel disease, or inactivity, can also make feet more prone to problems. Gentle massage and warm (never hot!) foot baths help increase circulation. You might want to invest in an electric footbath – you fill it with warm water and it delivers gentle vibrations while you soak your feet.

Consult your doctor

If you have diabetes or poor circulation in your lower legs and feet, you

Foot care tips

◆ Wash your feet with mild soap to reduce irritation and prevent dry skin. You can look for a soap that contains cold cream or other moisturizers or else rub in some moisturing lotion.

◆ Always dry your feet carefully, especially between the toes, and make sure toenails are regularly and properly trimmed straight across to prevent them from becoming ingrown and painful.

◆ Your toenails may be thicker now than they used to be, which can make them harder to cut. Regular visits to a podiatrist or other foot care specialist might be necessary. In some communities, foot care providers will even come to your home.

are especially susceptible to infection and should never treat minor foot problems yourself. Always see your doctor or a foot specialist (chiropodist or podiatrist) if you have corns, calluses, warts, bunions, or toenails that have become ingrown or extremely thick.

Treatment

Your doctor or a foot care specialist will examine your feet to determine whether corns, calluses and bunions are caused by an underlying bone deformity that requires special treatment. In some cases, he may prescribe or apply medications to treat corns and calluses and use techniques to cut away, burn or freeze off warts. An ingrown toenail is usually treated by removing part of the toenail and applying antibiotic cream to cure any infection. Some bunions may be cured through the use of special splints or a change of shoes, although when the joint is severely deformed, surgery may be necessary. For some conditions you may require special orthopedic shoes custom designed to fit the contours of your feet.

Headaches

If you suffered from headaches when you were younger, it's likely they'll become less of a problem in your later years. Although no one knows the reason, doctors who treat older adults say that headache complaints are less common in this age group. Even so, some people do continue to have frequent and severe headaches for the rest of their lives.

There are four basic kinds of headache. The most common is the *tension headache*, caused by the contraction of muscles in the scalp, face, jaw, neck and shoulders, usually in response to stress or fatigue. Poor posture and eyestrain can contribute to tension headaches. *Migraine headaches* seem to be related to chemical and other changes in the brain that affect blood flow. Both tension and migraine headaches are more common among women than men. The *cluster headache*, the rarest type, is not well understood but is more common in men over age 50. A fourth type of headache, the *sinus headache,* usually occurs with or after a sinus infection.

Symptoms

◆ *Tension headache:* mild to moderate pain that develops gradually and usually occurs on both sides of the head. It's often worse later in the day and can last for hours or days. There may be no warning signs or other symptoms.

◆ *Migraine headache:* moderate to severe pain, usually (but not always) on one side of the head, triggered by stress, fatigue, certain foods, alcohol, weather changes, bright lights and odors. The pain may last for hours but seldom longer than a few days. There may be no warning, although many sufferers describe an "aura" – visual flashes or blind spots, tingling or numbness on one side of the face or body, unusual moods or cravings – before the onset of pain.

◆ *Cluster headache:* excruciating pain on one side of the head that comes on suddenly, often during sleep and without any warning sign. The pain lasts from 20 to 90 minutes, and is accompanied by same-sided redness, tearing in one eye and stuffiness in one nostril.

◆ *Sinus headache:* a dull ache, which may be constant or intermittent, across the forehead and often felt around the eyes, nose and cheeks. There is often a feeling of fullness or heaviness as well.

What to try

The best way to control a headache is to figure out what triggered it and eliminate the trigger, if possible.

Because tension headache is caused by muscle tension, avoid sitting in one place or position for too long. Shrug your shoulders and do some gentle neck rolls every hour or so.

Deep breathing can also relieve muscle tension, as can other techniques for stress management (see page 81). Tension headaches can usually be relieved at home by taking a non-prescription analgesic such as acetaminophen (Tylenol), which is less irritating to your stomach than acetylsalicylic acid (Aspirin). A warm heating pad or compress on the back of the neck or a gentle massage can also help. If you have a muscle spasm, an ice pack may help relieve the pain.

If you've suffered from migraine headaches before, you probably know your triggers and try to avoid them. But if you're an older woman, you may not know that hormone replacement therapy can cause migraine headaches. Any headache that could be related to estrogen replacement should be reported to your doctor. If you have migraine or cluster headaches, never drink alcohol, which can trigger pain or make it worse.

Headaches can also be triggered by some

How to prevent and relieve tension headaches

These simple exercises can reduce muscle tension and may prevent or help relieve a tension headache. Just be careful not to roll your head around or from side to side in a single swift movement.

◆ Gently bend your head forward so your chin approaches your chest, pause, then gently roll it backwards.

◆ Turn your head slowly from side to side.

◆ Drop your left ear down to your left shoulder as far as you can go, then bring your right ear down to your right shoulder.

medications. These include over-the-counter pain relievers and decongestants taken more than twice a week, and nitroglycerin (taken for angina).

Consult your doctor

Let your doctor know about any new headache pain that isn't relieved by the maximum dosage of a non-prescription pain reliever within a day. You should also seek advice about headaches that occur more often than twice a week or last longer than usual (unless this has been a life-long pattern). Early morning headaches may indicate a medical problem. A persistent headache in the forehead or temples, accompanied by problems in chewing, could mean you have an acute or chronic inflammation of the blood vessel that runs up the side of your face (temporal arteritis). Sometimes a problem in the temporomandibular joints (in your jaw and the side of your face) can cause facial and headache pain.

Fortunately, fewer than 10 percent of headaches are caused by serious conditions such as an aneurysm, brain tumor, infection or stroke. Get immediate attention for any headache accompanied by loss of balance, momentary paralysis, loss of speech or double vision – this could signal a stroke. Headache with fever, and especially with a stiff or sore neck, could be an early sign of serious infection.

Treatment

Most tension headaches respond to the self-help treatments already mentioned. Migraines are usually treated with stronger pain-relieving medications and antimigraine drugs such as sumatriptan, available only by prescription. If a migraine is especially severe and accompanied by nausea, your doctor may give you an injection of sumatriptan. However, this drug may not be suitable if you have angina due to ischemic heart disease or if you suffer from uncontrolled hypertension.

In some cases, your doctor may prescribe other medication to prevent disabling migraine and cluster headaches. These include beta-blockers, antidepressants and calcium channel blocking drugs.

Hearing changes

You may have noticed a subtle change in your hearing ability when you were about 50 years old. By the time you reach your 70s, your chance of hearing loss is much greater.

Loss of hearing can seriously interfere with your health and well-being later in life. It cuts you off from the world around you, from other people, music, radio and television, which can lead to feelings of isolation and depression. Even though age-related hearing changes are extremely common, many older people deny them and avoid seeking help. Unfortunately, others may misinterpret their difficulty in hearing as a sign of cognitive disease, so it's important to have your hearing checked and explore possible remedies.

Symptoms

Loss of hearing in older people is usually due to age-related changes in the inner ear, which transmits sounds to the brain. You may begin to miss higher-frequency sounds, such as "k," "f" and "s" sounds in words, and have trouble making out normal conversation. If all sounds seem to be duller, or if you experience a sudden loss of hearing in one ear, there may be an obstruction in your ear canal.

What to try

Many people with hearing loss can be significantly helped by using a listening device. If your hearing loss has already been diagnosed and no treatments are available to restore adequate hearing, you must learn how to compensate. When someone is talking to you, ask the person to face you so you can read his or her lips, and suggest that the person speak more loudly, at a slower rate, and, if possible, at a lower pitch.

If you think you have a buildup of ear wax in your ear canal, never try to clean it out yourself with a Q-tip or other implement – this can push the wax plug deeper into your ear and you may damage delicate structures inside. Consult your doctor. If you are prone to ear wax, your doctor may suggest you rinse out your ears regularly with mineral oil to prevent a wax buildup.

Consult your doctor

Any sudden loss of hearing should be reported to your doctor immediately. After examining your ears and doing some simple hearing tests, he may decide to refer you to a hearing specialist for further testing and treatment. You should also let your doctor know about any gradual hearing loss. (You may not always notice this yourself, but other people may tell you that they've observed a change in your hearing.)

Treatment

If your doctor diagnoses a simple wax buildup, he will use an ear syringe and water to dislodge the obstruction and may suggest you come back regularly for cleaning.

If your hearing loss isn't exclusively related to nerve damage, you are probably a candidate for a hearing aid. There are many kinds of hearing aids, some which fit inside the ear, others which are worn behind the ear, and some which are attached to an amplifier carried in your pocket.

A hearing aid should always be fitted by an expert, who will teach you how to use the device properly. If your hearing aid bothers you in some way, don't abandon it and go back to living in muted tones and silence. Speak to your doctor or audiologist, who may be able to find an acceptable solution.

It usually takes time for people to adjust to a hearing aid, so be patient with yourself and ask others to be patient with you too.

Heart palpitations

Older people often experience heart palpitations. When they happen, they can be extremely upsetting. You may think that you're about to have a heart attack or worry that you're about to faint.

Symptoms

You may feel as though your heart has stopped or "missed a beat" or sense a fluttering in your chest. Some palpitations are more dramatic – your heart seems to pound or beat much more rapidly than normal. The symptoms, which can last from a few moments to a few hours, may be related to a sudden movement such as bending down or turning over in bed, or they may occur with no apparent cause.

What to try

If possible, lie down and wait to see if the palpitations ease or stop. Try to relax your mind – anxious thoughts can prolong some cases of heart palpitation. Some people who experience repeated attacks of palpitations can learn techniques to stop them.

Consult your doctor

Always report any new onset of palpitations to your doctor, and also report such symptoms if you have heart disease or high blood pressure. If palpitations occur suddenly and are accompanied by the following symptoms — pain in your chest, arm, shoulders, neck or jaw; sweating, vomiting, extreme dizziness or weakness; fainting — seek immediate help. Call your doctor

or if someone can drive you there, go to the nearest hospital emergency room, or dial 911.

Treatment

If your doctor suspects that palpitations are related to underlying heart disease, she will recommend an electrocardiogram or other tests. In many cases the palpitations stop before you get to your doctor, and she may suggest that you wear a device called a "Holter monitor." This portable device is worn for a day or longer and continuously monitors your heart rhythm. Palpitations are also associated with thyroid disease and anemia, and they may be a side effect of certain drugs such as antidepressants. Since palpitations are often caused by feelings of anxiety, your doctor may ask whether you are under stress and suggest ways for you to prevent or control stressful feelings. She may also ask you to reduce your intake of caffeine, found in coffee, tea, chocolate, cola drinks and some over-the-counter pain medications, because caffeine can contribute to palpitations.

Hemorrhoids

As you get older, you become more prone to developing hemorrhoids, also known as "piles." Hemorrhoids, which are really varicose veins of the rectum, can occur inside the anus, where you may not feel them, or outside the anus, where they are felt as a lump or protrusion. Hemorrhoids can be extremely painful and may also cause itching and burning in the rectal area, especially during bowel movements. This may lead to poor bowel habits, such as holding back stool, which can actually aggravate hemorrhoids.

Symptoms

Internal hemorrhoids are often symptomless, although they may bleed slightly, leaving streaks of blood on your underwear, in your stool or on the toilet tissue. Those that become large enough may protrude through the rectum, usually after a bowel movement, and are referred to as "prolapsed hemorrhoids." External hemorrhoids may also be painless, although they are prone to bleeding.

What to try

To prevent hemorrhoids from occurring, you should avoid becoming constipated (see page 99). Hemorrhoids may be caused or aggravated by any activity that puts pressure on your body – for example, prolonged sitting or standing and chronic coughing. Avoid wearing tight, synthetic underwear, which irritates the anal area, and practice good anal hygiene: always wipe your anal area well (but gently) after a bowel movement, and try using moistened paper or commercially available silicone-soaked cleansing pads rather than dry tissue.

You may be tempted to try various over-the-counter suppositories and ointments, which are supposed to shrink hemorrhoids and relieve pain, but check with your doctor before using them. Most suppositories contain local anesthetics such as lignocaine or benzocaine, and these can cause an allergic reaction or local irritation.

Some soothing strategies include: cold compresses to reduce pain, two or three daily warm sitz baths (taken in a specially designed basin which fits into the toilet bowl and allows you to bathe your rectal area) and non-prescription lotions, including witch hazel, to calm itching and pain. Another option is Anurex. This reusable, gel-filled probe is cooled in the freezer and inserted twice daily into the anus, where it provides relief and stops bleeding from internal hemorrhoids.

If an internal hemorrhoid has prolapsed, try to push it gently back into your rectum after a bowel movement to prevent it from becoming strangulated (caught outside the anus by a muscle spasm).

Consult your doctor

Any unexplained rectal bleeding should be reported to your doctor, who will want to make sure that it isn't being caused by something serious such as bowel cancer or colitis. You should also report a hemorrhoid that has become especially large, swollen and uncomfortable or that bleeds profusely.

Treatment

If your hemorrhoids have become a chronic problem or are causing acute discomfort, your doctor will probably recommend that they be removed. External hemorrhoids can be removed surgically under local anesthetic as an office procedure.

Internal hemorrhoids are usually removed by a relatively painless and extremely effective procedure called rubber band ligation. If you're in fairly good health, this can be done in a doctor's office. An elastic band is wrapped around the hemorrhoid to interfere with its blood supply, and both the elastic and the hemorrhoid slough off within two weeks. This procedure may be combined with local cryotherapy (freezing).

Indigestion

Indigestion is another complaint that becomes more common with age. There are many kinds of indigestion (also known as dyspepsia), and while it can be an early symptom of ulcers, gallbladder disease or even cancer, in most cases the problem is related to other less serious factors.

Symptoms

A common type of indigestion is heartburn, a burning sensation beneath the breastbone. It tends to occur after you've eaten a large meal or certain spicy foods, and is usually caused by irritation of the esophagus (the foodpipe between your mouth and stomach). Older people are more likely to get heartburn than younger people because the sphincter, a circular band of muscles between your stomach and esophagus, becomes weaker with age, causing food and stomach acid to back up into the esophagus. Heartburn and bloating can also occur as your stomach's ability to empty slows with aging.

Trapped gas, which causes crampy or shooting pains in your abdomen, chest or shoulders, is another type of indigestion. It also leads to constant burping up of air or the expulsion of gas (flatus).

Note: If symptoms of indigestion – heartburn, shooting pains, nausea – are unusual in any way and if they don't respond immediately to the self-help strategies listed below, consult your doctor right away to rule out any cardiac problems.

What to try

Preventing indigestion should be your first strategy. Cut out foods that may contribute to heartburn – spicy foods, fried and other high-fat foods, coffee, and citrus and tomato juice, which are very high in acid. Smoking and peppermint gum or candies can cause heartburn, as can certain drugs such as progesterone and some antibiotics. Other contributing factors include being overweight, eating too quickly, feeling stressed and wearing clothes or belts that constrict your chest or stomach.

Chew your food well and try to eat smaller, more frequent meals. Avoid lying down or reclining after you eat – try to stay upright and active for at least one or two hours.

If heartburn does occur, you can try taking a non-prescription antacid, which contains ingredients to neutralize stomach acid. Taking too much antacid can be hazardous, however – many of them contain magnesium and aluminum, which can be toxic at high levels in people with kidney problems. Because these preparations also usually contain sodium, they should be avoided if you have high blood pressure.

Gas, which causes bloating, burping and flatulence, is produced by many foods, including beans and other high-fiber vegetables. Rather than giving up these healthy foods, you can try using a non-prescription product like Beano (see page 25).

Avoid eating too quickly, sucking on candies, chewing gum or drinking beverages through a straw. Swallowing air also contributes to a buildup of gas.

As you age, your body may produce less lactase, the enzyme that breaks down lactose, the sugar found in milk and dairy products. In some people, this enzyme disappears completely. This leads to a condition known as "lactose intolerance." When you take in lactose, you experience gas, abdominal cramping and runny stools. One obvious solution is to reduce or eliminate your intake of dairy products, but they're an important source of calcium for older adults. Instead, try buying lactose-reduced milk and aged cheese, or try taking Lactaid tablets to prevent symptoms.

Consult your doctor

If none of these self-help strategies reduces your indigestion, see your doctor, who may wish to rule out underlying problems. For example, you may have an ulcer or a hiatus hernia, where abdominal contents, including stomach acid, protrude into the hiatus – the space in the diaphragm through which the esophagus or food tube connects to the stomach.

Treatment

Heartburn caused by excess stomach acid may be treated with prescription drugs such as cimetidine or ranitidine, which decrease acid production. If the problem is a slowing down of gastric emptying, your doctor may suggest drugs to improve this function – for example, metoclopramide or domperidone (also sold as Motilium).

If she suspects an ulcer or hiatus hernia, she will suggest a barium X-ray (see page 99) or other tests such as gastroscopy. This involves passing a lighted probe down the esophagus (your throat is anesthetized first to prevent the normal gag reflex from occurring), which allows direct examination of your esophagus and stomach.

Unlike pain from heartburn, ulcer pain may be worse when you haven't eaten. Treatment for ulcers usually involves a combination of antibiotics and antacid. If you have a hiatus hernia that is causing severe, uncontrollable symptoms, surgery may be considered.

Itching

Everyone has experienced itching due to allergies and insect bites. But as you get older, you become more susceptible to other types of itching. These can cause considerable distress and may, in some cases, be a sign of illness.

Symptoms

As you age, your skin becomes thinner and drier, and this can lead to itchiness, especially during the winter, when your skin is driest. The skin looks

Dry skin care

◆ Avoid showering or bathing every day – twice to three times a week should be enough.

◆ Don't soak in the tub or shower for longer than 15 minutes, and use warm rather than hot water, which dries out the skin.

◆ Use a mild, superfatted soap and stay away from deodorant and anti-bacterial soaps, which are drying.

◆ There's no need to soap your whole body – concentrate on your face, underarms, genitals, hands and feet.

◆ After washing, pat rather than rub the skin dry, and apply an inexpensive moisturizer.

◆ Bath oils are good for dry skin, but be careful when you use them – they make the bathtub slippery.

slightly rough and may show marks caused by scratching. Itchiness (sometimes accompanied by a rash) is also caused by allergies to food, to metals found in jewelry, to synthetic materials, and to some substances found in cosmetics, cleansers and laundry detergents.

The most common sites for itching are the genitals (often a symptom of a urinary tract or yeast infection), the anus (hemorrhoids) and between the toes (fungal infection).

What to try
Many of us were taught that cleanliness is next to godliness. But overwashing – showering or bathing every day – can cause mature skin to become dried out and itchy.

Some cases of genital or anal itching are caused by poor hygiene, or by overwiping the skin with abrasive toilet paper. Keep these areas clean with moistened paper or commercially available glycerine-soaked pads.

When you feel itchy, your first impulse is to scratch; some itching, though, is actually prolonged by too much scratching. If you can resist scratching the itchy area for a day or two, the itching may stop.

Consult your doctor
If itching persists for more than a week, your doctor may want to rule out underlying illnesses that can cause itching such as diabetes, some immune disorders or kidney disease.

Treatment
Some cases of itching due to local skin problems respond well to ointments containing cortisone. If the itching seems related to an allergy, your doctor may refer you to a specialist who will do tests to determine the kind of allergy. Itching caused by a urinary tract infection will stop when the infection is cleared up with antibiotics. Older women should know that a common source of vaginal itching – yeast infections – can actually be caused by antibiotic drugs that you're taking for another infection. Your doctor can recommend appropriate anti-fungal creams to stop the itching.

Leg pain

Pain in the legs is another fairly common complaint among older adults. In many cases it's a relatively minor problem, but in others it signals a potentially serious health problem.

Symptoms

Cramps in your calf muscles or feet, lasting a few seconds or several minutes, come on for no reason and may even wake you in the middle of the night. These painful contractions are caused by an unexplained firing of nerve signals or as a side effect of certain medication, particularly diuretics prescribed for heart failure. Diuretics may cause a rapid loss of important fluids, salt and other minerals, and this can occasionally result in muscle cramping.

Another common type of leg pain is the result of poor or blocked circulation, also known as intermittent claudication. The discomfort usually occurs during walking and is felt as a dragging or aching pain in your leg, usually in the same spot. If you stop and rest for a while, the pain goes away. This is a sign that the muscles in your legs aren't getting enough oxygen because of reduced blood flow or blockage due to atherosclerosis (so-called hardening of the arteries). If you have severe obstruction, you may also develop sores on your legs or feet that don't heal. In the most severe cases, the tissue may become gangrenous and amputation may be the only treatment.

If you have a localized pain in your leg and can feel a hardened or cordlike area that is extremely sensitive to pressure, you may be suffering from superficial phlebitis. This is an inflammation of a vein near the surface of the skin, often accompanied by the formation of a clot. Leg injury, infection, some clotting disorders and chemical irritation are the usual causes. The area surrounding the vein may be red and warm to the touch. In extreme cases, where deep veins are blocked, the entire leg may be pale, cold and swollen.

What to try

If you experience leg cramps at night, try to stand up and put weight on the affected muscle, or use your fingers to apply pressure against the painful area. This is often enough to stop the pain. If you are taking powerful diuretics, mention the cramps to your doctor, who may want to change your medication.

Leg pain due to poor circulation is often associated with certain risk factors which may be within your control. These include a history of smoking, diabetes, high blood pressure, high cholesterol levels, obesity, and a sedentary lifestyle. If your doctor says it's all right for you to exert yourself, you can improve blood flow in your legs by 30 minutes of regular exercise three to five days a week. The best activities for this problem are walking, climbing stairs or riding a stationary bicycle. Always stop if you feel pain.

If you are confined to bed for long periods of time because of illness, it's important that you make the effort to move your legs a few times each hour. For example, rotate each ankle, bend and flex your knees, raise your legs up and down. This will help maintain circulation.

As for leg pain due to phlebitis, the condition always requires prompt medical attention and treatment.

Consult your doctor

You shouldn't try to diagnose leg pain on your own. If the problem is poor circulation, you should begin treating it as soon as possible to avoid surgery.

Your doctor will examine your legs and feet carefully. She will measure the blood pressure in each foot and compare these readings with blood pressure measurements taken in your arms. If the pressure in your feet is significantly lower than in the rest of your body, this usually means a blockage. She may also order a special ultrasound scan to pinpoint the obstruction.

Treatment

Leg pain due to poor circulation is usually relieved when circulation improves. To accomplish this, try to reduce some of the risk factors mentioned above and make an effort to exercise your legs. If your symptoms don't improve, your doctor may suggest a drug called pentoxifylline (Trental), which can improve circulation.

About 15 percent of people with this condition require surgery to restore blood flow to their legs and feet. A commonly used technique is balloon angioplasty. A device containing a tiny balloon is threaded through the blocked blood vessel, inflated with sterile water, and withdrawn from the vessel, clearing away any obstruction. (A similar technique is sometimes used to clear blocked coronary vessels, which cause angina. See page 150.)

Phlebitis is usually treated with anti-clotting medication, moist heat applied to the affected area (if the blocked veins are near the skin surface), and – once the swelling has subsided – an exercise program.

Mouth problems

Mouth problems are usually minor, but they can make you feel quite miserable and shouldn't be ignored. Pain in a tooth or gum should be reported to your dentist as soon as possible, so he can investigate the source of the trouble and begin treatment if necessary. If you feel pain in the soft tissues of your mouth (tongue, inner cheeks, roof of the mouth), talk to your dentist or doctor immediately.

Mouth pain

Pain in the mouth can have many sources. One of the most common is dental caries, the decay of a tooth or its root. The root is normally covered and protected by gum tissue, but gum disease can cause this tissue to shrink, exposing the root surface and making it vulnerable to decay.

Pain may also be caused by gum (periodontal) diseases, which affect the bone and soft tissues that support your teeth. The most common ones are gingivitis (reversible inflammation of the gums caused by bacterial infection) and periodontitis (the same inflammation accompanied by changes in the structure of your gums and jaw). Once periodontitis occurs, your teeth may become loosened.

Pain may stem from injury to the soft tissues of your mouth, tongue and cheeks, often caused by jagged or crooked teeth and poorly fitting dentures.

Abnormalities in the nerves may cause pain or burning sensations in the mouth.

Oral lesions

You may develop sores, bumps or other growths in your mouth that may or may not be painful.

Many oral lesions are symptoms of an infection or disease such as thrush, herpes or an infected tooth.

Some lesions are caused by an antibiotic or another type of medication. Antibiotics can cause an overgrowth of a certain fungus called "candida albicans," which causes an infection of the mucous membranes called "thrush."

Another oral lesion found in older adults is associated with a condition called "leukoplakia." A whitish patch or patches appear inside the mouth (on the inside of the cheeks, on the roof of the mouth, on or under the tongue). Men are more prone to leukoplakia than women, and it's especially common among smokers – although non-smokers may also develop the problem. Any whitish patch should be checked out by your doctor. If untreated, about 5 percent of these whitish patches will become cancerous over time.

Oral cancer is the most serious type of lesion that appears in the mouth. You should be aware that its incidence increases with age and the use of tobacco and alcohol. The main symptom of oral cancer is the appearance of a raw or raised red or whitish sore in your mouth that may bleed and doesn't heal. You may also notice a painless lump or thickening in the soft tissues of your mouth.

You should examine your own mouth regularly for any changes, and expect your doctor and dentist to do the same during routine examinations. This is especially important if you are or have been a heavy smoker or drinker. It's also another excellent reason to give up these habits.

Dry mouth

Even though there's no evidence that age affects how well salivary glands produce saliva, many older people complain about chronic dry mouth – a condition referred to as "xerostomia." Besides being uncomfortable, dry mouth increases your chance of developing cavities, makes dentures difficult to wear and can make it harder to chew, swallow and digest.

If you suffer from dry mouth, it may be due to medications that are known to affect saliva output – the most common culprits are tricyclic antidepressants such as nortriptyline (Aventyl), some drugs used to treat incontinence such as oxybutynin (Ditropan), and some over-the-counter decongestants. Diuretics taken to treat high blood pressure or other problems can cause dehydration and dry mouth as well. Less common causes are infections of the salivary glands and some rare diseases affecting glandular secretions such as Sjögren's syndrome.

You can stimulate the production of saliva by chewing sugarless gum or sucking on tart-tasting, hard candy (preferably sugarless to protect your teeth and waistline). You can also keep some bottled water handy to moisten your mouth regularly.

Neck pain

As you get older, you will probably start to notice that you can't take your neck for granted anymore. Until your neck begins to trouble you, you rarely stop to think about just how important a healthy neck is.

Symptoms
You may notice that your neck tends to feel stiff or sore when you first get up in the morning or after you've been sitting in one position for a long time.

As with back pain, the most likely cause is osteoarthritis, which causes varying degrees of neck pain in about 85 percent of people over 70. This "wear-and-tear" arthritis occurs when the discs cushioning the bones or vertebrae in your neck become thinner and the small neck joints lose their cartilage. When this happens, the bones rub together, which can cause pain. You may then instinctively tense your neck muscles. This tends to strain them, producing more pain.

Pain in your neck, including the area between your shoulder blades, may mean that you've strained a muscle during a normal movement. In some cases, osteoarthritis or neck strain can also cause a headache, usually in the back of your head.

What to try
For some reason neck pain due to osteoarthritis tends to flare up and then get better. A non-prescription pain reliever such as acetaminophen (Tylenol) used according to instructions for several days can relieve discomfort. Resting your neck during the day by lying down or leaning back in a chair with head support can also help. As with back pain, though, too much rest can actually increase stiffness and pain. Try not to sleep on your stomach, and ask your doctor or an occupational therapist whether you should use a cervical pillow to give your neck added support during sleep.

When the pain is severe, apply a cold pack several times daily (a bag of frozen vegetables works fine) for no longer than 20 minutes at a time. If you have heart problems or a reduced sensitivity to temperature, ask your doctor to recommend an appropriate method for cold application. Once the acute pain has subsided, warmth from a heating pad, water bottle, warm shower or heat lamp can help relax muscles.

Consult your doctor
Always call your doctor for any neck pain related to an injury, for pain that occurs suddenly, or for pain that persists longer than three days. You should also call him if you feel tingling or numbness radiating to your arms or legs. This can signal a pinched nerve in your neck.

Treatment

✔ For severe neck pain that doesn't respond to self-help strategies, your doctor may prescribe more powerful pain relievers, muscle relaxants, or non-steroidal anti-inflammatory medication such as acetyl-salicylic acid (Aspirin), ibuprofen or naprox-en sodium. (Because these drugs can irritate your stomach and kidneys or interact with other medications, they should be taken only on the advice of your doctor.) Other treatments for neck pain include massage, injections of local anesthetic to specific areas and – in extreme cases – surgery to relieve pressure on a pinched nerve.

Your doctor may suggest that you be assessed by a physiotherapist, who may be able to pinpoint the problem and recommend exercises to ease your symptoms.

Some people consult chiropractors who attempt to treat neck and back pain through manipulation and other techniques. Although many users of this alternative therapy swear by chiropractic treatment, there's some debate about its effectiveness and safety – especially in older people. As you get older, your bones and other structures such as ligaments and tendons become less pliant and may be more prone to damage from manipulation. If you still want to try chiropractic therapy, it's a good idea to discuss it with your doctor first so you can understand the possible risks of manipulation.

Sensitivity to heat and cold

All of us have our own individual temperature preferences. Some people enjoy feeling warm and toasty while others prefer a cooler, airier environment. (Incidentally, it seems to be a law of nature that those who like it warm invariably live with those who like it cool!)

As people get older, they tend to become much more sensitive to heat and cold. While some people develop increased temperature sensitivity, others experience quite the opposite problem: they lose their sensitivity to heat and cold.

Symptoms

❗ People who are *sensitive to cold* typically complain of icy hands and feet. This happens because your autonomic nervous system, which controls your body's response to changes in temperature, is directing blood flow away from your limbs to keep vital organs such as your heart warm.

You should be aware of a potentially life-threatening condition known as "accidental hypothermia." This occurs when exposure to cold causes your body temperature to drop below 95° F (35° C) or lower. While accidental hypothermia can occur at any age, it often affects older people, especially those who are chronically ill and bedridden, those who are unable to afford adequate heating, those who have lost sensitivity to the cold and those who have problems with their metabolism. Symptoms include a slow or irregular heartbeat, slurred speech and confusion.

Accidental hypothermia is most likely to occur outdoors – for example, if you faint and are left lying on the cold or icy ground for too long. But this loss of body heat can also happen in a cold bedroom –that's why older people who are sensitive to cold should always dress warmly at night. Wear layered clothes (a sweater or robe over your pajamas or nightgown, and warm socks) in case you become uncovered during the night.

People who are *sensitive to heat* typically complain of perspiration and feeling sluggish or unwell. This happens when your autonomic nervous system causes small blood vessels in your skin to dilate (open wider), allowing more blood to flow to the skin's surface, where it cools.

There are two heat-related conditions you should know about. The most serious is *heatstroke*, which occurs when your body temperature rises above 104°F (40°C) or higher because of exposure to heat. Heatstroke occurs suddenly, and symptoms include faintness, dizziness, headache, confusion, nausea, rapid pulse and flushed skin. A milder condition, *heat exhaustion*, occurs more gradually. Symptoms, including weakness, sweating and queasiness, are caused by an overwhelming loss of water and salt. Untreated heat exhaustion may progress to heatstroke.

What to try

If your hands and feet always seem cold, wear clothes made from fabrics that hold in warmth – wool, down, silk or synthetics such as polypropylene. Layered clothing – for example, a silk blouse under a wool sweater – will keep you warmer because air trapped between the layers reduces heat loss. In the winter, always make sure your ears and head are covered when you go outside – most heat loss occurs through the head.

It's also important to eat properly, and to stay as physically active as possible, since activity increases blood flow to hands and feet. Avoid nicotine, caffeine and drugs such as phenylpropanolamine (found in some cold remedies), which can contribute to cold hands and feet. If you take propranolol or other beta blockers (used to treat high blood pressure), this can also contribute to chilly sensations. Try to avoid or control stress, which prompts your body to produce adrenaline, decreasing blood flow to your extremities.

If you always feel warm, especially during hot weather, wear lightweight, loose-fitting clothes in light colors. They will keep you cooler by reflecting the heat and allowing your perspiration to evaporate, which has a cooling effect. Drink plenty of liquids (except alcohol), and don't overexert yourself. Cool – not cold – baths or showers, cool compresses, and electric fans or air conditioners can also keep you comfortable. If your house or apartment is too warm, spend the hottest part of the day in an air-conditioned library, movie theater or shopping mall.

Consult your doctor

Feeling too cold or warm may be annoying, but it rarely signals any serious illness. Even so, your doctor may want to test you for anemia or a thyroid disorder. You should also inform your doctor if you notice that your hands turn white when exposed to cold and then turn blue and painful after warming. This may be a sign known as Raynaud's phenomenon. It is sometimes associated with immune disorders. You should also call if one hand or foot feels cold all the time, or if any fingers or toes appear blue. These could be symptoms of a blocked artery.

Treatment
Hypothermia and heatstroke are considered medical emergencies and should be treated as such. A case of heat exhaustion should always be reported to your doctor, who may suggest you go to the nearest hospital emergency room. Depending on the severity of your symptoms and your general health, you may require longer hospital care.

Shortness of breath

This complaint, which doctors call "dyspnea," is a common source of distress and anxiety for older people. It's more than just physically unpleasant – if you feel unable to breathe properly, you're likely to decrease your activity, and this can have a negative impact on your overall health.

Symptoms
You may find that you stop what you're doing to "catch your breath." Or you may be aware that you're breathing more rapidly than before and your chest feels tight or heavy.

What to try
How you deal with shortness of breath depends on what's causing it. A major factor at any age is poor physical fitness, which causes you to become breathless after exerting yourself – for example, after walking up a flight of stairs or hurrying to catch a bus. When you feel uncomfortably short of breath, your first impulse is to slow down. Until your doctor can determine the cause, this is probably a good idea. If you smoke, your heart and lungs may be warning you that it's time to stop.

Consult your doctor
If shortness of breath is an ongoing problem, or if it's accompanied by other symptoms such as wheezing, faintness, heart palpitations, fever, dizziness or chest pain, report it to your doctor right away. She will want to rule out an underlying lung problem – emphysema, asthma, bronchitis or even pneumonia – and also check for any underlying heart disease. A sudden onset of dyspnea is a potential emergency and requires immediate medical attention. Ask someone to drive you to the nearest hospital emergency room or dial 911.

Treatment
If your doctor determines that your shortness of breath is due to lack of physical exercise or other factors such as obesity and smoking, she will discuss ways you can improve your overall fitness. Even if you're in your 70s, 80s and even 90s, you can still benefit from increasing your activity level (see page 30).

Varicose veins

These are veins, usually located in the back of the leg between the top of your thigh and ankle, which become raised and may be painful. The condition is often triggered by hormonal changes and weight gain during pregnancy, making it more common among women than among men.

Symptoms

The veins in your legs appear raised or twisted because they have become overfilled with blood. They are most likely to become painful if you stand on your feet for long periods of time.

What to try

It's important to keep blood from pooling in your legs, so whenever possible, keep your feet raised. If you have to stand or walk a lot, you may want to try wearing elastic stockings or support hose (also available for men). Because being overweight places an added strain on varicose veins, it's prudent to see your doctor or a nutritionist about beginning a weight loss program.

Consult your doctor

You should mention varicose veins to your doctor if they become especially swollen or painful, if you notice bruising around the vein, or if you develop dry brown patches or ulcers (sores) on your lower leg.

Treatment

Various treatments exist for the discomfort caused by varicose veins. Properly fitted support hosiery worn during the day is usually enough to relieve symptoms, but in some people aching and swelling persist. One treatment called "sclerotherapy," usually done in the doctor's office without anesthetic, involves the injection of a solution directly into the veins. This produces inflammation and scar tissue, which reduces swelling by restricting blood flow to the vein. If this doesn't work, or if you have a great number of varicose veins, you may require surgery, usually done in hospital, to tie off or completely remove varicose veins.

Vision changes

About 80 percent of people over age 65 will experience age-related changes in vision that are severe enough to warrant glasses. A significant decrease or loss in vision is serious at any age, but it can be especially devastating when you're older. Impaired vision interferes with daily activities of living and makes you more vulnerable to accidents, especially falls, and may increase your sense of isolation.

Symptoms

The most common age-related change in vision is called *presbyopia*, which occurs when the lens of the eye loses its ability to bring objects into focus. You may notice that it's harder to focus on something close up – for example, the page of a book – and you have to move the object farther away from your eyes in order to see it clearly. Another condition common in older people is *macular degeneration*. The central portion of the retina, called the "macula," deteriorates, and you may have trouble reading or focusing on small objects.

As you age, the lens of the eye turns yellow, which makes it more difficult for you to perceive colors in the blue/green range. It also takes more time for your eyes to adjust from bright lights to darkness, and your ability to see in the dark decreases.

What to try

Too many older people grimly accept their visual impairment without seeking help. If glasses have already been prescribed for you, wear them. If they aren't comfortable or don't seem to help, you may need a different type of lens, so consult your eye doctor. However, if you suffer from loss of vision due to macular degeneration, changing glasses probably won't improve your condition substantially.

Making simple improvements in your environment can help if you suffer from age-related vision loss. If necessary, boost the lighting in your house or apartment, replacing low-watt bulbs in lamps and light fixtures with more powerful ones (make sure they can safely take the extra wattage). If you go out and expect to return home when it's dark, leave the lights on so you don't return to a darkened house. Place strips of fluorescent tape around your light switches, door handles, keyholes and electrical sockets so you can see them more easily in the dark.

Consult your doctor

Any sudden change in vision or eye pain should be reported to your doctor immediately – it could be an early sign of glaucoma, cataracts, retinal detachment or a blocked retinal artery. Vision problems can also occur as a complication of diabetes or a symptom of neurological disease.

Even if your vision seems all right, it's important to have your eyes examined periodically by your primary care doctor and preferably by an optometrist. Regular examinations can often pick up signs of disease that, if left untreated, could cause serious impairment and even blindness.

Treatment

If your vision problem can be improved by wearing glasses, your doctor will send you to an optometrist or an optician to determine the right type of lenses. Unfortunately no treatment exists to reverse the effects of macular degeneration. But magnifying glasses and other vision aids can make a difference, and large print books and books-on-tape are now widely available at libraries and stores.

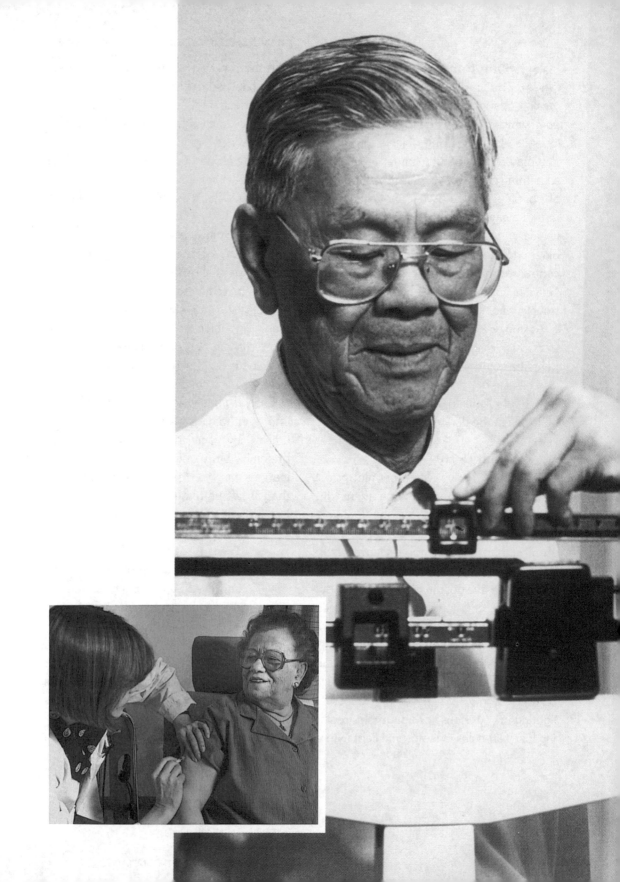

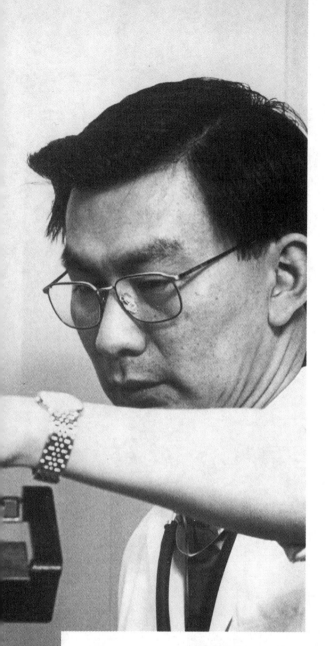

4

Illness is the night side of life. … Everyone who is born holds dual citizenship, in the kingdom of the well and in the kingdom of the sick. … Sooner or later each of us is obliged, at least for a spell, to identify ourselves as citizens of that other place.

SUSAN SONTAG

Common Health Problems after 65

EVEN THOUGH IT'S POSSIBLE TO LIVE to a good old age without serious illness, most people can expect to develop some kind of health problem later in life.

Despite the amazing strides made by medical researchers in your own lifetime, many of the physical, mental and emotional ailments common in older people still can't be cured. But many of these problems can now be managed and controlled effectively.

No one likes to think about getting sick, but the experience of acute or chronic illness can be especially upsetting later in life for many reasons:

◆ You may not have the physical and mental reserves that you had when you were younger to deal with illness.

◆ You worry about becoming dependent on others during the course of a long or difficult illness – especially family members who are already suffering from health problems of their own.

◆ You may no longer have a network of social supports – friends, co-workers, relatives – which is so vital to coping with illness.

◆ If you don't have a good health insurance plan or other coverage, you may worry about the expense of a major or chronic illness.

◆ The experience of serious illness later in life forces you to think about your own mortality, which is much closer now than when you were younger.

Illness provokes many emotions. Some of them are common to everyone who faces illness, while others are more specific to you. For example, if you've already suffered and recovered from other illnesses, you may be better equipped than someone who has never had a sick day before. If you experienced serious or chronic illness in your family – a seriously ill parent, a chronically ill sibling or child – becoming ill yourself can dredge up many buried feelings.

When you get sick, it's normal to feel anxious about yourself and upset about the changes occurring in your life. Anger is common – you may feel angry at your own body for "betraying" you by breaking down, angry at fate for what's happening, angry at your doctor. If you've ignored your health until now, chances are you'll feel guilty about the fact that you haven't taken care of yourself.

One of the best allies against illness, especially among older people, is information. You need to know that your body has changed and that you may not become sick or respond to treatment in the same way a younger person would.

"But surely my doctor knows all about these things?" you may ask.

In many cases this is true, but unfortunately some doctors still aren't fully aware of the special health needs of older adults. That's why it's important for you to understand some of the health problems that can occur later in life. Remember – you are a full partner in your own health care and must assume your share of the responsibility.

One way to do this is to become informed about those diseases and conditions that are most likely to affect you, your partner or your parents.

The next three chapters will provide you with some of the most recent information and expert advice about major health problems, including heart disease, stroke, diabetes, arthritis, osteoporosis, cancer, Alzheimer's disease and depression, as well as specific health problems affecting older women and those affecting older men. You'll also learn about difficult problems such as grief, hypochondria and alcohol dependency.

Arthritis

Even though arthritis is a widespread chronic disease, affecting about 15 percent of the population, many myths still surround it.

◆ *Myth:* Arthritis is always a disease of older age.

◆ *Fact:* Problems with the joints and bones can occur at any age – in fact, about half of all people with arthritis are aged 30 to 50. However, some types of arthritis are more common with advancing age, and many older people do suffer from arthritic symptoms.

◆ *Myth:* If your joints are sore, you have arthritis.

◆ *Fact:* Many other problems, including inflammation of the muscles, tendons, or cushioning sacs called "bursa," can cause arthritis-type pain.

◆ *Myth:* If you have arthritis you must expect to live with severe chronic pain and disability.

◆ *Fact:* Although arthritis can be painful, many people experience relatively mild discomfort that can be readily relieved with medication. It's true that certain types of arthritis cause permanent damage to joints and bones resulting in disability, but education about the disease along with early treatment can greatly reduce or prevent further damage.

◆ *Myth:* If you get arthritis, there's not much you can do about it.

◆ *Fact:* Arthritis can't be prevented, but proper treatment and management can ease pain, prevent or minimize disability and improve quality of life for most older people with this disease.

 What are the most common types of arthritis affecting older adults?

There are more than 100 diseases that fall under the general category of arthritis. Some of these conditions affect only the joints and bones, while others cause damage to other organs.

If you're over 65, you're most likely to be affected by the following types of arthritis, and it's not uncommon for older people to have more than one type:

◆ *Osteoarthritis*, a degenerative disease, occurs after years of wear and tear on bones and joints. The cartilage, a tough, elastic covering that cushions the ends of your bones and prevents them from rubbing against each other, develops small cracks and begins to wear away, causing pain and stiffness. The most common sites for osteoarthritis are in the weight-bearing joints – the spine, hips and knees.

Osteoarthritis is by far the most common type of arthritis, affecting equal numbers of women and men. About half of all people over age 65 and three-quarters of those over age 75 have this type of arthritis. While the condition can be extremely painful, osteoarthritis usually responds to treatment that reduces pain, improves mobility and prevents major disability.

◆ *Rheumatoid arthritis* occurs when the tissue lining your joints, called the "synovium," becomes inflamed, thickened and filled with fluid. The joint then becomes hot, tender and swollen. Because moving an inflamed joint is very painful, you tend to stop using it. This causes the surrounding muscles to become weakened, and over time the joint may become permanently immobile.

Rheumatoid arthritis usually develops in more than one joint and tends to affect the smaller joints in the hands, wrists, feet, neck and jaw. In addition to painful joints, you may also experience fatigue, fever, loss of appetite and problems with your heart and lungs.

This type of arthritis, which affects women more often than men, usually makes its presence known between ages 20 and 50, although the first attack can occur after age 65. Recently Australian researchers announced that they had identified a genetic mutation that may play a role in so-called autoimmune diseases such as rheumatoid arthritis. (Autoimmune diseases occur when your body's immune system reacts abnormally and begins to attack its own healthy tissues.)

◆ *Gout* is triggered by abnormally high blood levels of uric acid, a waste product excreted by your kidneys. For some reason, uric acid crystals are deposited in the joints, where they cause inflammation and pain. Gout usually affects joints in the feet, especially the big toe, which becomes swollen and extremely painful.

Although gout can strike at any age, it's most likely to occur later in life, and 80 percent of sufferers are men. An attack of gout can be triggered by excessive eating and drinking, by stress and certain medications such as diuretics that may produce increased levels of uric acid.

◆ *Fibromyalgia (also known as fibrositis)* is a fairly common disorder that some researchers now think is related to arthritis. Until recently it was poorly understood and many doctors were slow to believe that it existed. For some reason, most fibromyalgia sufferers are women.

Symptoms include chronic aches, pains or stiffness in the neck, back or other joints. Sleep disturbances, headaches, irritable bowels and fatigue are also common, and you may have certain tender areas – points of pain located in your knees, elbows and/or the back of your neck.

◆ *Polymyalgia rheumatica* is a treatable type of rheumatic disorder that's especially common in older adults. Symptoms include pain and stiffness of the hips and shoulders, especially in the morning. You may notice that you have to swing your legs over the edge of the bed and then rock the upper part of your body to be able to stand upright. Some people may experience swelling in the hands without redness or inflammation.

Polymyalgia rheumatica can easily be

misdiagnosed, and sufferers may be told they have osteoarthritis of the neck or spine or rheumatoid arthritis. But blood tests showing an elevated ESR (erythrocyte sedimentation rate) can help your doctor pinpoint the condition.

◆ *Temporal arteritis (also known as giant cell arteritis)* affects about 15 percent of people with polymyalgia rheumatica. This inflammatory disease damages the walls of arteries, including the temporal arteries. (You have two temporal arteries, one on either side of your head, and they supply blood to your face and scalp.) In addition to the pain and weakness of polymyalgia rheumatica, people with temporal arteritis may suffer from headache, fever, weight loss, tenderness and swelling of the temporal artery, painful chewing and dimming of vision – especially while walking.

Diagnosing temporal arteritis usually involves taking a biopsy of the temporal artery. Getting the right diagnosis is extremely important. If untreated, the condition can cause permanent damage to blood vessels in the eyes and lead to irreversible blindness.

❓ How is arthritis treated?

If you're like many older people with arthritis, you may have resigned yourself to living with pain. It's not uncommon for those who suffer chronic or recurring pain to become inactive or depressed, which may make your pain even worse.

If you suffer from arthritis, it's absolutely vital that your condition is properly diagnosed so that your doctor and other health care specialists can devise the best plan of treatment. Unfortunately, many older adults with arthritis fall into the trap of diagnosing their own aches and pains and treating themselves, often with over-the-counter pain relievers that can cause more problems than they solve.

Of course you know your own body better than anyone else, and if you find a remedy that seems to work for you, you should use it. But it's best to do this in cooperation with your doctor.

Most cases of osteoarthritis can be successfully diagnosed and treated by your family doctor. If your pain doesn't respond to treatment or if you suffer from a serious or complicated case of arthritis, you may be referred to a rheumatologist who specializes in arthritis.

Arthritis treatment falls into two basic categories: a lifestyle or non-drug approach and a medication approach. Your doctor will probably start off with the former. This may include assessment and advice from a physiotherapist and/or occupational therapist, who may recommend one or more of the following:

◆ keeping a pain diary for a few weeks or months, noting when your symptoms feel worse and better and how pain is related to certain activities, times or periods of stress;

◆ losing weight if necessary, which can help relieve or reduce pain by taking strain off your hip, knee, ankle and foot joints;

◆ an exercise program geared toward strengthening muscles so they are better able to take some of the pressure off your joints;

◆ changes in how you move and use your body, including strategies to conserve energy and protect vulnerable joints in your knees, hips, elbows, neck, back and hands;

◆ the use of splinting to immobilize painful joints, mechanical devices to support weak joints and muscles, and walking aids to help take the stress off painful joints.

Your therapists may also teach you relaxation techniques that will help you to manage flare-ups better and give you advice about ways to soothe pain. These may include the use of warm water pool therapy and the proper use of heat and ice: for example, many people don't realize that a hot, inflamed joint requires cooling rather than warmth.

In other cases arthritis sufferers may also require medication to relieve pain and/or control inflammation. In the past doctors often began treatment using anti-inflammatory medications, even for older people whose pain often didn't involve inflammation. Now doctors are adopting a different approach.

If you have pain with no inflammation, you may get significant relief from an over-the-counter painkiller such as acetaminophen, which has few troublesome side effects if taken properly.

If you have pain and inflammation, your doctor may prescribe an anti-inflammatory drug such as acetylsalicylic acid (ASA), or a non-steroidal anti-inflammatory drug (NSAID) (see page 130)

Other drugs used to treat symptoms of rheumatoid arthritis include corticosteroids (injections), gold salts (pills or injections), anti-malarial drugs such as chloroquine, and chemotherapeutic drugs such as methotrexate that suppress the body's immune response.

If you have gout, your doctor will proba-

bly prescribe an NSAID (but not ASA) to reduce an acute attack of pain and inflammation, and you may also need local injections of steroids into the joint. You may be asked to stop eating liver, kidney and other organ meats, which cause your body to produce high levels of uric acid. For recurring gout, a drug called allopurinol, which inhibits the production of uric acid, may be required on an ongoing basis.

If you suffer from fibromyalgia, you may benefit from aerobic and muscle-strengthening exercises, counseling, painkillers such as acetaminophen, massage and biofeedback. Low doses of antidepressant medications may be useful as well.

Polymyalgia rheumatica doesn't usually respond to non-steroidal anti-inflammatory drugs used to treat arthritis symptoms. The best treatment is a low daily dose of corticosteroid medication such as prednisone, which can often relieve stiffness very quickly, sometimes within a few days. Treatment for polymyalgia rheumatica involves a fairly long course of potent, corticosteroid medication.

Can surgery help arthritis?
Most people with arthritis will not require surgery, but if years of pain and inflammation have caused severe, irreversible damage to a particular joint or bone, it may be recommended. You may have lost a great deal of joint mobility, and at this stage, strategies such as drugs, rest and exercise will have little effect.

The goal of arthritis surgery is to relieve pain and inflammation and restore joint function and mobility. For some people this results in fairly modest improvement, while for others the benefit is dramatic: After years

A warning about NSAIDs

If you're over 65, non-steroidal anti-inflammatory drugs (NSAIDS), such as acetylsalicylic acid (ASA), ibuprofen, ketoprofen and naproxen can cause a range of unpleasant and even dangerous side effects. They should be taken only on the advice of your doctor and according to her instructions. Here's what you should know about NSAIDs:

◆ In low doses these drugs relieve pain; in higher doses they block your body's production of prostaglandins, which are known to be involved in the painful process of inflammation.

◆ NSAIDs should be used only when you're experiencing inflammation – heat, swelling and redness of joints. Once the inflammation subsides, you should try switching back to acetaminophen.

◆ NSAIDs can interact with many other prescription and non-prescription drugs – for example, diuretics and anticoagulants. Before taking an NSAID, make sure your doctor knows about all the drugs you're taking – including over-the-counter medications. If you're taking an NSAID, don't start taking anything new before checking with your doctor.

◆ Common side effects may include nausea, stomach upset, heartburn, diarrhea, and ringing in the ears. Less common ones are mild depression, headache, confusion, blurred vision and skin rashes.

◆ More serious side effects, especially among older people, are gastrointestinal ulcers and internal bleeding in your stomach or bowel. You should be alert to the symptoms of gastric bleeding. They include vomiting blood, nausea, pain in the abdomen, black stool and fainting. (Some gastric bleeding is hidden, producing no obvious symptoms until you've lost a lot of blood and become anemic.)

An acute episode of gastric bleeding is an emergency: If you experience any of these symptoms, you should call your doctor right away or go to a hospital emergency room. (If you are alone, don't drive yourself – ask someone else to drive you, call a cab, or if symptoms are severe, dial 911 for emergency assistance.)

◆ If you're taking an NSAID for arthritis, your doctor may recommend that you also take a drug called misopristol, which can protect your stomach and bowel from the harmful effects of NSAIDs.

of disability, they may be able to leave their walkers, canes and wheelchairs behind.

If you're considering surgery for arthritis, you should know that it requires a period of convalescence, and, in order to get the maximum benefit, you'll need intensive rehabilitation afterward.

Fusion is a surgical procedure that involves fusing joints – usually in the spine, hip or ankle – together. While this often relieves pain, it further limits your ability to move the joint. Before opting for fusion, it's important for you and your doctor to discuss whether the benefits of this procedure outweigh the risks for you.

Joint replacement involves removing the

damaged joint and replacing it with an artificial one made out of metal, ceramic and/or plastic. The procedure is considered quite safe, even for people in their 70s, 80s and 90s, and the benefits can be dramatic. Joints in the fingers, knees, wrists, ankles and hips can be surgically replaced. The procedure is done in the hospital under a general anesthetic.

Joint replacements typically last 10 to 15 years before wearing out, which means you may eventually need a second operation.

❓ What are some strategies for living with arthritis?

How you cope with this disease depends on many factors: how severe and frequent your symptoms are, your general physical and psychological well-being, how much disability the disease has caused, how much help you have, and whether you're living alone.

If you are living with arthritis, you need more than just medical help. You need information so that you can become the "manager" of your disease. Check in your library for books about coping with arthritis or contact the local chapter of your arthritis association. Your doctor can also put you in touch with a physiotherapy or occupational therapist who specializes in the management of arthritis.

Here are some other tips that may be helpful:

◆ Take care of yourself by eating properly, keeping a healthy body weight and getting adequate rest.

◆ Aim for a balanced attitude toward your pain. Learn to respect your pain. This means knowing when it's all right to continue an activity despite your pain, and when it's best to slow down.

◆ Learn how to use your body properly to protect your joints, ligaments and muscles. This means knowing the proper ways to sit, stand and sleep, and being careful when you perform tasks such as dressing, cooking and washing. For example, if your finger joints bother you, don't carry your purse or a shopping bag in one hand – move it up higher onto your forearm.

◆ Learn about equipment that is designed to make life easier for people with arthritis – for example, devices that raise the heights of chairs, beds and toilet seats; specially installed handrails beside stairs, which reduce strain on your knees and back; long-handled brushes and utensils; and devices to help you open jars. An occupational therapist or physiotherapist can tell you more about where to get and how to use these helpful devices.

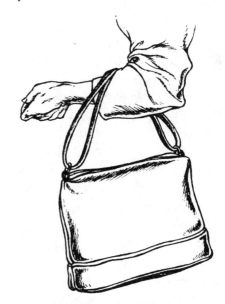

Cancer

If you're like most people, just reading the word "cancer" is probably enough to terrify you. There's no doubt that some cancers can be fatal – in fact, cancer is the second major cause of death and illness in older adults, after cardiovascular disease. But while a cancer diagnosis is frightening, it doesn't mean your life is over:

◆ Today some types of cancer can be completely cured, and many more can be effectively treated and managed, allowing you to live for many years in relatively good health.

◆ Many of the treatments now used to control cancer are far less radical than they were 20 years ago, and various techniques and drugs have been developed to minimize treatment-related discomfort.

◆ There's greater access than ever before to information and support groups that can help you and your family cope with cancer.

What is cancer?

You don't feel it happening, but each day millions of cells in your body die and are reproduced. In healthy people, this amazing process happens in a controlled fashion, but when cells begin to reproduce in a haphazard, uncontrolled way, the result is cancer. Eventually the cancerous cells begin to outnumber and damage the healthy ones, and some cells may travel from the original cancer site to other areas of the body, where they continue to multiply out of control – a process known as "metastasis." Unless this process is stopped or slowed, the disease can lead to further illness and death.

Certain factors have been implicated in the development of cancer. So far, they include an inherited vulnerability to certain cancers, a genetic mutation caused by exposure to radiation and certain chemicals, and a genetic mutation caused by repeated, long-term exposure to cancer-causing substances such as tobacco and ultraviolet radiation in sunlight.

Some researchers also believe that factors such as diet and stress may play a role in the development of cancer, but these links aren't conclusive.

Does cancer risk increase with age?

The longer you live, the more likely you are to develop cancer – in fact, more than half of all cancers are diagnosed in people aged 65 and older. Researchers offer two basic explanations for this:

◆ The longer you live, the longer your body has been exposed to cancer-causing substances in the environment and the more likely you are to finally develop cancer.

◆ Aging seems to have a negative effect on functions that probably protected you from cancer when you were younger – for example, certain genes that once helped your body control renegade cancer cells become less reliable with age.

What are the common cancers affecting older adults?

Cancer is really many different diseases, and it would be impossible to describe

A cancer prevention strategy for older adults

Many of the factors that increase your risk for cancer can't be controlled – for example, you may be genetically vulnerable to a certain type of cancer, or you may look back over a lifetime of high-risk habits that can't be undone.

But even if you're over 65, you may still be able to reduce your cancer risk by making a few changes:

◆ Control or eliminate risky behaviors such as exposure to ultraviolet light, tobacco use and alcohol intake.

◆ Some research suggests that lowering your dietary intake of saturated fat may reduce your risk for cancers of the breast, bowel and prostate. Other studies suggest that increasing consumption of fiber (found in whole grains and cereals), dried fruits and vegetables such as broccoli, cabbage and brussels sprouts may also be beneficial. Some research has also raised the possibility that fruits and vegetables high in vitamins A, C, E and beta carotene may somehow play a role in preventing cancer.

◆ Obesity has been linked to higher rates of breast cancer. If you need to lose weight, speak to your doctor about the most sensible approach. Some evidence also suggests that regular physical activity may play a role in reducing breast cancer risk.

◆ If you're over 65, don't let denial, fear or embarrassment prevent you from taking advantage of cancer screening procedures. Depending on your medical situation, these may include: regular Pap tests for cervical cancer; breast self-examination, professional breast exams and mammography to detect breast cancer; digital rectal examinations; stool analysis and/or sigmoidoscopy for colorectal cancer; and digital rectal examinations and/or prostate-specific antigen (PSA) testing for prostate cancer. *If your doctor isn't recommending these procedures, it's your responsibility to ask why not. If you aren't satisfied with the answer, you should discuss your concerns or seek another opinion.*

◆ Always report any changes or unusual symptoms to your doctor right away. Too many older people ignore or deny warning signs out of fear, or a sense that they would "rather not know" about a serious illness like cancer. If it isn't cancer, you'll be relieved to find out, and if it is cancer, you're much better off knowing about it so you and your doctor can begin treatment.

them all here. But certain cancers are more common later in life, and the following information about symptoms, risk factors, prevention, detection and treatment may be useful. Please remember: This is only a guide. If you have any questions or concerns about your own health or the health of someone you care about, speak to your doctor or seek information from your local cancer hospital or cancer society.

Breast cancer

Even though 45 percent of all breast cancers

How to examine your own breasts

You're never too old to start examining your breasts for early signs of cancer. Much of the recent advice about the benefit of breast self-examination (BSE) has been directed to younger women, even though women over 50 face the greatest risk of breast cancer.

Researchers are still divided about whether practicing regular BSE actually increases your chance for surviving breast cancer. But it makes sense that early detection allows you to get treatment sooner, which could extend or even save your life.

Unfortunately, most women still don't examine their breasts on a regular basis. If you are uncomfortable about looking at and touching your own breasts, make an effort to overcome these feelings. Look at your breasts when you're bathing or showering and examine them in the mirror. Healthy breasts are a natural and beautiful part of your body. They are also susceptible to serious disease, so don't let modesty get in the way of your health.

Many women say they don't examine their breasts because they're afraid of finding something that might turn out to be cancer. It's important to balance this fear with the facts: Some studies show that women who don't practice regular breast examination are more likely to be diagnosed with advanced breast cancer than those who do. You should also know that most breast lumps found on self-examination turn out to be harmless.

Women also say they don't do BSE because they're afraid of not doing it correctly. It's true that most women – and many doctors, too – aren't very skilled at finding lumps or other abnormalities in breast tissue. The best place to learn how to examine your breasts thoroughly and properly is at a women's health center or breast clinic, where a doctor or nurse can guide you. At some clinics you can practice on silicone breast models that contain various-sized lumps.

Women who have learned BSE using such models are able to detect lumps as small as a pearl or pea, while those using standard BSE techniques can only find lumps the size of a cherry. Women with no BSE training can't find lumps until they're already the size of a golfball.

You should examine your breasts once a month (pick the first or last day so you don't forget). Here's how to do it.

Look

◆ Look at your breasts in the mirror, noting any dimpling of skin, retraction or crusting of the nipples, or any watery, yellow, pink or bloody discharge.

occur in women over age 65, older women tend to be less well-educated about breast cancer risks and early detection than younger ones.

◆ *Symptoms:* Signs include a painful or painless lump or thickening in your breast or under your arm, a breast that suddenly appears asymmetrical in the mirror, a dimpling of your breast skin, and any type of discharge from your nipple, either spontaneously or when it's squeezed.

◆ Lean forward slightly to look for puckering of the skin.

◆ Raise your arms slowly and evenly above your head and press your hands together in front of your forehead, observing any changes.

◆ Place your hands on your hips and tighten your chest and arm muscles, again observing your breasts.

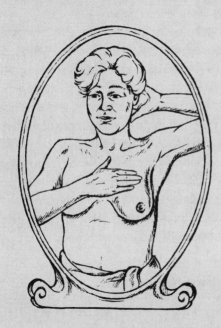

Feel
◆ Lie flat on your back. Raise one arm up and examine the breast on that side. Use the pads of your fingers (not the tips). Begin at the nipple and continue in a circular direction around the nipple toward the outer areas.

◆ Feel for any unusual lumps or thickening, or changes in the texture of your skin.

◆ Pay special attention to the following areas where cancers are most likely to occur: directly under the nipple; in the outer area between your nipple and armpit; under your armpit.

◆ Repeat with the other breast.

◆ Lower your arm to your side and perform the circular examination again, feeling carefully for lumps.

◆ Repeat with the other breast.

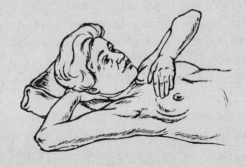

Report
Remember: The most important component of BSE is reporting any abnormality to your doctor as soon as possible.

◆ *Known risk factors*: These include a previous breast cancer; a family history of the disease, especially if it occurred before menopause in your mother, grandmother or sister; early menstruation (before age 11) and late menopause (after 55); never being pregnant or having your first pregnancy after age 30; obesity after age 50; having used the drug diethylstilbestrol (DES) to prevent miscarriage; regular alcohol consumption (more than one drink a day), which increases estrogen levels; exposure to moderate or high doses of ionizing radiation during treatment for other diseases or in the workplace. *But you should also know that approximately 80 percent of women with breast cancer have no known risk factors.*

◆ *Prevention/Detection:* There's no clear proof yet, but some recent research suggests that reducing your intake of saturated fat and increasing your consumption of fruits and vegetables may reduce your risk. Early detection can improve your chance for survival. Unfortunately, many older women feel shy or uncomfortable about examining their own breasts or letting a doctor or nurse do it; they may hesitate to be screened for the same reason. It's vital that you overcome these feelings and take care of yourself properly. You should learn and practice monthly breast self-examination to detect any changes in your breasts (see page 135), and you should also have regular professional breast exams by a nurse or doctor. If you started having regular screening mammograms in your 40s or 50s to detect very small cancers, keep it up; if you're over 65 and have never been screened, it's not too late to start! Ask your doctor to recommend an accredited breast screening center that uses the latest equipment.

◆ *Treatment:* If a lump or abnormality is found, your doctor will recommend a biopsy to examine the cells for malignancy. This may be done under a local anesthetic by needle aspiration in your doctor's office or a clinic, or else a surgical biopsy may be recommended. If the lump is found to be malignant, it will be removed surgically (lumpectomy), as will some lymph nodes under your arm. The nodes will be checked for the presence of malignant cells. If none are found, the lumpectomy will be followed by radiation therapy. But if cancerous cells have spread, if you have small breasts and a large tumor, or if the tumor is located directly under the nipple, the entire breast will be removed (mastectomy). Depending on the nature of the tumor and other factors, this will be followed by chemotherapy, radiation therapy and/or hormonal therapy with a drug such as tamoxifen.

While some older women who have had a mastectomy are content to live without a breast or to use a prosthesis, some opt for breast reconstruction. In the past, surgeons used foam-covered or silicone implants filled with gel, but these are no longer considered safe and are currently banned in some countries, pending further research. However, saline-filled implants are still available, and doctors have developed a new technique to create a breast using fat and tissue from other parts of the woman's body.

Colorectal cancer

This refers to cancer of the colon (large bowel) and the rectum.

◆ *Symptoms:* These include a sudden change in your normal bowel routine, including the frequency and consistency of your stool (sudden constipation and/or diarrhea); blood or pus in your stool that may be visible or invisible; pain in your lower abdomen; unexplained weight loss and fatigue.

◆ *Known risk factors*: Some types of colorectal cancer are known to be genetic, so a family history of the disease increases your risk. Other risk factors are a diet high in saturated fat and low in fiber-rich whole grains, fruits, vegetables and legumes.

◆ *Detection:* Your family doctor may recommend a periodic examination of your lower bowel using a lighted probe called a "sigmoidoscope," as well as a test that analyzes stool samples for the presence of extremely small – and therefore invisible to the eye – amounts of blood.

◆ *Treatment:* Treatment usually involves surgical removal of the malignant growth, providing your general health is good enough. If the cancer is located low in your bowel, close to the rectum, your doctor may recommend that you undergo a colostomy. This is a surgical procedure done in hospital under general anesthetic. A loop of the large bowel is brought through the muscle and skin of the abdomen, and an artificial opening is made; a flexible bag is worn over it to collect stool. A temporary colostomy is done to give your body time to heal after intestinal surgery; if the rectum itself has to be removed because of cancer, the colostomy is permanent. While you may be understandably upset over the prospect of living with a colostomy, many people who have them live perfectly normal lives, although you'll probably need some special instruction on how to manage your colostomy at first. If your cancer is too extensive to be surgically removed, radiation therapy combined with chemotherapy may improve symptoms and prolong your life.

Lung cancer

Lung cancer usually occurs after a lifetime of smoking. It's a major cause of death among older men because it used to be more socially acceptable for men to use tobacco. Unfortunately, women seem to be catching up, and as they continue to smoke, more of them are developing lung cancer later in life. While lung cancer is one of the most preventable cancers, it's also one of the most difficult to treat successfully, and mortality rates are relatively high – fewer than 15 percent of people with lung cancer will be alive five years after the disease is discovered.

◆ *Symptoms:* The early symptoms, especially chronic coughing, are often hard to recognize because they're so common among smokers. Later symptoms include blood in the sputum, recurrent bouts of pneumonia, fever, weight loss and weakness.

◆ *Known risk factors*: These include regular use of tobacco, including cigarettes, cigars and pipes; long-term exposure to second-hand smoke from living or working with a smoker; and exposure to high levels of pollution or certain carcinogens such as asbestos in the workplace.

◆ *Prevention/Detection:* The best way to prevent lung cancer is to stop smoking and/or to encourage those around you to give up tobacco. This can be extremely difficult, especially if you've been smoking for many years. But it's well worth the effort – after you quit, your risk of lung cancer drops by 50 percent during your first five nonsmoking years, and after 15 years, your risk is substantially lower. (Smoking is also a major risk factor for many other diseases, including other types of cancer, heart disease and osteoporosis.)

Early detection offers the best chance for surviving lung cancer, so, if you continue to smoke, if you live with a smoker, or if you were exposed to cancer-causing substances at work, your doctor may recommend regular chest X-rays. You should know, however, that by the time lung cancer shows up on an X-ray, treatment is unlikely to save your life.

If you want to quit smoking, speak to your doctor, who will be happy to advise you on the latest strategies for quitting. Even if you've tried and failed to quit many times before, don't give up!

♦ *Treatment*: Treatment for lung cancer will depend on the type and extent of your disease. If it's fairly localized, your doctor may suggest surgery to remove the primary tumor or, in some cases, all or part of the affected lung. Chemotherapy and radiation therapy may also help slow down the progress of the disease.

Prostate cancer

This is the second most common cancer affecting men (after lung cancer), and it's also a major cause of death among older men. The disease begins in the prostate, a walnut-sized gland located at the base of your bladder, which is responsible for the production of seminal fluid.

♦ *Symptoms*: As you get older, you're more likely to experience a benign enlargement of your prostate gland. Early symp-toms of prostate cancer, when they exist, may be quite similar to symptoms of benign enlargement (see page 184). They include a weak or interrupted urine flow; difficulty in starting to urinate; the need to urinate often, especially during the night; blood in the urine; or a urine stream that isn't straight. If the cancer has spread, you may develop pains in your back, thighs and/or pelvis.

♦ *Known risk factors*: These include a family history of prostate cancer in a father or brother (even on your mother's side of the family) and race – the prevalence of prostate cancer is 30 percent higher among men of African descent. Researchers are also studying whether dietary fat and substances found in red meat and vegetable seed oils may increase risk.

♦ *Prevention/Detection:* There's still no sure way to prevent prostate cancer, but early detection may offer some benefit for long-term survival, and it may also decrease your risk for serious complications. You should be screened at least once a year with a procedure known as a digital rectal exam (DRE). Your doctor inserts a gloved finger into your rectum to probe your prostate for firm nodules or other abnormalities that could indicate cancer. But this exam can miss small cancers, so some doctors are now recommending that you have a regular blood test called a prostate-specific antigen (PSA) test. This test detects levels of PSA, a protein produced by your prostate, which tend to increase when cancer is present. Because PSA levels also rise normally as you get older, your doctor will have to determine what's a normal level for you according to your age.

The benefits of PSA screening are still controversial, and some studies have failed to find any real benefit for men over age 75. That's because prostate cancer in this age group tends to be slow growing and is unlikely to cause death (the idea is that you'll die from something else before the cancer kills you). Most doctors agree, however, that an annual DRE is of value for older men.

If a rectal examination and/or a PSA test detects an abnormality, your doctor may suggest ultrasound to give a picture of the prostate, or he may recommend a biopsy, a relatively painless procedure done without anesthesia in a hospital or your doctor's office. A thin needle guided by ultrasound is inserted through the rectum, and a small tissue sample is withdrawn for laboratory analysis.

◆ *Treatment:* This depends on many factors, including the size and location of the cancer, whether the malignancy has spread beyond the prostate gland, your age and general health. The options range from watchful waiting to more aggressive approaches, including radiation therapy to destroy the cancer and surgical removal of the gland (prostatectomy). You may also be treated with female hormones or drugs that can block the effects of male hormones and slow the cancer's progress.

Skin cancer

The most common cancers affecting older people are non-melanoma cancers of the skin. Fortunately, these are also the most treatable types of cancer. About 80 percent of all these skin cancers develop on the head, face and neck, which are exposed more often than other parts of the body to the effects of ultraviolet radiation.

◆ *Symptoms:* Non-melanoma cancers include *basal cell cancers* (smooth, waxy or pearly bumps) and *squamous cell* cancers (firm or flat-looking growths with a crusted, ulcerated or scaly surface). *Melanoma* is a less common type of skin cancer, but it's more serious because it can spread to other parts of your body. Melanomas appear as partially raised blue, black or brown growths. They're unevenly shaped with irregular borders and they may change in size and color.

◆ *Known risk factors:* These include a lifetime of unprotected exposure to the sun and a history of blistering sunburn, especially in childhood or adolescence. Your risk also increases if you're Caucasian, fair-skinned with blonde or reddish hair, and if you tend to freckle or burn easily in the sun.

◆ *Prevention/Detection:* If you still lie out in the sun to develop a tanned appearance, don't! In fact, stay out of the sun as much as possible, and always wear a sunscreen with a sun protection factor (SPF) of at least 15 when you go outside during the day – even in the winter. Sunscreen should be worn on all exposed areas of your body, including the face, back of the neck and ears. When you're out in the sun, wear light, tightly woven clothing with long sleeves and choose a broadbrimmed hat. If you can manage it, use a hand mirror to check your own skin regularly for any suspicious-looking spots or changes, or ask your partner, a friend or your doctor to do it for you.

A cancer glossary

◆ *Benign:* this means non-cancerous (the opposite of malignant). A benign tumor won't spread anywhere else in your body and isn't life-threatening, unless its presence puts pressure on vital organs. Because it may grow larger and crowd healthy structures, your doctor may recommend that it be surgically removed.

◆ *Biopsy:* a test in which cancer cells are removed, either surgically or using a needle (called "needle aspiration biopsy") to draw out a tiny sample from a suspected tumor. The cells are then studied in a laboratory for malignancy.

◆ *Carcinogen:* any substance known to cause cancer – for example, tobacco smoke, asbestos and a wide variety of chemicals.

◆ *Chemotherapy:* a course of potent, anti-cancer drugs, given by mouth or intravenously. Your oncologist will determine the type of drugs used and how often you take them, based on your age, general health and the stage and type of cancer you have. These drugs are designed to kill cancerous cells, but they also tend to wipe out healthy cells. This can cause side effects such as temporary hair loss, fatigue, nausea and vomiting. Fortunately, new anti-nausea medications are quite effective at reducing or preventing discomfort.

Chemotherapy may be used alone or in conjunction with surgery and radiation therapy. Sometimes chemotherapy is given before surgery to shrink large tumors. In other cases, the surgeon removes as much of the tumor as possible before chemotherapy, which may increase the chance that the drugs will be more effective on a smaller amount of tumor.

◆ *Lumpectomy:* the surgical removal of a breast tumor along with a thin margin of healthy tissue.

◆ *Lymph nodes:* these tiny structures in your body's lymphatic system filter and destroy invading bacteria as part of your immune system, and also drain fluid from tissues. When cancer spreads, it often does so through the lymphatic system. Malignant cells tend to show up in the nodes, especially those under the arms, in the groin and in the abdomen.

◆ *Malignant:* the opposite of benign. A

◆ *Treatment*: Treatment for non-melanoma cancers usually involves excision (surgical removal), curettage and electrodesiccation (the cancer is scraped away and remaining cells destroyed using an electric needle), or specialized Mohs surgery (the cancerous skin is shaved layer by layer and checked microscopically until no abnormal cells are left).

Mohs surgery is usually used for non-melanoma cancers that have penetrated deep into areas such as the nose, ears and around the eyes. If you have malignant melanoma, your doctor may also suggest chemotherapy and/or radiation therapy to kill any cells that may have spread from the original tumor.

malignant tumor can be life-threatening because it has the ability to invade and destroy healthy tissue and to spread from its original site to other parts of your body.

◆ *Mammography:* a specialized type of breast X-ray. Diagnostic mammography is used to give doctors a clearer picture of a lump or other abnormality, while screening mammography is used to screen healthy women for early signs of breast cancer.

◆ *Mastectomy:* the surgical removal of the entire breast. In the past, surgeons sometimes removed underlying muscles as well, but this isn't done any longer.

◆ *Metastasis:* the transfer of malignant cells from the original or "primary" cancer through your bloodstream or lymphatic system to another part of the body.

◆ *Oncology:* the area of medicine that specializes in the diagnosis and treatment of cancer.

◆ *Pap test:* developed in 1928 by Dr. George Papanicolaou, the Pap test or smear can detect cervical cancer. A special instrument is inserted into the vagina to take a scraping of cells from the cervix. The cells are examined in a laboratory for abnormalities.

◆ *Radiation therapy:* during this therapy, cancer cells are exposed to radiation, which destroys them or slows down their rate of growth. New techniques allow doctors to target cancer cells more precisely, preventing damage to healthy tissue. The course of therapy, which is usually done on an outpatient basis, depends on many factors, including the type and stage of cancer and your general health. Side effects may include temporary fatigue and local skin redness. Radiation therapy, often combined with chemotherapy, can sometimes cure cancer, but the treatment is also used to shrink tumors and reduce pain in people with advanced cancer.

◆ *Tamoxifen:* a drug used to treat breast cancers that, after laboratory analysis, are shown to be stimulated by the female hormone estrogen. Tamoxifen is also used to prevent breast cancer from recurring in women who have already had the disease.

◆ *Tumor:* a tumor is a growth of tissue that can be benign or malignant. Also called a neoplasm.

How does age affect cancer detection and treatment?

Until recently doctors didn't know much about the relationship between cancer and aging, other than the fact that cancer is much more common later in life. But in some ways, getting cancer at age 80 is quite different from getting it at age 50.

If you're over 65, you're more likely to be suffering from other illnesses that can affect how well you tolerate treatment such as chemotherapy and radiation therapy. There's no evidence, however, that healthy older adults can't tolerate cancer treatment or are less likely to benefit from it.

In general older adults aren't screened for certain types of cancer as often as younger ones – for example, women over 70 are less likely to have regular mammograms to detect breast cancer or Pap tests to screen for cervical cancer. Why is this? There are several reasons. Some older people refuse to be screened, some doctors and other health experts are less aggressive in promoting screening for older people, and for certain malignancies, the benefit of screening decreases in older age.

Some surgeons are less likely to recommend major cancer surgery for older patients with cancer, even though studies have shown that people as old as 90 can survive and benefit from these procedures. This may be because many doctors fear that older people don't have the physical and emotional reserves to come through such surgery. Doctors also tend to be less aggressive in recommending chemotherapy and radiation therapy for older patients for the same reason.

But there may be good reasons for doctors to be less aggressive in treating certain older patients for some kinds of cancer. For example, if your cancer is slow-growing and treatment will neither prolong your life nor improve the quality of your remaining years, watchful waiting or less aggressive approaches may be the treatment of choice.

? What are some ways to cope with cancer later in life?
As more people survive into their 70s, 80s, and 90s, they will have to confront cancer in themselves or in someone they love.

If you're like most older adults, you probably grew up in a time when a diagnosis of cancer was considered a death sentence and cancer treatment was painful and disfigur-

ing. This may make it even harder for you to face a diagnosis of cancer now. But the fact is that as detection and treatment improve, you are more likely to find yourself living with cancer than dying from it.

Even so, a diagnosis of cancer is hard to face, and you should expect to go through various stages, including shock, denial, grief, depression and anger.

How well you cope with cancer depends on many factors, and not all of them are in your control. Is your cancer curable or at least treatable? Will you require surgery and rehabilitation? Do you have ready access to good doctors and treatment facilities? Are you insured against the cost of treatment and medication? Do you have other health problems that are causing you physical and/or emotional stress? Are you a caregiver who is looking after a disabled spouse or elderly parent? Do you have people around you to offer emotional and physical support during treatment and recovery? These issues will have a major impact on how well you cope with your cancer and may even affect your physical recovery. Unfortunately, many older people, especially those who are retired, widowed or who live far away from family members, don't have a strong social support network. Always remember that information and help are available:

◆ Speak to your doctor or to a social worker affiliated with the hospital where you are receiving treatment. They can put you in touch with services that provide supportive nursing care, respite care and household help.

◆ Go to the library or bookstore and check out the wide assortment of books and videotapes on living with cancer.

◆ Take advantage of the many cancer support and educational programs that exist in your community. They can put you in touch with other older people who understand what it's like to live with cancer and who can give you much-needed advice and encouragement.

Diabetes

Diabetes (also known as "diabetes mellitus") is often misunderstood by many people, even those who have this difficult disease.

Because there may not be any dramatic symptoms – at least in the early stages – it's easy to think of diabetes as a fairly harmless condition. In general, it isn't as immediately life-threatening as a heart attack or stroke. But untreated diabetes can seriously threaten your health and well-being later in life.

If you're over age 65, you probably remember a time when people with diabetes died or else lived in an extremely restricted way. Although living with diabetes still presents certain challenges, most older people with this disease continue to lead active and enjoyable lives.

? What is diabetes?

Diabetes is a disease that affects your ability to absorb and use a nutrient called "glucose." During digestion, the food you eat is converted into glucose – your body's most important immediate source of energy. To maintain a healthy balance of glucose in your blood, your pancreas normally produces a hormone called "insulin." But if your body doesn't produce enough insulin, or fails to use it properly, the levels of glucose in your blood and tissues start to rise, creating all kinds of short-term and long-term health hazards.

Type II, or mature-onset diabetes, accounts for about 85 percent of all cases in older adults. This type of diabetes, which affects more than 10 percent of people over age 65, begins gradually after age 40. While some people with this type of diabetes may need insulin therapy, in most cases the condition can be managed with lifestyle changes and/or medication.

Type I, or juvenile onset diabetes, usually develops suddenly in childhood or early adulthood, and requires lifelong insulin therapy. Doctors now think this type of diabetes is, at least in part, an autoimmune disorder that occurs when antibodies attack special cells in the pancreas that are necessary to produce insulin. Not long ago, Type I diabetes was looked upon as a life-threatening disease, and sufferers faced a daily struggle to keep their illness under control. Since the discovery of insulin, however, this is no longer the case.

? What are the dangers of diabetes?

The main danger of diabetes lies

in not being aware that you have it. If you don't know there's a problem, you can't take steps to protect yourself and prevent complications down the road.

If you're over 65 or 70 and have been newly diagnosed with diabetes, here are some important facts:

◆ Diabetes that begins later in life has an impact on your long-term health.

◆ Because you may not have any dramatic symptoms, it's tempting to dismiss a diagnosis of diabetes and deny the importance of getting started on proper treatment.

◆ Since there's still no cure for diabetes, your goal is to keep blood sugar (also called "blood glucose") levels at a healthy level or "in control." If you don't, you face a variety of short-term and long-term health risks.

◆ *Short-term dangers:* Hypoglycemia occurs when your blood glucose level becomes too low, either because you've missed a meal or because you've taken too much medication. Typical symptoms of this condition include trembling, faintness, clammy hands, mood swings, sweating, headache, dizziness, blurred speech and drowsiness. This can be relieved by drinking sweetened orange juice or another glucose-rich drink.

Another less common complication of diabetes in people over age 65 is a serious condition called "hyperosmolar coma." This occurs when your blood glucose level sky-rockets out of control, often because you are ill or dehydrated for some reason. It often happens to older people who don't even know they are diabetic. You lose conscious-

ness, and if the brain becomes starved of glucose, you may go into a coma or develop paralysis. This is a medical emergency that must be treated in hospital. You will be given intravenous fluids to help bring your blood glucose down to a more normal level.

◆ *Long-term dangers:* If your blood sugar level remains abnormally high over many years, you can develop a host of complications that affect many parts of your body.

What are the possible complications of diabetes?

Many complications of diabetes occur because high glucose levels are associated with problems that lead to a build up of fatty deposits in blood vessels. This can constrict blood flow to some parts of your body. In the past, most people, including doctors, believed that blindness, kidney failure, nerve damage and other complications were inevitable. But studies show that, if diabetes is diagnosed early and treated properly, many of these complications can be prevented, postponed or at least controlled.

◆ *Eye damage:* About half of all people with diabetes will develop eye damage, also known as retinopathy, about 15 years after the onset of the disease. In some cases, this can lead to partial or total blindness later in life. However, not everyone with diabetes is doomed to loss of vision. If you develop diabetes after age 60 and keep it under good control in the first few years after onset, your risk of serious complications later in life is greatly reduced.

There are two types of eye damage related to diabetes.

The most common problem found in

older people with diabetes is cataracts. If you already have cataracts, you should know that they tend to advance more quickly when diabetes is present, but otherwise the condition is usually treated just as it would be in a non-diabetic person.

Some older people experience damage due to the leakage of blood from tiny vessels in the eye. If such leakage is detected early on a routine eye exam, laser treatment can be used to seal off the ruptured vessels and decrease the risk of further damage.

◆ *Kidney disease:* If your diabetes isn't well controlled, your kidneys may not function properly, and waste products can build up in your blood. Common symptoms of kidney problems related to diabetes are more frequent urination, swelling (edema) in your hands or feet, and the leakage of protein into your urine, which can be detected by laboratory tests.

◆ *Blood vessel damage:* The buildup of fatty deposits in blood vessels associated with chronically high glucose levels can increase your risk for heart attack and stroke. It can also lead to a condition called "peripheral vascular disease." Blood vessels in your legs and feet become extremely narrowed or blocked, which can cause a variety of foot ailments (see page 102). In extreme cases this may lead to amputation of a toe, foot or leg.

◆ *Nerve damage:* People with chronic, poorly controlled diabetes may suffer various kinds of nerve damage. One of these is neuropathy – a progressive loss of pain and touch sensation, particularly in the feet, which can contribute to ulcers and foot

How to prevent diabetic complications

◆ Regular medical exams are absolutely vital. Your doctor will tell you how often she wants to see you to check your blood glucose and weight. You'll probably see her often at first, and then once your diabetes is under control, you may only have to see her once or twice a year.

◆ You should consult an ophthalmologist for periodic eye exams, which can detect signs of damage related to diabetes.

◆ Because you're more prone to infections as well as nerve and blood vessel problems that can damage your feet, you should consult a foot specialist (either a chiropodist or a podiatrist) regularly – especially if you're unable to care for your feet properly.

problems. Another type of nerve damage is diabetic amyotrophy, which develops over a period of weeks or months, usually in older people with extremely high levels of blood glucose. The symptoms are pain, weakness and wasting, first in one thigh and then in the other, and the person may develop trouble walking. Once glucose levels are brought down, the condition is often reversible.

◆ *Other complications*: If you have diabetes you're also more prone to infections, including urinary tract infections and tuberculosis.

What are the risk factors for diabetes?

◆ *Obesity:* Many doctors now believe that obesity is the single highest risk factor for diabetes. Although most people who develop diabetes are overweight, don't think you are immune because you're thin – lean people can and do get diabetes!

◆ *Lack of physical activity:* People who don't get regular physical exercise are more prone to diabetes, partly because exercise itself has a beneficial effect on how your body uses glucose, and partly because it helps keep your weight under control.

◆ *Age:* Growing older may increase your risk for diabetes simply because your body can't process glucose as efficiently as it did when you were younger. Other factors that may be related to age – such as obesity and lack of regular physical activity – are known to increase your risk for diabetes.

◆ *Family history:* If a close relative such as a parent, grandparent or sibling was diagnosed with either type of diabetes, this increases your risk.

◆ *Other risk factors:* Diabetic symptoms can be triggered by a serious illness such as a heart attack or pneumonia, or by taking certain drugs such as prednisone. These symptoms may disappear after the illness is gone or when the medication is discontinued, but the risk for diabetes may persist.

What are the early warning signs of diabetes?

If you're like many older people, you may not realize that you have diabetes. The disease often occurs without any obvious symptoms, at least in the early stages. It's also common for older adults to blame symptoms such as fatigue and frequent urination on other health problems.

Here are some signs that *may be* an early warning of diabetes and should be promptly reported to your doctor:

◆ abnormal hunger or thirst;

◆ more frequent urination;

◆ unexplained weight loss;

◆ blurred vision;

◆ fatigue;

◆ slow healing of cuts, bruises and sores;

◆ tingling or numbness in hands or feet;

◆ itchiness;

◆ unexplained nausea, vomiting or abdominal pain;

◆ sweet-smelling breath and/or urine.

How is diabetes diagnosed?

Even if you don't have any obvious symptoms of diabetes, your doctor may detect abnormal levels of glucose in your blood and urine during routine laboratory tests. If she suspects diabetes, she will recommend that you undergo further testing to measure your blood glucose levels. She may also recommend that you have an eye examination to check for abnormalities related to diabetes.

How is diabetes treated?

In the past, many doctors weren't aggressive about treating diabetes in older adults. They didn't know about the benefits of treatment and thought that diabetes was just a common aspect of aging, something that older adults had to live with.

While many of these beliefs have been discarded because of new information, even today your doctor may not realize how vital optimal treatment is in preventing diabetic complications in people over age 65.

Here's what you should know about treatment for diabetes:

◆ *Diet:* In recent years, doctors and dietitians have been revising their ideas about what people with diabetes should and shouldn't eat. Experts used to recommend very strict diets that severely limited the intake of both sugar and complex carbohydrates, found in pasta, bread, fruits and vegetables.

Now many doctors and dietitians who specialize in diabetes are recommending a "non-dieting" approach. They feel the traditional diabetic diet may actually be counterproductive. If you feel deprived, chances are you won't be able to follow the diet on a long-term basis. The newer diabetic eating plan is based on the following principles:

Your diet should be individually tailored, taking into account the type and severity of your diabetes, how long you've had diabetes, your weight, your food preferences and how easy it is for you to shop for food and prepare meals.

If you're overweight, you should try to lose weight by cutting back calories – especially from foods high in saturated fat – and by increasing your level of exercise. But you should avoid severely restricting your intake of foods, because this can have many negative health consequences. Most public health departments and hospitals can refer you to a qualified dietitian who will be able to advise you.

Many people with diabetes are told that reducing their intake of dietary cholesterol found in eggs, meat and dairy products may help them control their condition by keeping their weight under control. However, it's still not clear whether such advice is as relevant for older people with diabetes as it is for those under age 65.

You may not have to give up simple sugar altogether. Depending on how severe your diabetes is, a dietitian may be able to work some sugar and sweets into your diet, especially if they are taken as part of a meal. This will add to your enjoyment of food and make it easier for you to stick to your meal plan.

You should eat regularly and avoid skipping meals since this can lower your blood glucose levels too much and cause you to overeat later.

If you enjoy foods containing artificial sweeteners such as aspartame, that's fine. But avoid buying special diabetic foods, which are expensive and usually unnecessary. You should be able to get all the nutrients you need from ordinary foods.

◆ *Exercise:* Regular physical activity can help you manage diabetes by burning up calories and helping you to shed extra body weight. Recent studies have found that physical exercise also improves your body's ability to use insulin. This effect lasts as long as you continue to exercise regularly.

Before you embark on any exercise program, speak to your doctor first to make sure it's safe (see page 30). Because diabetes makes you more prone to foot problems, it's vital that you wear properly fitted shoes and check your feet for injury after exercising.

◆ *Medication:* Recent studies have found that *many cases of diabetes that develop after age 65 can be controlled by diet*

Foot care tips for diabetics

◆ To avoid injury, don't go barefoot.

◆ Wash feet daily and dry them well.

◆ Use a moisturizing cream to prevent the skin from drying and cracking.

◆ Inspect your feet daily and report any blisters, cracking, sores or redness to your doctor.

◆ Take extra care in cutting toenails to avoid injuries (if you can't manage this, you should consult a foot specialist), and never cut your cuticles.

◆ Wear clean socks each day.

◆ Buy and wear properly fitted shoes that protect your feet from pressure and injury; to avoid putting pressure on the same spots day after day, don't wear the same pair too many days in a row.

◆ Finally, be sure to let your dentist know that you have diabetes, since this increases your risk for dental infections and means you have to take better care of your teeth.

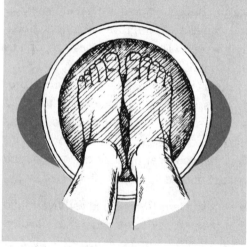

alone for 10 to 20 years – as long as people are willing and able to make substantial dietary changes. If such efforts don't lead to good control of the disease, you may require some type of medication.

The first step is usually to try *oral antidiabetic drugs* such as sulfonylurea, which stimulates your pancreas to make more insulin, or biguanides, which increases your body's sensitivity to insulin and helps your cells take up glucose more quickly. If you comply with your doctor's advice about diet and weight control, oral medication may be enough to keep your condition stable for many years.

If oral antidiabetic drugs don't work or become less effective over time, you may need daily *insulin* injections. In the past, this was a complex procedure, but today, easy-to-use home glucose monitoring systems and preloaded insulin injector pens make it much simpler for you to keep track of your blood glucose and deliver the right amount of insulin.

The idea of testing your own blood and injecting yourself with insulin may be daunting to many older people, and not everyone can manage it, especially at first. Help is available from many sources, including your doctor, some public health departments, visiting nurses and special clinics.

? **What are some strategies for living with diabetes later in life?**
Your doctor or other specialists can advise you about medication, diet and weight control, but in many ways, diabetes is a self-help disease: It's up to you to take control of the situation. This can be especially difficult for older adults:

- You probably feel anxious about having diabetes and wonder whether you're going to face the frightening prospect of diabetic complications such as loss of vision or amputation.

- You may feel overwhelmed at the prospect of changing your shopping, cooking and eating habits. If you enjoy sweets, you may feel depressed at the thought of giving them up.

- Other health problems may be sapping your physical and mental energy, making it more difficult for you to follow your doctor's advice.

- If you live alone, you may no longer enjoy preparing nutritious foods, and you may not have enough emotional support to help you cope.

Such problems can interfere with your ability to follow your doctor's advice. It's important that you speak to your doctor honestly and find some way to resolve these problems.

The best way to approach living with diabetes is to educate yourself about your condition. Your doctor, nurse and nutritionist can certainly help by answering questions, and you can also obtain relevant, easy-to-understand information from books and magazines written especially for diabetics.

Heart disease

Heart disease is the main cause of death and disability in older adults. In fact, about half of all people over age 65 show some evidence of heart disease, although not everyone develops symptoms serious enough to warrant treatment.

If you or someone you love is diagnosed with a heart condition, it doesn't mean that your life or theirs is over. With the proper treatment and a willingness to follow doctors' advice, many older people, including those with serious heart disease, can still live reasonably full and enjoyable lives!

The good news is that aging alone doesn't seem to cause any significant changes in your heart or its function. If you've watched your diet, exercised regularly and avoided smoking, there's no reason why your heart shouldn't remain healthy. The only exception here may be a genetic tendency toward heart disease, which may have a major effect on whether you develop serious heart disease.

While older people generally suffer from the same cardiac ailments as younger ones, their disease may be more severe by the time it shows up, simply because damage to the heart and blood vessels has been taking place over many more years.

The symptoms of heart disease later in life may be somewhat different than they are among younger people. If you don't know this, you may overlook warning signs and not get prompt and proper treatment.

While younger men face a greater risk for heart disease than younger women, this changes once women reach menopause and stop producing female hormones. But even though older women are just as prone to heart disease as men, their symptoms may be more subtle and don't always receive the same attention. That's because until recently, most of the research done into heart disease – including risk factors, diagnosis and treatment – has focused on men. Older women and those who care about them need to become more educated about female heart disease, as do many health professionals.

❓ What are the most common types of heart disease affecting older people?

One of the major types of heart disease begins with a gradual process called *atherosclerosis*. This occurs when fatty deposits called plaque build up in the arteries or blood vessels that carry blood and life-sustaining oxygen to and from your heart muscle. If these vessels become too narrowed by plaque, the flow of blood is reduced and the risk of blockage increases – a condition called *coronary occlusion.*

When the occlusion or blockage reaches a level of 50 to 60 percent, the decreased flow of blood and oxygen may begin to damage your heart or cause symptoms – a condition known as *ischemia*. In many cases this process occurs without symptoms, although it can show up on an electrocardiogram or a special test that stresses the heart's function through physical activity (known as a "stress test"). Some research suggests that the stress test may have less value in accurately predicting heart disease in women than in men.

Here are some of the most common heart conditions affecting older people, along with advice on treatment:

Angina (angina pectoris)

This occurs when your heart needs more oxygen than your coronary arteries are able to deliver due to atherosclerosis.

◆ *Symptoms:* These include pain, pressure, burning, tightness or heaviness in the chest, especially behind the breastbone. You may also feel pain in one or both of your arms, in your hand, neck, jaw or back. Angina pain usually lasts for a few minutes, although it can last much longer. It can be triggered by physical exertion, emotional distress, exposure to cold, eating a large meal or illness.

In some cases angina is stable – that means it occurs regularly and predictably and is quickly relieved by rest or medication. But if you suffer from so-called unstable angina, the pain is more severe, is more easily triggered or occurs spontaneously, and treatment may not bring immediate relief.

◆ *Treatment:* If you've never had chest pains before, don't assume they are caused by angina. You could be having a heart attack and you should act promptly (see page 154).

If the condition is diagnosed as stable angina, your doctor will recommend treatment. This includes medication that reduces your heart's need for oxygen by lowering blood pressure and heart rate (for example, calcium channel blockers or beta blockers). Nitroglycerine, which causes your coronary arteries to dilate or widen, increasing blood flow to your heart, may also be prescribed. You will be encouraged to prevent attacks by modifying your physical activity, avoiding emotional upsets and changing your eating habits.

If you have severe, unstable angina, which is seriously affecting your quality of life and which doesn't respond to medication, you may be a candidate for surgery (see page 155).

Heart attack (myocardial infarction)

This occurs when a clot in the coronary arteries severely reduces or cuts off blood and oxygen to your heart. A heart attack can lead to damage of the heart muscle that ranges from mild to severe.

◆ *Symptoms:* The classic symptoms of a heart attack are an uncomfortable pain, pressure or squeezing in the center of your chest that lasts for two minutes or longer. The pain may worsen, and it can spread to the entire chest, down one or both arms, or to the shoulders, neck and jaw. There may also be sweating, shortness of breath, nausea, vomiting, faintness, dizziness, weakness and palpitations.

If you're over 65, you can experience any of these symptoms, but in older people, heart attack may be less obvious. Typical symptoms in older adults are shortness of breath, fainting, weakness, confusion, and pressure or pain in the stomach, which may be interpreted as indigestion.

◆ *Treatment:* If your heart has stopped pumping (cardiac arrest) as a result of the heart attack, the medical team at the hospital will use emergency procedures to get it started again. An immediate diagnosis of the nature of the heart attack is vital because the cause will determine how you're treated.

If doctors suspect the attack was caused by a blood clot, they will order diagnostic procedures such as an electrocardiogram and blood tests to detect enzymes released by a damaged heart. If the diagnosis is confirmed, you may get an immediate injection of streptokinase, or the newer "clot-busting" drug called "tissue plasminogen activator" (TPA). These drugs can reduce damage to your heart and improve your chances of survival.

Most heart attack sufferers spend 24 to 36 hours in the coronary care unit, where they are closely monitored. They are then moved to a step-down unit or medical floor where they remain for several days or weeks, depending on the severity of the damage and their overall health.

Recovery time after heart attack varies, but older people may find it takes longer for them to recover strength and function. In the past, heart attack patients were treated with weeks of bedrest, but now you will probably be encouraged to move around slowly and gradually.

In general, the heart takes about three months to heal following a heart attack. You can certainly resume many activities during that period, but you shouldn't overdo it when you get home. Your doctor should be able to tell you how soon you may resume various activities. He will also discuss the need for medications, dietary changes and exercise.

It's not uncommon to feel vulnerable, anxious and a bit depressed after a heart attack. You may worry that the slightest stress will trigger another attack, and you may notice those around you acting over-solicitously or anxiously. Such feelings are quite normal. If they persist, you should share them with your doctor.

It's never too late to prevent heart disease

If you've reached 75 or older without signs of overt, serious heart disease, chances are there's something working in your favor!

In the past many people (and their doctors) believed that older adults were doomed to death or disability from heart disease. But research has shown that this simply isn't true. Even if you already suffer from atherosclerosis or an existing heart condition, you can still benefit from controlling certain risk factors for heart disease. This may not give you back the healthy heart you had at 20, but it can prevent or delay further damage and significantly improve your quality of life.

One risk factor you can't control is a *family history of heart disease*, including heart attack and stroke. Such a history is a risk factor for men (especially if your mother or father developed heart disease before age 55) and for women (if it developed in a par-

ent before age 65). Of course, heredity is only one risk factor.

Even if you have a hereditary predisposition to heart disease, that doesn't mean you should give up. Here are some risk factors you can control:

◆ *Obesity* places an extra strain on your heart and may also have an effect on blood levels of cholesterol (see below). If your doctor advises you to lose excess pounds, it's worth making an effort. But in order for your weight loss efforts to succeed, you need a safe diet and exercise plan you can live with (see pages 19 and 30).

◆ *Smoking* causes you to inhale nicotine, which makes your heart beat faster and cuts its oxygen supply. This increases your risk for heart disease. If you've been smoking for many years, you are addicted and need

Congestive heart failure

This occurs when your heart has become weakened by disease and can no longer pump enough blood to meet your body's demands. Congestive heart failure, a progressive and potentially life-threatening condition, is a major cause of hospitalization and death among people over age 65.

◆ *Symptoms:* When your heart isn't working properly, fluid builds up in your body and you feel weak and tired. When this fluid

accumulates in your lungs, you feel short of breath. In the early stages of congestive heart failure, this breathlessness, known as "dyspnea," happens after physical exertion, but it can progress into a terrifying condition known as "acute pulmonary edema." You cough and wheeze and may feel completely unable to breathe, almost as though you were drowning. Fluid may also collect in other body tissues, particularly your lower legs and feet, making them puffy, swollen and uncomfortable.

help. Even if you've already tried to quit and failed, it's never too late to stop exposing your body to the harmful effects of tobacco. Ask your doctor to recommend a smoking cessation program.

◆ *High blood pressure* is a major risk factor for heart disease, and you should take steps to protect yourself from its effects (see page 172).

◆ *Diet* plays an important role in many ailments, especially heart disease. Cut down on your intake of saturated fats while increasing the amount of fruits, vegetables, legumes and whole grains you eat.

Many older people have been told to reduce blood levels of cholesterol, either by reducing fat and cholesterol in their diets (see page 24) or by taking prescription medications that lower cholesterol. However, some researchers are now beginning to question whether having high cholesterol levels is as dangerous for people over 70 as it is for those who are younger. The reasons aren't clear, but studies have found that people ages 71 to 104 who had high cholesterol levels suffered no more heart attacks or deaths than people the same age with normal cholesterol levels. If your doctor has advised you to lower your cholesterol, you should continue to follow his advice, but you may want to discuss this research information with him at your next appointment.

On the other hand, if you're over 65 and have already had a heart attack, controlling your cholesterol is still a good idea.

◆ *Lack of regular exercise* increases your risk for heart disease, so do whatever you can to start moving. If you haven't exercised before and want to get started, you should speak to your doctor first. (For tips on exercising later in life, see page 36.)

◆ *Diabetes* also increases your risk for heart disease, so be aware of the warning signs (see page 146) and report them to your doctor if they occur. If you have diabetes, protect your heart by taking an active part in the treatment and management of your condition (see page 146).

◆ *Treatment:* If you suddenly develop symptoms of heart failure, call immediately for emergency assistance.

Although congestive heart failure is a serious condition, in the early stages it can be treated with changes in lifestyle and medication. Your doctor will probably advise you to dramatically decrease the amount of salt in your diet, since salt causes you to retain fluid. You may be given diuretic drugs that reduce fluid buildup by causing you to urinate more often. Other drugs used to manage heart failure are digoxin and angiotensin-converting enzyme (ACE) inhibitors such as captopril, enalapril and similar drugs that increase your heart's ability to pump effectively.

If congestive heart failure is being caused by abnormalities in your heart's rhythm, your doctor may recommend that this be treated by medication and/or by the surgical insertion of a pacemaker (see page 155).

Your doctor will also advise you to help your heart by decreasing your level of

What to do when a heart attack happens

What should you do when you suspect that you or someone else is having a heart attack? Immediate medical attention is absolutely vital. Even a few minutes' delay can mean the difference between life and death. And the sooner you receive treatment, the more likely you are to decrease the amount of damage to your heart muscle.

◆ If you're alone and think you're having a heart attack, dial emergency assistance (usually 911) and give your address right away, telling the operator that you're having a heart attack. She will call fire, paramedic or ambulance services, which can transport you to a hospital quickly. *Never try to drive yourself to the hospital.* If possible, try to unlock the front door.

◆ If you're with someone who is having a heart attack, try to stay calm. Have the person sit or lie down, loosen any clothing around his or her neck or midriff to allow easier breathing, then call for help right away. While you're waiting, provide comfort and reassurance.

◆ Each year many people die because they won't admit that they're having a heart attack. It's frightening to think that this may be happening to you, but if you delay seeking treatment out of fear and denial, the consequences could be far worse. You may also delay getting help because you genuinely doubt that your symptoms indicate a heart attack. However, as you've learned, older people don't always have classic symptoms, so it's better to be safe than sorry.

physical exertion. If breathlessness bothers you at night, try propping yourself up on several pillows to sleep.

Rhythm disorders (cardiac arrhythmias)

A regular heart rhythm is vital because it keeps blood flowing smoothly to the rest of your body. The normal heart beats an average of 72 times per minute, speeding up and slowing down according to a variety of factors. For example, it beats more quickly during exertion or emotional stress, and slows down during periods of rest or sleep. When your heartbeat increases to more than 100 beats per minute, this is called "tachycardia"; if it drops to below 60 beats per minute, the condition is called "bradycardia."

Although these normal changes in rhythm won't hurt a healthy heart, they can cause problems if your heart is already weak. Abnormal changes in rhythm are more serious, however, and may require treatment.

◆ *Symptoms:* You may feel that your heart is beating too quickly – a fluttering sensation inside the chest known as palpitations (see page 107). Or it may seem to beat too slowly when you take your pulse. You may also feel as though your heart has produced an extra beat or missed a beat. Such fibrillations are known as "ventricular" or "atrial" premature contractions, depending on whether they are produced in the upper or lower chambers of the heart.

Some rhythm disorders are much more subtle. You may not notice any change in your heart rate or rhythm but may experience episodes of lightheadedness, dizziness or even fainting. If blood flow to the brain is reduced because of a rhythm disorder, you may become confused, or suffer from nightmares, and your personality may even be affected.

A fairly common type of rhythm disorder is called "atrial fibrillation" (AF). This condition is potentially dangerous. A blood clot from your heart can be thrown off into your bloodstream and create a blockage in one of the carotid arteries leading up the sides of your neck to your brain, resulting in a stroke (see page 169). Or else the clot can travel to an artery in your leg, where it can cause a serious blockage (see page 114).

A more serious rhythm disorder occurs when your heart's ability to beat effectively is completely disrupted. This life-threatening condition is known as "ventricular fibrillation." When it occurs, your heart can no longer pump out blood, which builds up rapidly in the organ. Ventricular fibrillation is a medical emergency: Unless the normal heartbeat is restored quickly, death will occur within moments.

◆ *Treatment:* In many cases, abnormal heart rhythms aren't medically serious, but you should always report them to your doctor, who may decide to investigate further. For example, you may be asked to wear a Holter monitor, a portable device that records your heartbeat over a period of 24 hours or longer. If your doctor doesn't find a serious disorder, no medical treatment may be necessary – although you may be advised to reduce your stress level (see page 81).

A more serious arrhythmia may be treated with drugs that can help normalize heart rhythms. You may also have to wear a pacemaker. This small, battery-operated device produces electrical impulses to help regulate your heartbeat. You will be admitted to hospital, where the pacemaker will be surgically inserted in a pocket under the skin of your chest or upper abdomen, with two leads attached to your heart.

An artificial pacemaker can be a lifesaver if you have a rhythm disorder that results in a serious slowing of your heart. The use of this device, which is worn by thousands of people, can allow you to enjoy most normal activities.

If you have a pacemaker, your doctor will ask you to monitor your pulse regularly and report any changes or other symptoms immediately. You should wear a medical alert bracelet that states that you wear a pacemaker and includes the model number, the year of insertion and which hospital performed the surgery. Modern pacemakers are designed to last up to 15 years.

Are you a candidate for heart surgery?

It would be impossible to list and describe the many surgical procedures available to people with different types of heart disease. In the past doctors hesitated to perform heart surgery on people over 65 or 70. They wondered whether older patients could survive such surgery or benefit from it.

Now surgeons are much more willing to operate on older patients, but the risks and benefits of such surgery are not always clear. If your doctor recommends that you see a surgeon to discuss a heart operation, it's probably because there's good evidence that the procedure will improve the length or quality of your life. If the situation isn't clear, it may be a good idea to get a second opinion before agreeing to heart surgery.

Taking ASA (aspirin) to prevent heart disease

Recent studies have shown that small, regular doses of acetylsalicylic acid (ASA) can reduce the incidence of heart attack and stroke in some people. That's because ASA is known to prevent blood from becoming sticky.

Your doctor may have already suggested that you take a regular dose of ASA. Studies suggest that older people may not need as much ASA as younger ones – as little as one-third of a regular, 325-milligram tablet of ASA every day may be enough. Lower doses may also reduce the chance that ASA will irritate your stomach or cause internal bleeding. Never take ASA without your doctor's permission, because it can interact with other medication and aggravate other health problems (see page 71).

Angioplasty

It's not uncommon for the arteries that bring blood to your heart to become narrowed due to atherosclerosis. When this happens you may experience chest pains (angina), fatigue and other unpleasant symptoms that interfere with your ability to function and enjoy life. Narrowed coronary arteries also increase your risk for a serious heart attack.

In many cases the narrowing can be improved with changes in diet, exercise and the use of drugs. If the narrowing is surgically accessible, or if your doctor doesn't think you're a candidate for more drastic

coronary bypass surgery (see below), then another procedure known as coronary angioplasty may be recommended.

Angioplasty is a hospital procedure. The patient is given a general anesthetic, then a special catheter attached to a tiny balloon is threaded into the narrowed artery. When it's in place, the balloon is inflated in order to stretch the obstructed artery and compress the fatty plaque that is blocking it.

While angioplasty helps many people with blocked coronary arteries, it carries certain risks: in a small percentage of cases, a heart attack occurs during or just after the procedure; In another small percentage, the patient will need emergency bypass surgery; in about one-third of patients, the blood vessel will become clogged again, but these patients may be treated successfully with a second procedure.

Coronary bypass surgery

The most common type of heart surgery recommended for older adults with ischemic heart disease is coronary bypass surgery. While some studies have shown that bypass surgery can prolong life, prevent heart attacks and increase quality of life for many people with heart disease, other research has suggested that, in some situations, the procedure has been overdone.

The goal of this surgery is to "bypass" the blocked and narrowed arteries and improve blood flow to your heart. The surgeon can create a bypass around the obstruction in two ways.

A vein from your leg can be removed and attached to one end of the artery before the narrowing; the other end of the leg vein is then attached to a point beyond the obstruction. Or an artery from your chest wall may be redirected to the heart muscle.

Although this is a major operation that requires a hospital stay of several days, most older adults have an excellent chance for recovery!

Both you and your doctor should consider bypass surgery if other strategies – for example, lifestyle changes and medication – haven't worked. You may be a candidate for surgery if:

◆ you have unstable angina that hasn't responded to medication;

◆ you have angina pains that are seriously compromising your quality of life;

◆ you continue to have chest pains after suffering a heart attack;

◆ you have already suffered several heart attacks;

◆ you have already undergone coronary angioplasty without adequate relief of symptoms;

◆ your general physical and psychological health are good enough for you to withstand the surgery and recovery period.

If your doctor thinks bypass surgery is an option for you, you will be referred to a surgeon. You should read as much as you can about the surgery beforehand and come prepared with a list of written questions. It's useful to have another person accompany you. Don't feel rushed or pressured into making a quick decision either way, unless your doctor has warned you against waiting too long. It's also a good idea to talk to someone else who has had the surgery so you have a better idea about what to expect afterward.

What are some strategies for living with heart disease?

Your ability to recover from a heart attack and to live with chronic heart disease depends on many factors, including the amount of damage to your heart and your general health.

It's not unusual for people who have had a heart attack to become anxious and depressed for a period of time. Go easy on yourself and try to follow your doctor's advice. If you are told that it's safe and even advisable to begin resuming your normal activities, do so. If you have specific concerns about exercise or sex, share them with your doctor.

If you're living with someone who has had a heart attack or who suffers from heart disease, it's also common to feel upset and anxious yourself. Husbands of older women with heart disease seem to be at particular risk for anxiety and depression, because they may be less likely to express their fears. If you don't feel comfortable talking to your partner about how you feel, speak to your doctor or a counselor, who may be able to reassure you.

Incontinence

Imagine a condition affecting about one in every five adults over age 65 and about 37 percent of older women. Besides being embarrassing and upsetting, this condition can lead to a number of serious problems, including social withdrawal and isolation. It may even result in the premature need for institutionalization. About 80 percent of sufferers could be significantly helped or even completely cured – yet fewer than 20 percent ever seek treatment.

The problem is urinary incontinence, which doctors define as an involuntary loss of urine. When this urine loss is copious or frequent enough to cause distress, then you are suffering from incontinence.

There are many reasons why older people are so reluctant to seek help for urinary incontinence:

◆ You may believe incontinence is a normal part of growing older.

◆ You hope the problem will eventually resolve itself.

◆ You may think you have to live with incontinence because of other common health problems or conditions. For example, older women may feel they have to live with the consequences of pelvic muscles weakened by pregnancy and childbirth. Or older men may think that incontinence automatically goes along with prostate problems.

◆ You may feel embarrassed about losing control or "wetting," which you may associate with childishness or dependence.

◆ You may think it's normal or at least acceptable to live with incontinence – an attitude reinforced by the recent surge in the marketing of adult disposable diapers. (While these products are useful if you suffer from incontinence despite treatment, it's too easy to rely on them and avoid seeking potentially helpful treatment.)

◆ You may feel uncomfortable discussing the matter with your doctor and may never have been asked about it.

What is incontinence?

First, it's important to understand that incontinence is not a disease in itself, but rather a symptom of other problems. There are several kinds of incontinence, and it's not unusual to suffer from more than one kind at the same time.

Usually reversible, temporary incontinence tends to come on suddenly, and is often triggered by other factors such as urinary tract infections, high fever and delirium, heart failure, or even extreme constipation that puts pressure on the bladder.

Long-term incontinence tends to develop more slowly and persists without treatment. There are three types of long-term incontinence:

◆ *Stress incontinence* is the most common type of incontinence, and it's also the type most likely to affect older women. Any sudden movement or stress – bending over, lifting, coughing or laughing – puts stress on the bladder and on the sphincter that controls the urethra, causing a sudden leakage of urine.

Stress incontinence arises when the muscles that control urine flow become weakened. If you're a woman, this can happen as a result of childbirth. In severe cases the urethra can protrude into your vagina (a urethrocele) or your bladder can sag into the vaginal opening (a cystocele). If you're a man, these muscles may be damaged by prostate surgery.

◆ *Urge incontinence*, the next most common type, occurs when muscles controlling your bladder don't work properly. An uncontrollable contraction or spasm of the bladder muscle occurs, and you feel a sudden, overwhelming urge to urinate – all too often, you don't make it to the bathroom in time.

◆ *Overflow incontinence*, which is more common among men, occurs when the bladder becomes filled beyond its normal capacity – often because it doesn't empty completely during urination. It then overflows, resulting in a slow, continuous leakage or periodic loss of urine. This type of incontinence is often related to an enlarged prostate gland, which causes a blockage or narrowing of the urethra.

? **Are older people more prone to incontinence?**
Although incontinence can occur at any age, certain factors associated with growing older do increase your risk.

◆ *Age-related changes:* As you get older, there are certain normal changes in how your urinary system functions – for example, your bladder holds less urine than it did when you were younger, your urethra is less flexible and the muscles supporting your bladder are weaker. These changes may mean that you urinate more frequently now, especially at night.

◆ *Other health problems:* Many diseases and conditions common in later life can cause or contribute to incontinence. These include urinary tract infections and diabetes (which can damage nerves controlling your bladder). Some studies suggest that, in women, reduced levels of estrogen after menopause may cause reduced muscle tone, which contributes to certain types of incontinence. Other health problems – arthritis, osteoporosis, heart failure, poor vision, paralysis due to stroke or other neurological problems – may reduce your mobility, making it more difficult for you to reach the bathroom in time. People with brain damage due to Alzheimer's disease and other dementing illnesses often become incontinent because they no longer respond to sensory cues that signal a full bladder.

◆ *Medications:* When you're older, you may be taking drugs that can trigger or aggravate incontinence. For example, if you take diuretics to control high blood pressure or congestive heart failure, your body may produce urine more quickly than usual, and you may not be able to make it to the bathroom in time. Sedatives or tranquilizers can also make you sleep so soundly that you don't realize you need to urinate during the night or during a daytime nap.

? **How is incontinence diagnosed?**
Before you and your doctor can begin to treat the problem, it must be

correctly diagnosed. You should undergo a complete physical examination and medical history to rule out any underlying illnesses or medication effects that might be causing your incontinence. Once such problems are treated or addressed, your incontinence may improve or completely disappear.

You will be asked to keep a detailed "bladder diary" for several days or a week, noting how much you drink, when you drink, when you urinate and how much; how often you are actually incontinent; how much urine is leaking; and what you were doing when the incontinence occurred. This chart is an important diagnostic tool that can give your doctor vital clues about the nature of your incontinence.

If the source of the problem is still unclear, or if he feels it's warranted, he may refer you to a urologist (for men) or a urogynecologist (for women). You may be asked to undergo various urodynamic tests to measure how well your urinary system is working.

? **Why is treatment so important?** If you or someone you know is suffering from incontinence, it's very important to get treatment. For older adults especially, the consequences of not treating this problem may be far-reaching and serious, affecting your sense of self-esteem, your physical independence, and your social and psychological well-being. Consequences include the following:

◆ The continuous release of urine makes it difficult for you to keep yourself clean, particularly if you have trouble changing or washing and thus remain in wet clothes. Because bacteria are likely to grow in this situation, you're more prone to developing a urinary tract infection. The constant wetness and acidity of the urine can also be extremely irritating to your skin, causing rashes or infections.

◆ The sudden urge to urinate, combined with anxiety about "not making it," can cause you to rush to the washroom, increasing your risk for falls and injuries.

◆ Fear of incontinence can undermine your self-confidence and self-esteem. You worry about unpleasant odors and stained clothing, and anxiety about your problem may prevent you from enjoying sex. These concerns can also lead you to withdraw from enjoyable social activities, and this can have many negative effects on your physical, mental and emotional well-being.

◆ Untreated incontinence is a major cause of dependence and may be an important factor in the decision to seek institutional care, simply because family members find it so difficult to look after an incontinent spouse or parent.

? **How is incontinence treated?** How your incontinence is treated depends on many factors, including the type and severity of the problem and your general health. Doctors agree that it's best to begin with the least invasive therapy, and if that doesn't work, move on to the next option.

◆ *Changing your diet:* Many foods and beverages can stimulate your bladder or the production of urine. They include alcohol, tea, coffee, cola drinks, chocolate, acidic fruits or fruit juices, tomatoes, highly spicy foods, dairy products and sugar. Your doctor may suggest eliminating them from your diet for a few weeks to see if you improve. If you're overweight, this can put added stress on your bladder, so your doctor may recommend a sensible weight loss program as part of incontinence treatment.

◆ *Exercise:* Your doctor may recommend special exercises, known as Kegel exercises, which help control stress and urge incontinence by strengthening certain muscles in your pelvic area. This helps keep your bladder sphincter closed and prevents your bladder from contracting involuntarily. In the past these exercises were recommended for women, but recent studies suggest that they can also help men achieve better urinary control (see page 162).

◆ *Behavior:* Some types of incontinence can be improved by changing when and how you urinate, a process known as bladder retraining. The goal is to set up a predictable pattern of urinating and then stick to that schedule. For example, if you have to urinate once an hour (or if you're incontinent that often), you'll be encouraged to urinate every hour, whether or not you feel the need. The amount of time between bathroom visits is gradually increased, until you can wait two hours or even longer.

Sometimes a change in position while you urinate may also be helpful. If you're a woman, leaning forward while urinating helps empty your bladder completely. If you're a man, a switch from standing to sitting may help.

You may think that cutting down on fluids will help you beat night time incontinence, but this is risky. As you get older, you need plenty of water and other beverages to stay

The other kind of incontinence

While many older people feel embarrassed about discussing urinary incontinence, those who experience the other kind of incontinence almost never mention it.

Fecal incontinence refers to the involuntary loss of feces or stool. This can happen occasionally or develop into a chronic problem that creates great stress. You must cope with soiled clothing and feelings of shame and embarrassment, and you may stop going out for fear of having an unpleasant accident.

Fecal incontinence can be caused by a number of factors:

◆ an underlying neurological problem that has caused you to lose muscle tone in your lower bowel and rectum (most commonly due to a stroke or nerve damage from diabetes);

◆ the overuse of laxative medications;

◆ constipation or diarrhea – both conditions can lead to an overflow of stool, and incontinence may occur if you can't reach the bathroom in time.

If you or someone you know is having problems with occasional or chronic fecal incontinence, don't be afraid to mention it to your doctor. You may benefit from changes in diet and medication, and a program of bowel training – similar to bladder retraining (see page 162) – may also be helpful.

How to do Kegel exercises

These exercises involve repeated tightening and relaxing of a particular loop of muscles around your urethra. It's absolutely vital to locate the right muscles, or else you may end up contracting your abdominal muscles, which won't help reduce or control leakage of urine.

You can try to locate the muscles you want to strengthen on your own: Just stop your urine flow in midstream and notice which muscles are being used to control urination. If you can't figure it out, your doctor may be able to help.

Once you've identified the right muscles, you can begin by doing Kegels during urination. This means stopping and starting your flow of urine briefly two or three times each time you urinate. You should also do the following exercise routine two or three times a day:

◆ Contract your pelvic muscles and hold for three seconds.

Then relax for three seconds. Do this three times.

◆ Gradually increase the length of each contraction, until you're holding the muscles tightly for 10 seconds each time. Also increase the number of contractions until you're doing 10 contractions three times a day.

For Kegel exercises to be effective, you must do them routinely and consistently. The good news is that Kegels can be done anywhere – standing up, sitting or lying down, at home or on the bus, while you're watching television, drying dishes or reading. Because no one can tell that you're doing them, you can even exercise during a conversation if your concentration is good enough!

healthy. Cutting down on fluids also causes your urine to become more concentrated and may make you prone to urinary tract infections. However, if night time incontinence is a problem, it might be a good idea to avoid drinking tea or milk right before bedtime. If you cut down on fluids in the evening to prevent nighttime incontinence, don't forget to make up for it by drinking more the next day!

◆ *Medication:* In some cases your doctor may recommend medication to help with an incontinence problem. Recent studies have found that older women with stress or urge incontinence are helped by the application of estrogen-containing cream to the vagina or by complete hormone replacement therapy (HRT) (see page 180). Drugs such as oxybutynin and some antidepressants can ease urge incontinence by helping your bladder relax, thereby preventing extra contractions. Other drugs such as pseudoephedrine can strengthen the sphincter muscles that control urine flow. But these drugs should only be used under medical supervision – they have side effects and aren't advisable if you have certain kinds of heart disease or high blood pressure.

◆ *Devices:* Some older women develop incontinence due to the displacement or dropping of the bladder or uterus. This tends to occur as an after-effect of childbearing, obesity and simple gravity. While such a problem can be corrected surgically, your overall health may make surgery too risky. Your doctor may recommend a pessary – a specially fitted, ring-shaped rubber device similar to a diaphragm, which is inserted into the vagina to help support your bladder and uterus.

Another device used for some types of incontinence delivers tiny amounts of electrical stimulation to your pelvic muscles, making them contract in the same way as Kegel exercises (see page 162).

◆ *Injections:* This relatively new solution helps some people suffering from stress incontinence – the kind caused by weakening of the sphincter that controls the outflow of urine from your bladder. It involves injecting a small amount of collagen (a fibrous substance found in your skin) into the tissues of the urethra to strengthen the sphincter and prevent leakage. The procedure is done under local anesthetic or intravenous sedation on an outpatient basis. Because your body absorbs some of the water in the collagen, you'll probably need at least one more injection about three months after the first one. This technique is still being studied and is available on a limited basis.

The process doesn't help every kind of incontinence, and you have to be tested to make sure you aren't allergic to collagen. But studies show that two-thirds of women and half the men treated with collagen injections had either improved or been cured of their problem.

◆ *Surgery:* If your incontinence doesn't respond to lifestyle changes, exercise and medication, and if your general health is good, your doctor may recommend surgery. Although surgery can help, procedures to correct incontinence are done in the hospital under an anesthetic, and recovery may take several weeks or longer. They should be considered a last resort.

Bladder neck suspension surgery is recommended for mild to moderate stress incontinence and involves repositioning the neck of the bladder and urethra. The *sling procedure*, which can help in severe stress incontinence, involves surgically attaching a piece of tissue – your own or a synthetic mesh – to your urethra, rather like a sling. This helps your bladder stay closed while it fills, reducing the chance that a sudden move or sneeze will result in an outflow of urine.

Osteoporosis

Osteoporosis is a condition that affects your bones, making them fragile and prone to fractures. If it isn't diagnosed and treated properly, osteoporosis can have major health consequences and seriously jeopardize your quality of life in your later years.

Although the disease can occur at any age, it's especially common among older women – in fact, some studies show that 25 percent of all women past menopause suffer from some degree of osteoporosis. Older men, especially those over age 75, can also develop osteoporosis.

Most people tend to underestimate the serious potential of osteoporosis – at least until they or someone they know develops this condition. While it's true that some people can function fairly well with the disease, it remains a major cause of pain and disability later in life, and in extreme cases, it can actually contribute to death.

What is osteoporosis?

If you're like most people, you probably take your bones for granted. But bones are complex structures. They not only provide structure and support for your body, but also store calcium and other important minerals vital to your overall health.

Your bones consist of two layers: cells in the hard outer layer, or cortical bone, die off continuously, while the soft inner layer, or trabecular bone, is constantly being formed using calcium from your bloodstream. When the loss of bone cells in the outer layer becomes greater than the formation of new ones in the inner layer, bones lose their density and strength, becoming more porous and vulnerable to fractures.

Most people's bones reach their peak density at around age 30. After that they gradually become more porous. But just because you lose bone cells as you age, you won't automatically develop osteoporosis.

Compare your bones to your bank account. If you have $50,000 in the bank, losing $5,000 on a bad investment won't make you poor. On the other hand, if you started out with only $10,000, you're bound to feel the loss of $5,000. In the same way, a person who starts out with dense, healthy bones that aren't jeopardized by risk factors (see page 166) won't feel the effects of age-related bone loss as quickly or as much as someone with fewer reserves.

Although osteoporosis itself doesn't hurt, it makes you susceptible to fractures that can cause pain, loss of mobility, disfigurement and even death. Your bones can become so fragile that a simple sneeze is enough to cause a rib fracture, and turning over in bed can cause bone fractures in your spine.

About 30 percent of women over age 65 will suffer fractures of their spinal bones or vertebrae. Repeated spinal fractures can be extremely painful or completely painless. They can cause your back to bend, leading to a loss of height, a stooped-over posture and in extreme cases, a spinal deformity of the upper back once known as a "dowager's hump." This stooped posture may cause painful muscle cramping, interfere with normal neck movement and lead to compression of your lungs, which can make it difficult for you to breathe.

About one-third of women and one-sixth of men over age 65 will fracture their hips in falls. In the past it was thought that the bones of an osteoporotic hip were so porous that they broke on contact with a hard surface. But now some researchers think that, on occasion, these fragile bones actually fracture spontaneously, causing the sufferer to fall. Whatever the cause, there's no doubt that hip fractures pose a major health threat to older adults.

Studies show that between 25 and 40 percent of older people who break their hips never walk without help again – they need the support of crutches, a cane, a walker or a wheelchair.

Between 15 and 30 percent of people with hip fractures need so much help that they must spend the rest of their lives in a long-term care facility.

Between 15 and 30 percent actually die of pneumonia and other complications – from being inactive or bedridden – within a year of their hip fracture.

Two types of osteoporosis occur after age 65. One kind, which affects mainly the spongy or trabecular bone, is seen mainly in women between ages 55 and 65. The other, which involves the harder, cortical layer, is age-related and seems to affect women and men over age 75 in fairly equal numbers.

? How do you know if you have osteoporosis?

In the early stages, osteoporosis is usually symptomless. That's why it's often referred to as the "silent thief." It creeps up on older people, robbing them of their strength and vitality. In fact, you may not know that you have osteoporosis until you experience a painful fracture – for example, a sudden stab of pain in your ribs or back that occurs spontaneously or during a routine chore. Many painless fractures may have already occurred.

If your doctor suspects a cracked or broken bone, he will recommend an X-ray, but this is only useful in diagnosing the fracture. When it comes to diagnosing osteoporosis, conventional X-rays aren't useful until you've already lost about 30 percent of your bone density.

The first step in diagnosing osteoporosis is a thorough physical examination. It will probably include blood and urine tests and a medical history, including a dietary assessment.

Your doctor may then recommend a series of painless, non-invasive bone scans that can accurately measure bone density in particular areas such as the wrist and spine.

? Can osteoporosis be prevented?

Once you've developed osteoporosis, no therapy can fully restore the bone you've lost. Your best protection is prevention – that is, preventing or minimizing the amount of bone you lose.

Research has shown that the seeds of osteoporosis – not enough calcium in your diet, lack of exercise, regular use of tobacco – were planted much earlier in your life. But even if you didn't pay much attention to your bone health when you were younger, there's still a lot you can do now to prevent or delay the onset of osteoporosis.

◆ *Calcium intake:* Although there's no evidence that calcium alone can prevent bone loss, a lack of calcium can certainly contribute to osteoporosis. This mineral is essential for many body functions – from muscle contraction to blood clotting to bone formation. If you don't get enough calcium in your diet, your body will begin to draw it out of your bones.

As you grow older, it's easy to become deficient in calcium, partly because your body's ability to absorb it from foods can decrease with age. Many older people also suffer from an inability to digest lactose in milk. This may cause them to stop eating dairy products, which are an important source of calcium.

Many experts say that if you're over 65 – and this advice holds true for men as well as women – you should aim to get about 1,200 milligrams of calcium daily.

The best source of calcium is your diet. High-calcium foods include dairy products, canned fish with bones, fortified orange juice, tofu, almonds, beans, spinach, broccoli and rhubarb. If you don't like the taste of milk, you can still get calcium by adding nonfat milk powder to baked goods, meat loaves and casseroles. Five teaspoons of nonfat milk powder contain the same amount of calcium as one large glass of milk. If you're avoiding dairy products because you can't digest lactose, try using lactose-reduced milk, which is available in most supermarkets.

Some experts believe it's better to obtain calcium from your diet than from supplements, since calcium is absorbed more easily from foods. But if you can't get enough calcium in your diet, ask your doctor whether you should take a non-prescription calcium supplement such as calcium carbonate or calcium citrate.

Taking too much calcium can be hazardous – excess amounts of the mineral can form deposits around your joints or cause kidney stones. If your doctor recommends a calcium supplement, you shouldn't take more than 500 milligrams at one time, and take each dose with food to maximize absorption.

◆ *Vitamin D:* This vitamin – which your body produces when exposed to sunlight – plays a critical role in preventing osteoporosis because it helps you absorb calcium. If you're over 65, you should be getting about 800 International Units (IUs) of

Are you at risk for osteoporosis?

Researchers have identified a number of factors that seem to increase your risk for osteoporosis.

Risk factors that you can't control

◆ being past menopause (for women);

◆ being over age 75 (for men);

◆ being Caucasian or Asian;

◆ a family history of osteoporosis;

◆ being slim or small-boned;

◆ a diet low in calcium and/or vitamin D in adolescence or early adulthood;

◆ an early menopause or a surgical menopause (removal of ovaries due to underlying disease);

◆ medical disorders such as diabetes, hyperthyroidism or anorexia nervosa;

◆ long-term use of medications such as prednisone, heparin and some anti-cancer drugs.

Risk factors that you can control

◆ smoking cigarettes;

◆ heavy alcohol consumption;

◆ excessive dieting;

◆ lack of regular, weight-bearing exercise.

The best food sources of calcium

Food	Serving size	Milligrams of calcium
Low-fat plain yogurt	1 cup	415
Low-fat milk	1 cup	300
Canned sardines	3.5 oz.	295
Hard cheese	1 oz.	204
Low-fat cottage cheese	1 cup	146
Navy beans, cooked	1 cup	128
Broccoli, cooked	1 cup	72

vitamin D – found in fortified milk, eggs, canned sardines in oil and canned salmon – each day. Spending 5 to 15 minutes a day in full sunlight will also cause your body to produce an adequate amount of vitamin D. Not everyone can get enough vitamin D from their diet and may require exposure to sunshine to make up the difference. However, this can be a problem if you live in a northern climate where hours of sunshine are limited, or if you're confined to home because of health problems. If you aren't sure whether your vitamin D intake is sufficient, a supplement may be very important in helping you prevent bone disease.

◆ *Exercise:* Just like muscles, bones become weak when they aren't used. Astronauts who go into the confines and weightlessness of space often experience a temporary loss of bone density, as do people who must be immobilized following a serious injury or surgery.

Some studies have shown that a program of regular, weight-bearing exercise can stop and even reverse bone loss of osteoporosis by stimulating the formation of new bone cells. You should be able to benefit from regular weight-bearing exercise regardless of your current activity level.

If you're active, try tennis, dancing, bicycling and exercising with weights.

If you're less active, try walking, swimming, bowling, housework, stair climbing and gardening.

If you aren't physically active because of health or other problems, you can still put weight on your bones. If you spend a lot of time in bed, try sitting up for an hour or two. If you spend a lot of time sitting, try standing up for several minutes every hour.

◆ *Hormone replacement:* In women, bone loss accelerates around the time of menopause, partly because your body has stopped producing estrogen, a hormone known to be important for strong bones. Some studies have found that estrogen replacement therapy (ERT) started soon after menopause can reduce fractures by more than 50 percent. If you're at high risk for osteoporosis or already have the disease, you should discuss the benefits and risks of ERT with your doctor (see page 180).

◆ *Screening:* If you're over 65, your doctor should measure your height at least once a year. Recent studies have found that a height loss of 1.25 to 2 inches (3 to 5 cm) or more over several years is associated with lower bone density and osteoporosis. If you're at higher-than-average risk for osteoporosis, your doctor may suggest that you undergo regular bone density measurements to keep closer track of your condition.

? How is osteoporosis treated?

If you've been diagnosed with osteoporosis, your doctor will recommend a treatment plan to slow down the rate of bone loss and minimize the chance of damaging fractures.

◆ Make sure that you're getting adequate amounts of calcium and vitamin D.

◆ Begin a sensible program of weight-bearing exercise, recommended by and under the supervision of a qualified recreational therapist or a physiotherapist, if you have access to one. Otherwise your doctor may be able to recommend the right activities for you. The program, which can be tailored to meet your current health and fitness level, will help increase your bone mass, strengthen supporting muscles, improve your posture, prevent deformity, and relieve back pain. Some experts recommend exercising with weights attached to your hands and wrists to increase the weight-bearing effect. If you notice pain in your joints or elsewhere during or after exercising, stop and let your supervising therapist know.

◆ Try to maintain a healthy weight. Now isn't the time for dieting, however. In fact, a weight gain of 10 to 20 pounds (5 to 10 kilograms) after menopause is common and may actually protect you against osteoporosis. Body fat contains estrogen, which is good for your bones, and the extra weight stimulates the formation of new bone cells. Research has shown that two-thirds of women with osteoporosis have never weighed more than 140 pounds (63 kilograms).

◆ If you're a woman, you should discuss the benefits of estrogen replacement therapy with your doctor (see page 180).

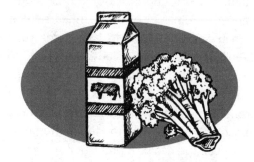

◆ Other kinds of therapy may help decrease the rate of bone loss in people with osteoporosis. They include injections of a hormone called "calcitonin" and a regimen involving oral doses of a substance called "etidronate disodium." Another type of therapy involves oral doses of sodium fluoride, the same substance that is added to toothpaste and drinking water to prevent tooth decay. It has been shown to stimulate the development of new bone. However, the quality of the new bone may not be the same, and such therapies are considered to be experimental until more research is done into their safety and effectiveness.

What are some strategies for managing pain due to osteoporosis?

How well you live with osteoporosis depends on many factors: in particular, how severe and advanced your disease is and how many fractures you've sustained.

Pain is usually at its worst immediately after a fracture. Your doctor will recommend pain-relieving strategies, including rest, immobilization and pain-killing medication.

Pain that occurs without any fracture can be alleviated by a number of methods. Non-drug methods include heating pads or warm water bottles applied to the sore area, especially designed exercises you can do at home and physiotherapy. You may also obtain relief from massage and ultrasound.

Medication is often necessary to control osteoporosis pain, but don't make the mistake of prescribing for yourself. Ask your doctor what type and strength of analgesic would be best for you (see page 77).

You may notice that you become very stiff at night and find it difficult to get moving in the morning. If you wake up early, ask your doctor if you should take a painkiller an hour or so before getting up (keep one dose of your medication and a glass of water on your bedside table). An early bath or shower can also help relieve pain and stiffness.

Stroke

A stroke occurs when the blood flow to the brain is blocked or when a ruptured vessel causes bleeding into the brain. If brain cells are deprived of vital oxygen, they can become irreversibly damaged, and in extreme cases, the sufferer can die.

There are two major types of stroke: Strokes due to blockage occur when a blood clot develops in an artery inside or leading to the brain (a cerebral thrombosis), or when a clot in an artery somewhere else in the body travels to the brain and blocks an artery there (a cerebral embolism); strokes due to bleeding occur when a blood vessel in the brain ruptures.

What are the early warning signs of stroke?

It's important to recognize the following signs and symptoms, which could mean that you're having a stroke:

◆ sudden weakness or numbness of the face, arm, hand or leg on one side of your body;

◆ sudden loss of speech, or difficulty forming or understanding words;

◆ sudden loss or decrease in vision, especially in one eye;

◆ sudden unexplained dizziness or feelings of unsteadiness that may cause you to fall, especially when associated with numbness, tingling or limb weakness.

If you experience these symptoms, it's crucial that you seek immediate medical treatment. Many people still believe that a stroke is less serious than a heart attack. They may also think that once a stroke occurs, nothing can be done.

In fact, like a heart attack, a stroke is a life-threatening event, and you should follow the same emergency procedures as you would for a heart attack.

If you're alone and think you might be having a stroke, dial emergency assistance (usually 911). If you can speak, give your address right away – if not, keep the phone off the hook so your call can be traced. The operator will call fire, paramedic or ambulance services, which can transport you to a hospital quickly. *Never try to drive yourself to the hospital.*

If you're with someone who is having a stroke, try to stay calm. Make sure the person is comfortable and call for help right away. While you're waiting, provide reassurance.

Each year many people die or are left with more severe brain damage than was necessary because they didn't admit they might be having a stroke. If treatment begins soon enough, doctors can save your life and may be able to minimize the amount of damage to your brain.

Many people who have major strokes experience an early warning signal known as a "transient ischemic attack" or TIA. This is a small, reversible interruption in the brain's blood supply due to a temporary blockage in a blood vessel in the brain. Symptoms of a TIA are the same as for stroke, except that they usually last from a few moments to minutes to hours and are followed by a total recovery. *Even if you feel fine, it's vital that you report a TIA to your doctor immediately,* so you can be examined and, if necessary, receive treatment that may prevent a major stroke from occurring. This usually involves medication such as aspirin, ticlopidine or warfarin, which lower the risk of stroke by making your blood less sticky and less likely to clot.

How is stroke treated?

When you arrive at the hospital with symptoms of a stroke, you will undergo tests to help doctors determine the nature and severity of the stroke. First, the doctor will assess how you're functioning: Can you move? Are your physical reflexes normal? Is your speech affected?

This will be followed by other tests such as a CAT (Computerized Axial Tomography) scan or MRI (Magnetic Resonance Imaging) scan that can reveal areas of damage in the brain.

If it's determined that the stroke is due to a blocked artery, you may be started on aspirin or anticoagulant medication. If it's found that the stroke is due to a hemorrhage, doctors will try to find the reason and treat the cause.

Can stroke be prevented?

Certain people are known to be at higher-than-average risk for stroke. Factors that increase your risk are:

◆ a previous stroke;

◆ other conditions such as heart disease, high blood pressure and diabetes;

◆ age (80 percent of those who suffer strokes are over age 65);

◆ being male (until age 75 when the risk for women catches up);

◆ a family history of cardiovascular disease.

But even if you're past 65 and have one or more of these risk factors, there's still a lot you can do.

Since many strokes are caused by atherosclerosis – a fatty buildup in your blood vessels – you should follow your doctor's advice about diet, exercise and smoking (see page 152).

A major risk factor for stroke is high blood pressure. Have your blood pressure checked regularly and follow your doctor's advice about treatment (see page 172).

Another risk factor is heart disease, particularly atrial fibrillation (AF) (see page 155). If you have this condition, it should be properly diagnosed and treated with a drug called warfarin, to prevent blood clots being thrown from the heart to the brain.

If you experience symptoms of a TIA, report them to your doctor immediately. A neurological assessment will be done to check for any permanent damage or signs that might explain the source of the symptoms. She will also use a stethoscope to listen for "bruits" in your neck – sounds made by the blood as it flows through your carotid arteries (located on either side of your neck) toward your brain. Abnormal sounds may indicate that these arteries have become narrowed. Your doctor may also decide to refer you for more specialized tests that use sound waves to detect areas of narrowing or blockage.

If tests show that your carotid arteries are blocked, your doctor may suggest surgery to clear the obstructions. The procedure, a carotid endarterectomy, involves scraping out built-up plaque from one or both carotid arteries while you're under a general anesthetic. Because complications can occur, this procedure isn't advisable unless tests show that your arteries are severely obstructed (at least 70 percent blocked). However, researchers are reassessing whether the risk of this procedure outweighs the benefit for people with less severe blockage.

What are the after-effects of a stroke?

Some people who have strokes don't suffer any serious or lasting problems. Others experience certain symptoms – paralysis, lack of coordination, difficulty swallowing, and/or loss of speech – immediately afterward. Even though these problems tend to improve over the first few weeks, it may take a while before you and your doctor know the full after-effects of a stroke. However, most of the recovery that will occur tends to take place in the first few months.

Although the brain cells that died as a result of the stroke won't regenerate, other parts of your brain may begin to take over in time, and it's possible that some or even all of your strength and speech will eventually return.

There may be more permanent damage.

High blood pressure – the silent killer

If you're over 65, it's important to have your blood pressure checked regularly. Studies show that about one in every five people suffers from high blood pressure – a condition known as "hypertension" – yet many of them are unaware of it.

Untreated high blood pressure can damage your body in many ways. It causes blood vessel walls to thicken, places a strain on the heart and kidneys, and may damage delicate structures in the eyes.

Blood pressure is measured with a device called a "sphygmomanometer," an inflatable cuff connected to a pressure gauge. The cuff is inflated and released while the doctor listens to your pulse through a stethoscope. The pressure is measured at two stages – when your heart is contracting (this is your systolic pressure) and when it's relaxing between beats (this is your diastolic pressure). The pressure is expressed as two numbers – for example, 120 (systolic) over 80 (diastolic).

Your doctor will decide what a "normal" blood pressure is for you, taking several factors into account – your general health, your previous blood pressure levels, what medications you're taking and whether you are overweight.

You should have your blood pressure checked at least once a year, and more often if you have other health problems such as diabetes or kidney disease. Because blood pressure tends to fluctuate as a result of physical exertion, emotional distress and even body position, your doctor will want to measure it more than once. He may take it while you're sitting, standing and lying down, and he may measure it in both arms.

Your blood pressure can shoot up if you

The type of damage that occurs after a stroke depends on what area of your brain was affected:

◆ *Strokes on either side of the brain* can cause weakness or paralysis on the opposite side of your body (including a widening of the eye or a drooping of the corner of your mouth).

◆ *Strokes on the right side of the brain* can sometimes lead to a condition known as "hemineglect." Your ability to see and perceive objects on the left side is impaired, so that you pay attention only to the right half of everything: For example, you don't notice a person approaching you from the left side or you miss food on the left side of your plate. If you don't understand this condition and take steps to compensate, hemineglect can be extremely upsetting for you and your caregiver. A right brain stroke can also result in poor judgment and insight, poor spatial ori-

feel nervous in the doctor's presence, or if you're worried about having your pressure checked. This is so common that doctors have a name for it: "white coat hypertension" (your pressure rises at the sight of the doctor's white coat!). If you feel tense, be sure to mention it to the doctor or nurse. It may be possible for you to take your blood pressure at home to see if it drops when you're in more familiar surroundings.

The exact causes of high blood pressure still aren't clear. There is some genetic connection, since hypertension is known to run in families. Other risk factors are obesity, lack of exercise and overuse of alcohol. Some people with high blood pressure also seem to be sensitive to salt (sodium) in their diets, and there's evidence that too much stress may play a role for certain people.

How your doctor treats you will depend on many factors. He may start by asking you to change your lifestyle – this may mean losing weight, increasing your exercise level if it's safe to do so, and restricting your intake of salt (see page 28). He may also recommend relaxation exercises to see if this lowers your blood pressure.

If these strategies aren't enough to bring your pressure down, he will prescribe a regimen of antihypertensive drugs. This may include diuretics, beta blockers, and other drugs that affect the heart and blood vessels in ways that decrease blood pressure.

Many of these drugs have side effects. These range from minor discomforts such as diarrhea or dryness of the mouth to more serious problems such as fainting, insomnia, nightmares, depression and sexual impotence in men. But with careful choice of drugs and dosage, most older people should be able to tolerate treatment.

You should never stop taking medication for high blood pressure without telling your doctor. If you do, you're putting your health in jeopardy. Report any unpleasant side effects to your doctor, who may suggest changing the dosage or else switching you to a different medication with fewer side effects.

entation, and non-verbal memory problems.

◆ *Strokes on the left side of the brain* can cause speech problems known as "aphasia" because in most people, the major centers controlling speech are found on the left side of the brain. Aphasia involves difficulty producing and/or understanding language, including reading or writing. If speech is affected, it's easy for caregivers to think that your intellectual capacity has been impaired, but in fact, this isn't usually the case. Your capacity hasn't changed, but your mind may not work as efficiently as it did before the stroke. This type of stroke can also lead to verbal memory problems.

Depression following a stroke is extremely common. While some doctors think this depression is an emotional reaction to serious illness, others now believe that the stroke causes certain biochemical changes in the brain that lead to mood disorders.

When someone you know has had a stroke

◆ Speak to the person's doctor and try to get a clear picture of what your partner, relative or friend will be able to achieve after a stroke. This will allow you to be encouraging and positive without being unrealistic.

◆ A person who has had a stroke needs more time to do things now, so try to be relaxed and unhurried when helping out. You may need to speak more simply and slowly, but don't speak to the person as if he were a child, and unless there were hearing problems before the stroke, there's no need to raise your voice.

◆ Encourage her to talk, and avoid interrupting or "helping" her along by supplying words. If speech is a problem, make room for alternative methods of communication – for example, pointing or other gestures, showing pictures of familiar objects or writing messages on a pad or white board.

◆ Encourage the stroke survivor to dress independently and maintain a normal, well-groomed appearance, which is important to self-esteem.

◆ Watch for changes in mood. If he seems depressed, this should be reported to the doctor because the depression may very well be treatable. In some people, a stroke can cause cognitive impairment such as memory loss and confusion, and these should also be reported.

How do you recover from a stroke?

You are the most important member of the recovery team, which includes doctors, nurses and a variety of rehabilitation specialists.

◆ *Dietitians* will help adapt your diet in case of swallowing problems or other eating difficulties.

◆ *Family members and other caregivers* are vital members of the rehabilitation team. Your spouse, adult children, other friends and relatives can do a lot to help you adjust to the effects of a stroke.

◆ *Occupational therapists* will help you learn how to safely manage such activities as dressing, using the bathroom, eating and cooking. They can also teach you how to use many adaptive devices designed for people who are recovering from stroke (see above).

◆ *Physiotherapists* will help you achieve maximum mobility and strength through special exercises and other treatments aimed at restoring as much function as possible.

◆ *Psychologists* will assess various functions, including speech and memory, and help develop strategies for rehabilitation and compensation.

◆ *Recreationists* will help you relearn old skills and learn new ones, and also encourage you to become involved in enjoyable leisure activities during your recovery.

◆ *Social workers* will offer helpful advice to you and your family, including how to manage your emotions during a difficult time. They can also help arrange for rehabilitation after you've been discharged from the hospital and will put you in touch with special programs and services in your community for people recovering from stroke.

◆ *Speech-language pathologists* will help you improve speech, assist with problems related to swallowing and teach alternative methods for communicating.

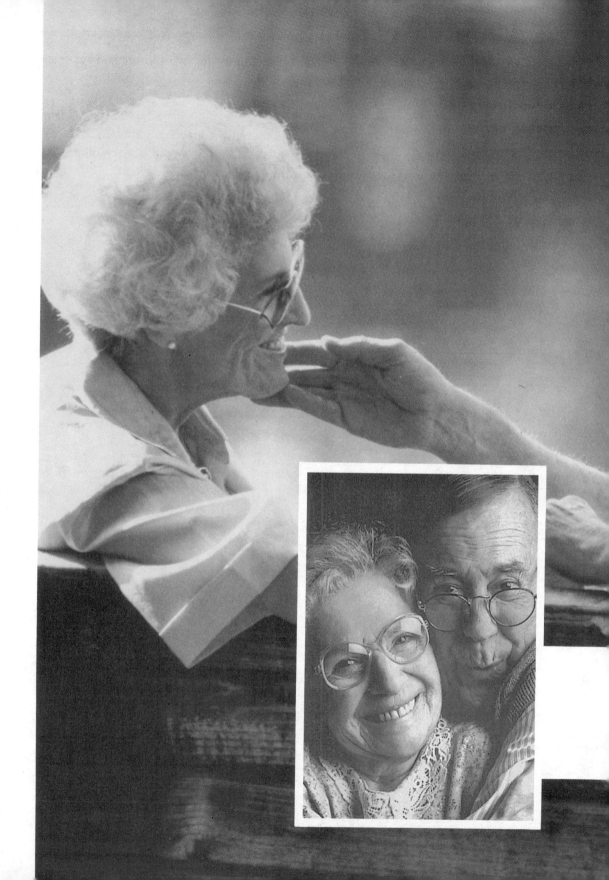

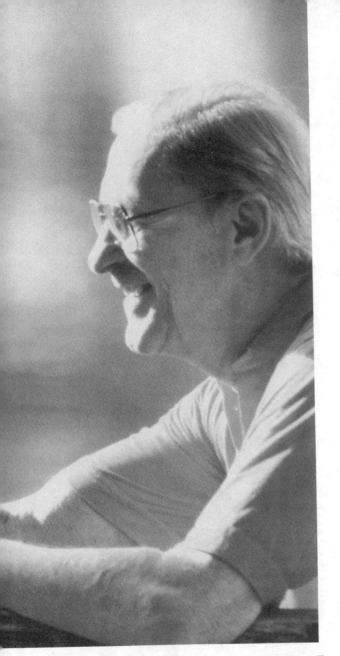

5

It would be a thousand pities if women wrote like men, or lived like men, or looked like men, for if two sexes are quite inadequate, considering the vastness and variety of the world, how should we manage with only one?

VIRGINIA WOOLF

Just for Older Women, Just for Older Men

SOME COMMON HEALTH CONCERNS of older adults affect just women or just men. Of course this doesn't mean that women shouldn't take an interest in problems that may be facing their male partners, nor should men avoid educating themselves about the special concerns affecting the women in their lives.

While this should be true at all stages of our lives, it's even more important now that you're older. After all, the health of you and your partner (if you have one) is probably the major factor determining the quality of life in your later years.

Just for older women

If you're a woman over age 65, you're probably accustomed to taking an interest in the physical and emotional well-being of others. But this focus on caring for others may cause some older women to take their own health for granted.

Here are some special concerns of interest to you now.

Menopause

If you're over 65, you have already passed through menopause – the so-called change of life that occurs when the amount of estrogen produced by your ovaries declines sharply and continues to dwindle. This process usually begins sometime between ages 45 and 55.

Many older women don't think about menopause, especially if they didn't experience any obvious or troublesome physical symptoms. However, it's never too late to educate yourself about this process and particularly about the benefits of hormone replacement therapy, which can reduce your risk for serious illness later in life (see page 180).

Just a few generations ago, when life expectancy was much shorter than it is now, most women lived just a decade or so after menopause. But that's changed: The average North American woman now starts menopause at around age 50 and has a life expectancy of about 80 years. That means many women can look forward to living between 25 and 30 years after menopause!

Look back and consider your own menopause for a moment. It's important to understand that there's no "right" or "normal" way to experience menopause – different women have different responses.

Many women pass through menopause with very few problems or no problems at all. They enjoy the prospect of entering a new stage of life, free from the pressures of menstruation, contraception and child-rearing. Many women see life after menopause as "their time" – a time when they can finally start to focus on their own needs and interests. These women give up "PMS" – premenstrual syndrome – for what anthropologist Margaret Mead called "PMZ" – postmenopausal zest!

Hormone replacement therapy

Hormone replacement therapy (HRT) refers to using estrogen and progesterone supplements to replace your body's natural supply after menopause. HRT can often reduce unpleasant symptoms such as hot flashes, insomnia, mood swings, headaches and vaginal dryness, which some women experience during menopause.

If you're over 65, chances are these symptoms have disappeared. But symptom control isn't the only reason for you to consider HRT. Studies have shown that many health problems affecting older women – particularly heart disease, stroke and osteoporosis – can be prevented or delayed by HRT. *If you're a woman over 65, you should take these problems seriously – they can threaten the quality of your later years, increase your risk of illness and disability, and shorten your life. (For more information on heart disease, see page 149; for information on stroke, see page 169; and for information on osteoporosis, see page 163.)*

Is it too late to consider starting HRT if you're in your late 60s? Although very little research has been done into this question, it may be worth discussing HRT with your doctor, who will help you weigh the benefits of HRT against the risks. For example, if you have a history of breast or uterine cancer, a family history of breast cancer, or a blood clotting disorder, the risks may outweigh the benefits.

If your doctor recommends HRT, you can take the hormone in pill form or in a hormone-containing skin patch worn on your buttocks, sides, lower back or pelvic area and changed twice a week. Some older women use estrogen in the form of a vaginal cream. This provides local relief for symptoms such as vaginal dryness but doesn't affect the rest of the body.

Until recently, women who took hormones after menopause took only estrogen. New studies have found that unless you take it with another hormone called "progesterone," estrogen can increase your risk of developing uterine cancer (unless you've had a hysterectomy) and breast cancer. That's why most doctors now recommend a combination of estrogen-progesterone therapy in cycles or on an organized, continuous basis.

Because the long-term health benefits of HRT end once you stop taking the hormones, you should consider it a lifelong program – although your doctor may recommend that you take an HRT "break" every so often, depending on your general health.

If you take a combination of estrogen and progesterone, the progesterone does cause some degree of bleeding each month. This is not a true menstrual period and doesn't signify a return to fertility! The flow may be similar to what you experienced before menopause, and you may also experience some premenstrual symptoms such as cramps or bloating. The symptoms may disappear after a few months, or your doctor may relieve them by changing your treatment regimen.

HRT can also cause temporary side effects such as water retention, headaches, weight gain and irritability in some women. A small number of women may be sensitive to certain types of synthetic estrogen or have a local skin reaction to the estrogen patch. You should report these symptoms to your doctor, who may decide to modify your treatment program to reduce unpleasant side effects.

Many other women do experience certain physical, mental and emotional changes during menopause, but these tend to be relatively minor and are usually temporary. Common physical symptoms include hot flashes, night sweats, and soreness, dryness or thinning of the vagina, which can make intercourse painful. (If vaginal discomfort lingers, speak to your doctor, who can suggest treatment.) Women may also experience emotional changes such as moodiness, tearfulness, irritability, memory lapses and loss of self-esteem. It's not clear how much of this is related to hormonal changes and how much to other factors such as fear of aging, marital problems, dissatisfaction with retirement, financial troubles and other health problems.

Whether your menopause was easy or difficult, you've probably put it behind you by now. But even as you reach your 70s and 80s, certain unexplored attitudes toward menopause can have a negative effect on your health and well-being.

You may have been raised in an era when menopause wasn't discussed at all, and may not know much about how this normal decline in estrogen can affect your body. For example, declining estrogen levels make you more vulnerable to some types of heart disease and to osteoporosis, a condition characterized by brittle bones and a high risk of fractures (see page 163). Because of this, you may want to talk to your doctor about the benefits and risks of hormone replacement therapy (see opposite).

You may believe that menopause is to blame for certain problems affecting you now such as depression and loss of sexual desire. While hormonal changes may play a role in these problems, they usually aren't the only factor to consider.

You may equate menopause with a loss of femininity, attractiveness and creativity. This is often a response to social pressures that have convinced women (and men) that smooth, unlined skin and a slender, youthful figure are the benchmarks of female worth. In reality, there are just two things you could do before menopause that you can't do now: menstruate and become pregnant.

Hysterectomy

Some studies have found that about one in every four women over age 50 has had a hysterectomy, which is the surgical removal of the uterus. In some cases, surgery may include removal of the ovaries and fallopian tubes.

In the past, some hysterectomies were done as a measure to prevent cancer of the uterus in healthy women past their childbearing years. Even today some doctors continue to recommend hysterectomy to solve relatively simple problems – for example, as a way to remove benign growths or fibroids in the uterus.

Many older women and a growing number of doctors are beginning to challenge the widespread use of hysterectomy, saying that the surgery is not a harmless procedure and should be performed only for more serious reasons. The fact is, even though your uterus no longer serves its primary function – as a place for a fetus to grow – it's part of your body, and, unless some serious disease is present, there's no reason why you should lose it and face the risks of major surgery.

If your doctor does recommend a

hysterectomy, it's important that you understand why. If you feel unsure about his reasons, it may be worthwhile to get a second opinion.

In general, a hysterectomy is probably advisable for the following reasons:

◆ to remove cancer in the vagina, cervix, uterus, fallopian tubes and ovaries;

◆ to control severe pelvic infections that don't respond to treatment;

◆ to stop severe, uncontrollable bleeding.

Your doctor may also recommend hysterectomy for the following conditions:

◆ to treat large or multiple fibroid tumors of the uterus that bleed or cause dangerous pressure on other organs;

◆ to treat extensive and very painful endometriosis – a condition where uterine tissue grows outside the lining of the uterus – in women who are still menstruating;

◆ to treat abnormalities of the uterus that are serious enough to interfere with the proper functioning of your bladder or bowel.

A hysterectomy is major surgery that is done in the hospital under a general anesthetic. There are two basic types of surgery. *Total abdominal hysterectomy* and *vaginal hysterectomy* involve removal of your uterus and cervix through an incision in the lower abdomen or vagina. *Complete hysterectomy* involves removal of your uterus, cervix, fallopian tubes and ovaries through an incision in the lower abdomen.

You should expect to remain in hospital for a week to 10 days, depending on your overall health. Recovery can continue at home, as long as you don't have to bend or lift anything for the first three weeks.

Some common sexual problems in older women

It's difficult to generalize about sex later in life. It would be pleasant to think that, as you age, you can continue to enjoy sexual activity with a loving partner – after all, the risk of pregnancy is over, you may feel more comfortable with yourself now, you know what pleases you and you're less afraid of saying so.

Many older women do enjoy sex after age 65, but many others face problems. For example, you may not have had an enjoyable sex life when you were younger. Your current partner may not be compatible sexually or emotionally. Or perhaps you don't have a partner at all (see page 49).

If you are still having a sexual relationship or relationships, you should be aware of certain problems that can interfere with your enjoyment of sex. These problems may have bothered you when you were younger, or they may have developed for the first time in your later years. Because it usually takes two for healthy, happy sex, you should also be aware of any problems your partner may be having (see page 186).

Inhibited sexual desire

You have no desire for sex – either sex with a partner or sexual release through masturbation. If you're alone, or if you and your partner don't really miss sex, then inhibited sexual desire isn't a problem. But if your partner is still interested, you may continue to have sex to please him or her, which can lead to feelings of resentment over time.

Many older people (and younger ones, too) find it extremely difficult to discuss sexual problems openly. However, it may be worth mentioning such problems to your doctor. She may want to examine you for any underlying physical conditions or medication side effects that could be interfering with healthy sexual feelings. If the problem is emotional, she may suggest that you speak to a therapist who specializes in helping people overcome sexual problems.

Arousal problems

You feel the desire for sex but have trouble becoming physically aroused. In women this often means that the vagina doesn't become sufficiently lubricated. This can lead to dyspareunia or painful intercourse (see below).

If your lubrication problem is related to hormonal changes, you may need to use a non-prescription lubricant jelly (see page 47) or an estrogen-containing vaginal cream prescribed by your doctor.

Arousal problems often have a psychological component. Your partner may not stimulate you long enough or in a way that arouses you. Maybe you feel distracted by worries or concerns, or perhaps there are unspoken problems in your relationship that interfere with arousal.

Dyspareunia

This is a term used to describe painful intercourse, which may have started when you were much younger, or which may have developed later in life. In some cases, pain occurs all the time during intercourse, while in others, it only occurs sometimes – for example, with a certain partner or in a certain position.

Dyspareunia has many causes and many treatments. If the problem is related to poor lubrication, you may benefit from using a non-petroleum based vaginal lubricant. If the problem is caused by anatomical problems such as excess tissue blocking the vagina, you may be a candidate for surgery.

There may be complex psychological reasons for pain during intercourse. You may have a negative attitude toward sex because you were raised in a strict family and during an era when women's sexual pleasure was never considered or discussed. Or you may have other reasons for disliking sex – perhaps you had unpleasant or even violent sexual experiences when you were younger. This can interfere with normal sexual arousal and even make your vaginal muscles constrict painfully during intercourse.

Such problems are difficult to overcome, especially if they've gone on for many years and if you haven't been honest about them with yourself and with your partner. Even though it's frightening and difficult to talk about these issues now, try raising the subject with your doctor, who may be able to help.

Just for older men

If you're a man over the age of 65, chances are you didn't pay much attention to your health when you were younger. Studies have shown that, in general, men are less likely than women to seek medical attention, they aren't well informed about health issues and they are often reluctant to admit to health problems. Men also tend to rely on women – first their mothers, then their wives – to "take care" of health-related business.

But it's especially important for older men to take responsibility for their own health. As certain illnesses and conditions develop, you'll be able to recognize them and report them to your doctor. This can be a real advantage in terms of effective diagnosis and treatment.

It's not a pleasant thought, but you should be prepared to take care of yourself in case your partner becomes ill or dies. Studies have shown that older men who lose a spouse tend to suffer more physical and emotional problems than women who experience the loss of a husband. One reason may be that men over 65 simply aren't prepared to take charge of their own health.

Here are some special health concerns of interest to you now:

Prostate problems

If you're over 65, there's a good chance that you have already had or can expect to have trouble with your prostate. This walnut-sized gland rests under your bladder just above your scrotum and is involved in the production of seminal fluid.

Because your prostate is situated so close to your bladder and your urethra, any inflammation or enlargement of the gland can interfere with urination.

The following are the most common conditions affecting your prostate:

Enlarged prostate

As you get older, it's normal for your prostate gland to increase in size. By the time men reach 70, about half of them have some prostate enlargement (benign prostatic hypertrophy, or BPH), and after 80, virtually all men do.

Although an enlarged prostate won't necessarily cause trouble, when the gland becomes very big – for example, swelling from the size of a walnut to the size of a grapefruit – problems can and do occur. You may have trouble emptying your bladder, which can lead to an unhealthy buildup of urine. This may result in bladder infection, incontinence, kidney problems and – in extreme cases – kidney failure. An enlarged prostate can also cause a total obstruction of the urinary tract, an extremely painful condition known as "acute retention." This is considered a medical emergency and must be treated in a hospital.

An enlarged prostate is usually diagnosed during a routine prostate examination, which should be done on a regular basis (see page 138). If there are no problems, your doctor may decide not to treat the enlargement and monitor your condition.

If an enlarged prostate is causing problems, your doctor will recommend treatment based on the severity of symptoms and your general health. This may include the use of drugs such as finasteride or terazosin. Some doctors have also used radiation or microwave therapy to shrink the gland.

About 30 percent of men with troublesome, enlarged prostates will need surgery. In the past, doctors removed the entire gland through a full surgical incision, and this may still be recommended if you have an extremely large prostate. Today, however, most men undergo a procedure called "transurethral" prostatectomy or TURP.

TURP involves the removal of the part of the prostate that is compressing the urethra, rather than the entire prostate gland. The surgeon inserts a thin tube or catheter with a telescopic viewer and a cauterizing device through the tip of the penis into the urethra and then into the prostate gland itself. The device burns or cauterizes the tissue forming the obstruction.

The advantages of TURP over traditional surgery is that the procedure is less drastic, there's less chance of damage to nerves that regulate erections and recovery time is shorter. A minority of men experience postoperative complications, including infection and incontinence, but these can often be cured or effectively managed. Some men also find they have trouble achieving or maintaining erections after prostate surgery. In some cases this may be related to anxiety or other emotional problems rather than to the surgery itself.

Prostatitis

About half of all men will have at least one bout of prostatitis – an inflammation of the prostate gland – sometime in their lives. Although this condition is more common among young men, it can occur at any age.

♦ *Non-bacterial prostatitis* is the most common type. Symptoms include discomfort in your groin, pain on ejaculation, trouble with erections and possibly pain in your abdomen or back. You may notice a burning sensation when you urinate and/or an unusual discharge. You may also feel the need to urinate more often, especially at night.

Doctors aren't sure what causes this type of prostatitis. The condition is generally considered more of a nuisance than anything else. In many cases it clears up on its own. Your doctor may recommend warm sitz baths (immersing the area in a special tub filled with warm water that is placed on the toilet). If this doesn't work, he may recommend a prolonged course of antibiotics.

♦ *Acute bacterial prostatitis* is less common, but more serious. It occurs when bacteria in your bladder or urethra cause an infection of the prostate gland. Common symptoms include swelling, heat and pain in the area of the prostate, burning on urination, a cloudy discharge from the penis, murky-looking urine and a fever that may be fairly high and is often accompanied by flu-like aches and pains.

Is there a male menopause?

If "menopause" is defined as a dramatic decrease in estrogen produced by the ovaries, then it's quite clear that men – who don't have ovaries and who produce only very small amounts of estrogen in their bodies – don't experience menopause.

But men do experience subtle hormonal changes as they grow older, and there's some evidence that these changes may affect your health and well-being later in life.

Recent studies have shown that levels of the male hormone testosterone begin to decline when you're in your 40s. Testosterone, which is produced in your testicles and regulated by the pituitary gland at the base of your brain, serves a number of functions: It plays a role in stimulating sexual desire and is involved in maintaining your muscle strength and bone density. Another substance, growth hormone, also declines with age and this may be partly to blame for decreasing muscle tone or "flabbiness," which is common in older men.

Does this mean that older men would benefit from hormone replacement therapy? Some research has shown that healthy men over 70 who were given testosterone injections experienced increases in muscle strength and said they felt more interested in sex. But other researchers point out that most healthy men continue to produce all the testosterone they need until past the age of 90. They say decreased muscular strength and problems with sexual desire in older men have less to do with hormonal changes than with other physical and/or psychological factors (see opposite).

If it isn't treated promptly and properly, acute bacterial prostatitis can lead to an abscess or a serious blood infection. Treatment usually involves a course of antibiotics to kill the bacteria, and in some cases, it may be necessary to have a catheter or voiding tube inserted temporarily to help you empty your bladder.

Prostate cancer (see page 138)

Some common sexual problems in older men

Many men enjoy healthy, active, satisfying sexual activity well into their 70s, 80s and even 90s. In fact, the main reasons for sexual inactivity later in life aren't related to sexual dysfunction at all, but to the presence of other health problems and the lack of a willing partner.

If you are still having a sexual relationship or relationships, you should be aware of certain problems that can interfere with your ability to participate in and enjoy sex. Sometimes these problems bothered you when you were younger, or they may have developed for the first time in your later years. Because it usually takes two for healthy, happy sex, you should also be aware of any problems your partner may be having (see page 182).

Inhibited sexual desire

You have no real desire for sex – either sex with a partner or sexual release through masturbation. If you're alone, or if you and your partner don't really miss sex, then this shouldn't be a problem. But if your partner is still interested, you may feel pressured to have sex to please her or him and this can lead to feelings of resentment over time.

Many older people (and younger ones, too) feel uncomfortable discussing sexual problems openly. This is especially true for men who have been made to feel that they must "perform" sexually. However, if you're having problems, it may be worthwhile discussing them with your doctor. He will want to examine you for any underlying physical conditions or medication side effects that could be interfering with healthy sexual function. If the problem is emotional, he may recommend that you speak to a therapist who helps men overcome sexual problems.

Arousal problems

You feel interested in sex but have trouble achieving or maintaining an erection. Some doctors still refer to this condition as "impotence," although the term has negative connotations that are making it less popular.

Erectile difficulty is an extremely common, even universal condition, and most men will experience it at some time during their lives. The problem is often temporary, but men become extremely anxious about it, and anxiety only makes the situation worse. As you already know, the surest way to delay, prevent or interrupt an erection is to worry about it!

Problems with erection can be caused by many factors, and it's rare to have just one factor involved. A psychological component – for example, anxiety about work, money or the relationship itself – is more common among younger men. If you're over 65, chances are greater that your trouble is due to some physical problem.

The most common culprits are diabetes, atherosclerosis (which affects blood supply to the erectile tissue in the penis), smoking, alcohol consumption, obesity and the use of certain drugs, including those to control high blood pressure.

Early or premature ejaculation

This inability to delay ejaculation affects about one-third of all men at some time in their lives. It becomes a problem when your sexual enjoyment is decreased because the act simply doesn't last as long as you might like. Or it can cause problems if it interrupts your partner's ability to enjoy sexual intercourse.

If you suffer from this problem and it's interfering with enjoyable sex, speak to your doctor, who may suggest some techniques that might help. Or he may recommend that you and your partner seek counseling from a therapist.

But older men may find that being able to control ejaculation isn't as important to satisfying sex as they once thought it was. There are many avenues to sexual pleasure for you and your partner that don't rely on male stamina and lengthy, athletic episodes of sexual intercourse (see page 48).

Breast disease: Not just for women

Most people think that breast disease is a female problem, but this isn't true: Older men can also develop breast problems.

Gynecomastia

Benign enlargement of the breast is the most common breast abnormality affecting men. Studies show that between 35 and 65 percent of adult men show signs of gynecomastia. This may be a gradual, painless enlargement of one or both breasts, or you may develop a painful, tender mass in the breast area, particularly under your nipple.

If you notice any changes in how your breasts look or feel, mention it to your doctor. He will want to rule out the possibility of male breast cancer.

Although the cause of gynecomastia isn't known, in about 25 percent of all cases doctors think that an imbalance between the female hormone estrogen (which is present in men's bodies too) and the male hormones is involved. This condition can also occur as a side effect of many commonly prescribed drugs – certain antibiotics, anti-ulcer medications, drugs used during chemotherapy to fight cancer, cardiovascular medications, tranquilizers and antidepressants. Other factors related to gynecomastia are malnutrition, cirrhosis of the liver, testicular tumors and thyroid disease.

Most cases of gynecomastia don't need to be treated, once more serious disease has been ruled out. But if the condition is painful or if the size of your breasts is causing you to feel upset or embarrassed, your doctor may suggest treatment, including the withdrawal of drugs that may be causing the problem. Other treatment involves the use of drugs such as clomiphene. If this doesn't work, surgical removal of excess breast tissue may be considered.

Breast enlargement may also be due to cysts, benign fatty growths, abnormalities of blood and lymphatic vessels, and breast cancer.

Male breast cancer

This fairly rare disease accounts for fewer than 1 percent of all breast cancers. Compared with female breast cancer, relatively little is known about breast cancer in men. Your risk seems to increase with age, and the disease is more common among white Jewish men. Some researchers now believe there may be a genetic component, but more research is needed in this area.

Male breast cancer also seems to be related to prostate cancer. Older men who are being treated with estrogen have developed it – either as a direct result of taking the female hormones or because the cancer has spread from the prostate to the breast.

Even though it's rare, breast cancer in men is a serious disease. Because men haven't been encouraged to examine their breasts regularly or to go for breast screening, the condition is often missed by men and their doctors until it's in a later stage.

The most common symptoms of breast cancer are a lump or thickening (which may be painless or painful) in the breast or under the arm, dimpling of the skin and a discharge from the nipple. If you develop any of these symptoms, you should report them promptly to your doctor.

Breast cancer in men is diagnosed and treated in much the same way as it is in women. If your doctor suspects a problem, he will refer you for a special breast X-ray or ultrasound. You may also need to have a biopsy – either using a fine needle to remove cells or surgical removal of the lump – to check for malignancy (see page 136).

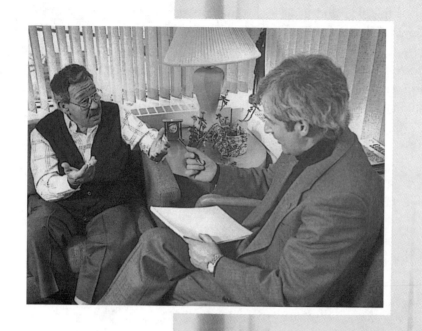

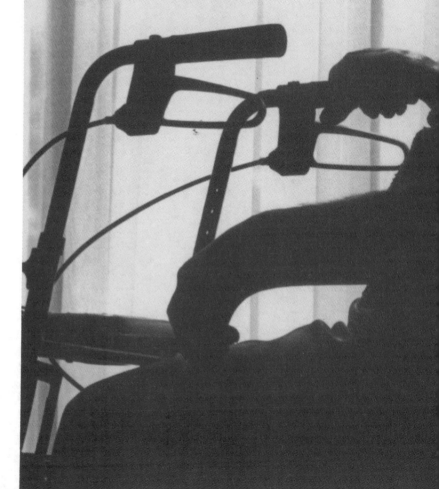

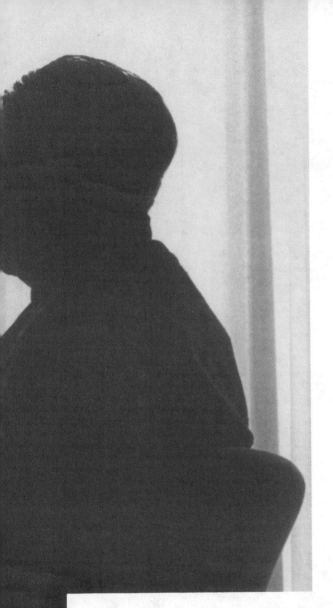

6

*The brain – is wider
than the Sky.*

EMILY DICKINSON

Problems of the Brain, Behavior and Emotions

THIS CHAPTER WILL DISCUSS A GROUP of disorders that cause great pain and suffering for many older people and their families. While these ailments certainly occur in people under 65, they tend to become more common with advancing age and can seriously affect both the quality and the length of your later years.

Doctors used to believe that these afflictions were purely psychological (in the mind), and therefore quite different from diseases such as cancer or heart disease, which were considered to be purely physiological (in the body).

Today we know that this belief is incorrect. Over the past 20 years, researchers have uncovered the complex connection that exists between mind and body. For example, it's been shown that psychological stress can weaken the immune system, leaving you more vulnerable to infection. If you suffer from a so-called physical disease such as asthma or arthritis, you already know that worry and stress have the power to make your symptoms worse.

Researchers have also learned that many so-called diseases of the mind – depression, dementia and schizophrenia, among others – are primarily biological disorders. They affect the structure and chemistry of the brain, producing abnormalities in thought, behavior and emotion.

This is an important piece of information, especially if you or someone in your family is affected by one of these disorders. In the past, these illnesses possessed a tremendous stigma, and people associated them with being "crazy" or "mentally ill." Feelings of shame, guilt and anger were common, and people often told themselves or the sufferer that if only he or she "tried harder," the symptoms would go away.

Even if you know that such reactions are wrong, it can be difficult to shed old prejudices and fears when it comes to mental or emotional illness. The good news is that many of these problems can be identified and some – particularly various mood disorders – can be controlled or even cured.

The best time to read about these problems is now – before they happen. That way you can avoid needless worrying and recognize genuine early signs if they occur. You'll also be better prepared to handle what lies ahead.

Choosing a doctor for your mental or emotional concerns

Like most people, you probably feel more confident about finding a good cardiologist or dermatologist than choosing someone to help you with a mental or emotional problem. If you or someone you love is suffering from any of the disorders mentioned here,

A consumer's guide to psychotherapy

Psychotherapy refers to various types of talking therapy that can help you gain insight into yourself and your behavior. The result of this insight is that you're better able to cope with problems and you experience fewer symptoms.

Some mental and emotional problems respond well to psychotherapy alone. But there's a growing trend toward seeing psychotherapy as just one aspect of successful treatment. It's now known that many disorders such as depression and anxiety may also require medication.

Psychotherapy may be *individual* (just you and the therapist), *family* (you and your spouse or other relatives), or *group* (you and other people with the same problem). How often you go for therapy (monthly, weekly, several times a week) is usually determined in consultation with the therapist. Here are some of the most common types of psychotherapy:

◆ *Cognitive-behavioral therapy* is used to help you correct negative thinking that can contribute to problems such as depression and anxiety. For example, you may tend to "catastrophize" everything that happens, making problems seem much worse than they really are. Or you may generalize – "I'm not good at this, so therefore I'm terrible at everything I do."

◆ *Psychodynamic therapy* works by helping you understand what certain problems mean to you in the context of your individual personality and early development. For example, if you often feel incapable of handling stress, you may discover that your parents were extremely critical of you early in life and you have no real sense of self-worth. The therapist is there to empathize and help you recognize these patterns and replace negative thoughts with more positive ones.

◆ *Behavior therapy* helps you gain control over certain problems by teaching you how to change unwanted behaviors and reactions. For example, you may learn that your anxious feelings can be prevented through controlled breathing or other self-relaxation techniques. Or you may discover that a certain aspect of your environment – for example, being alone all day – triggers unpleasant thoughts or physical symptoms. Therapy encourages you to recognize and accept these patterns of behavior and take greater control – in this case, you may be encouraged to interact more with people during the day.

the best place to start is with your primary care doctor or family physician.

If your doctor decides to refer you to a specialist, tell him you would prefer, if possible, to consult someone who is experienced in treating older adults. There are many reasons for this.

You need someone who understands the specific problems, including the psychological and social issues, of older adults.

You need someone who is skilled in prescribing medication for older patients, who are probably taking drugs for other health problems. Doctors who don't treat many older people may not understand that a 79-year-old patient often reacts differently to psychotherapy and drugs than does a 39-year-old patient.

You need someone who is comfortable dealing with questions, including concerns raised by family members.

You may be referred to one of the following specialists:

◆ *Psychiatrists* are medical doctors who specialize in the treatment of mental disorders such as depression, anxiety disorders and psychosis. In addition to diagnosing these conditions, psychiatrists may prescribe medication and treat patients through various forms of psychotherapy or "talk therapy."

◆ *Geriatric psychiatrists* are psychiatrists who have extra training and experience in treating older adults.

◆ *Neurologists* are medical doctors who specialize in diseases of the nervous system such as Parkinson's disease, Alzheimer's disease and stroke.

◆ *Behavioral neurologists* are specially trained neurologists who specialize in diagnosing and treating disorders such as Alzheimer's disease and other causes of dementia. They perform specialized, in-depth neurological assessments and may order various brain-scanning techniques to investigate problems.

◆ *Psychologists* are professionals with post-graduate training that equips them to undertake special testing of mental functions and to provide various types of therapy. Neuropsychologists specialize in assessing people for disorders of the brain such as Alzheimer's disease, while clinical psychologists test and counsel people with mental and emotional disorders. In some cases, these services may not be fully covered by your health insurance.

◆ *Social workers* are professionals who are trained to provide individual or group counseling. If you are facing a difficult situation such as a physical or emotional illness, or if you are facing family conflicts, they can provide support and guidance. They also help an individual or family facing a crisis or some difficult decision – for example, when a spouse or parent can no longer live independently (see page 259).

◆ *Occupational therapists* and *speech language pathologists* may also be involved in your treatment, depending on the nature of your difficulties.

◆ *Pastoral counselors* are members of the clergy who help people and their families cope with personal problems and crises.

Many older people are reluctant to follow their doctor's advice to seek specialized help for problems such as depression or anxiety. They may be eager for the doctor to prescribe tranquilizers or other similar medications that they hope will magically make their symptoms vanish.

There are many reasons for this kind of hesitation. Perhaps you grew up believing that such troubles should be kept private and are "nobody else's business." You may be reacting to the stigma that still surrounds mental and emotional illness. Older men may feel especially ashamed of owning up to emotional problems, which they see as a kind of weakness, and they may also have more trouble than women when it comes to talking about their feelings.

You should never avoid getting help for any of these reasons. Today we understand that many mental and emotional problems are just as real and treatable as physiological problems. Remember – if your doctor recommends specialized treatment, it's because she believes it can help you feel better.

However, don't be passive about staying with a therapist if you don't notice any improvement after a reasonable length of time. Let your doctor know how you feel. Sometimes a different approach or a change of therapist is necessary.

Aging and memory – "Your face is familiar but ..."

By the time you've reached 65, you may have noticed that your memory isn't what it used to be. You're constantly forgetting where you put your glasses, you can't recall

How to keep or improve your memory

If you want to keep your memory sharp for as long as you possibly can, here's what you should do:

◆ Maintain a healthy lifestyle. Poor nutrition, smoking, stress and lack of physical activity can all contribute to memory problems by depleting your energy. If you lack energy, it's harder to be mentally active and alert.

◆ Develop habits for lifelong learning. This means keeping mentally active by reading challenging material, writing in a journal, taking a course, learning a new skill, attending lectures or doing puzzles.

◆ Spend time with people who are interested in new ideas and enjoy challenging conversations. Studies have shown that just living with a bright, mentally active person can actually benefit your own mental abilities.

◆ Live in a way that encourages a sense of mastery and control. Research has shown

that people who feel in charge of their lives function at a higher level than those who feel they're at the mercy of circumstance.

If your memory isn't what it used to be, and the problem isn't related to illness or medication use, here are some strategies to help improve it:

◆ Avoid doing too many things at once – for example, don't talk on the telephone and try to follow a complicated recipe at the same time.

◆ Use lists to keep track of day-to-day information. These lists should be accessible and written on large pieces of paper or in a notebook rather than on tiny, easily lost scraps.

◆ Free your mind from too many details by keeping an appointment diary and calendar. Note appointments, tasks and birthdays, marking them in red on a large month-by-month calendar. Then each week, transfer

the name of your grandson's newest girl-friend or you leave home and find yourself fretting about whether or not you remembered to lock the front door.

Forgetfulness like this can happen at any age. But when you're older, you may worry that such lapses are an early sign of Alzheimer's disease or another kind of dementia. Excessive worrying can actually make a relatively minor memory problem worse, which only causes you and those around you to worry even more.

How does your memory work?

Memory is an amazingly complex process. Each day your brain is bombarded by countless bits of information that must be registered, stored and retrieved. How these bits are stored determines how easily they will be retrieved or remembered later. For instance, anything interfering with the storage process – being distracted or not paying attention – will probably make the memories more difficult to access later on.

Researchers have identified two basic types of memory. Short-term memory is what you can hold in your mind at any given moment – for example, a new name or a seven-digit telephone number. Long-term memory involves three types of remembering: *semantic memory* (being able to summon up knowledge of geography and history), *procedural memory* (recalling how to drive a car or play the piano) and *episodic*

---

the information to a smaller, week-at-a-glance diary. Each morning check your list, crossing off what you've done and adding anything else that comes up during the day. Anything that's left over can then be added to the next day's list.

◆ Use other memory aids such as timers, watches with alarms or buzzers, and specially designed medication trays that you fill once each week so you don't forget to take your pills.

◆ Develop regular checking routines and reinforce them by talking out loud. For instance, when you leave home, routinely check to see that the appliances are turned off, that the door is locked, and that you have everything you need in your purse or pocket. Tick off each action when you do it by saying: "I've shut off the stove," or "The front door is locked."

◆ Use exaggeration, imagination and humor to improve your memory. Let's say you're introduced to someone named Norma Greenberg and you don't want to forget her name. Listen to the name and repeat it to yourself once or twice. Try to associate the name with something significant or memorable – in this case, imagine the actress Norma Shearer and then visualize a green iceberg. Presto – Norma Greenberg!

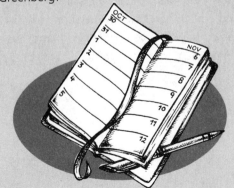

memory (recalling everyday events such as where you left your keys).

Aging doesn't seem to affect very short-term memory – for example, being able to remember the phone number you just looked up. But when you reach 60, your everyday, episodic memory does begin to decline.

Researchers have discovered some fascinating facts about how memory works. They've found that events that provoke an emotional response seem to become more deeply ingrained in our memories. That's why you can still recall certain "firsts" in your life – your first kiss, your first car – even though they happened more than 50 years ago. Smell is another powerful memory trigger. The scent of baby shampoo may bring back a forgotten moment with your children, while a whiff of a stranger's perfume may remind you of a friend or lover you haven't thought about for many years.

 What are the most common causes of memory loss in people over age 65?

Although aging is clearly a factor in certain types of memory loss, it's not uncommon for people to retain excellent memories well into their 70s, 80s and even 90s. Studies have shown that older people are still able to learn and remember new information. In some cases, they can even be taught to improve a failing memory. Here are some factors that may be involved in poor memory function:

♦ overmedication, especially with sedatives and tranquilizers, or interactions between drugs, including over-the-counter medication;

♦ alcohol abuse;

♦ depression or other mood disorders;

♦ a history of multiple small strokes;

♦ chemical imbalances such as low levels of vitamin B_{12} and abnormal levels of blood sugar or thyroid hormones;

♦ physical illness such as bacterial infection, flu or pneumonia;

♦ malnutrition and/or dehydration caused by a poor diet and inadequate fluid intake;

♦ social isolation caused by illness, poverty and other social factors.

Recently researchers have discovered other possible causes of memory loss. These include a history of mild head injury that may cause subtle brain damage, and chronic, untreated high blood pressure, which seems to damage small arteries in the brain, making oxygen supply less efficient.

Of course, sometimes memory loss can be an early sign of a more serious problem such as Alzheimer's disease and other illnesses that cause dementia (see opposite). If you or someone you know is experiencing ongoing memory problems, it's vital to consult your doctor.

Alzheimer's disease and other dementias

When you were younger, you might have heard someone refer to a grandparent or another elderly person as "senile." Until fairly recently, most people – including doctors – believed that confusion and memory loss were just a normal part of aging, something to be expected if you lived beyond age 75 or 80.

Not only was this belief false, but it almost certainly contributed to a widespread fear of growing older. Fortunately, doctors don't talk about senility anymore. They now understand that such symptoms aren't a natural consequence of long life and are due instead to a group of disorders known as "dementias."

Dementia

Dementia is a term used to describe what happens when disease causes the progressive deterioration of brain structures and functions such as language, perception, memory and awareness. As these vital abilities deteriorate, the sufferer finds it increasingly difficult to function independently.

Often there is an emotional component to dementia, and the sufferer may become agitated, anxious, depressed or withdrawn. These emotional changes may be part of the actual disease process, but they can also be understood as a normal reaction to difficult circumstances. For example, imagine that you can no longer understand what people are saying to you, yet they keep saying it over and over again. This would probably make you feel angry or upset. Or think about being unable to dress yourself, read a book or watch television. This would almost certainly make you feel unhappy and withdrawn.

 What are the common types of dementia affecting older adults?

To say that you are suffering from dementia is like saying you have a pain in your stomach. Stomach pain can have many causes – some of them are serious and irreversible, while others are fairly benign and usually reversible.

Likewise, some types of dementia are irreversible, while others may respond to certain types of intervention and be halted or improved. Some older people develop dementia-like symptoms due to drugs or combinations of drugs, and if they are correctly diagnosed, they are almost always reversible.

A recent study surveyed people age 65 and over and found that about 8 percent suffered from some kind of dementia. Researchers also found that the prevalence of dementing illness increased with age:

- 18 percent of cases were 65 to 74;
- 43 percent of cases were 75 to 84;
- 39 percent of cases were 85 and older.

A case history of Alzheimer's disease

At age 62 Helen* seemed quite healthy except for mild diabetes. She worked part-time as a secretary for a small office supply company and was normally a diligent and reliable worker. However, her supervisor began to notice that Helen was typing the same letters for him to sign two and even three times. She would also go to the mail room to pick up his mail, then return to her desk having forgotten to bring along the stack of letters.

At home her husband discovered that she was putting folded laundry into the wrong drawers, mixing up her clothing with his, and hanging damp shirts in his closet because she hadn't put them in the dryer. He started finding little scraps of paper around the house with lists and notes Helen had left herself about such everyday activities as using the stove.

Over the next six months Helen began to show subtle changes in her personality and behavior. Normally a soft-spoken, tidy person who took great pride in her appearance, she started having arguments with her two grown daughters and often wore the same clothes two or three days in a row. She was still functioning at her job, but only because a helpful co-worker was checking her work.

By this time Helen's husband and daughters were becoming concerned. When they asked if anything was bothering her, she denied it, blaming her mistakes at work and at home on "being tired." When her daughter suggested she see the doctor for a checkup, Helen became hysterical, accusing her family of spying on her. Finally, one of Helen's daughters made an appointment and simply took her mother to see her family physician. The doctor examined Helen and found her healthy except for the fact that her diabetes had worsened. He told Helen's family that her symptoms were probably related to an unstable blood sugar level and he changed her medication. This stabilized her blood sugar, but there was no change in her mental state.

A month later Helen's company told her that she was no longer needed, and she decided to retire from work. She no longer seemed to enjoy reading or gardening but instead began to spend most of her time alone in her bedroom. Her husband was now doing most of the shopping and cooking, and some mornings he would find Helen standing in the bathroom, her hair covered with soap that she had neglected to rinse off in the shower.

She refused to see the doctor again, insisting she was fine. While her husband was at work, she would wander around the neighborhood mall, greeting people she knew and even strangers with the same phrase, "Hello, my but you look nice." Sometimes she would repeat the words "nice, nice, nice."

One day Helen didn't come home from the mall at all, and her frantic husband called the police. She was brought home by a police officer who had found her sitting in a Laundromat at midnight.

Finally Helen's daughters convinced her to see a neurologist, and after a week of testing, the doctor told her family she was probably suffering from Alzheimer's disease.

* Note: "Helen" is a pseudonym and the details of her story are not based on the actual experience of any one patient. This case history is a composite that shows the typical progression of Alzheimer's symptoms.

Alzheimer's disease is by far the most common type of dementia. It accounts for more than two-thirds of all dementing illness among people over age 65 (see below). Other less common types of true dementia are vascular dementia, dementia associated with Parkinson's disease and dementia associated with depression.

Sometimes dementia-like symptoms can be caused by metabolic disturbances, such as infection, malnutrition and thyroid disorder. They may also occur as a side effect of certain drugs or combinations of drugs. Older people who must adjust to a new living environment, such as a nursing home, sometimes develop memory problems or other signs of mental confusion. That's because, in the past, they relied on the familiar surroundings of their home or apartment to help them compensate for memory loss. In a new setting, they find it much harder to function. Confusion, memory and other dementia-like symptoms can also occur in older people experiencing psychological trauma from abuse.

Alzheimer's disease

If you're like most people over 65, you're probably worried about the possibility that you, your partner or an elderly parent will begin to show signs of Alzheimer's disease. This anxiety is so common that perfectly healthy people who misplace their keys a few times will make an anxious call to their doctor, asking if they have Alzheimer's disease.

Fortunately, most complaints like this about memory loss don't turn out to be Alzheimer's disease. But even so, it's a good idea to learn as much as you can about the disease now, so that you are able to recognize genuine early warning signs if they

occur (see page 202). You will also be better prepared for what will happen should you or a loved one develop this difficult illness. Finally, if you know something about the condition, you're less likely to engage in useless worrying about normal memory changes that occur with aging.

What is Alzheimer's disease?

Alzheimer's disease involves a gradual but dramatic deterioration affecting nerve cells in the brain. Cells die off, causing the brain to function abnormally and shrink in size. Researchers who study the brains of Alzheimer's victims have noted the presence of abnormalities – so-called plaques and tangles – in the brain tissue, as well as unnatural clumps of a substance called beta amyloid protein.

This degeneration interferes with the brain's vital functions. The result is a variety of disorders, including impaired language and memory, lack of awareness and changes in personality and behavior. The disease is progressive, which means it gets worse over time, and eventually most sufferers become so impaired that they need round-the-clock supervision and care. The disease always ends in death, either directly or indirectly, usually five to ten years after onset, although some people die much sooner and a few survive longer.

What are the stages of Alzheimer's disease?

Alzheimer's disease follows a generally typical course.

The onset of symptoms is usually gradual, and the changes may not be obvious to the casual observer. Symptoms progress at a fairly steady rate, and while they may

Common changes in behavior and personality in Alzheimer's disease

◆ repetitive behavior or speech;

◆ tendency to lose personal belongings;

◆ depression and withdrawal;

◆ agitation and/or angry outbursts;

◆ restlessness, wandering (especially at night);

◆ disturbed sleep-wake habits;

◆ mood swings from crying to laughter and back again;

◆ lack of recognition of familiar places or people;

◆ loss of judgment and awareness, which may result in inappropriate social behavior.

sometimes fluctuate and improve, such improvements are only temporary. The early signs may include loss of memory and changes in language and expression.

As the disease progresses, memory becomes more impaired. For example, the person may be able to recall a past event, but the details are missing. Changes in behavior and habits become more obvious, especially to family members. As the person loses the ability to navigate, episodes of wandering may occur and she may become lost in familiar surroundings.

In the later stages of the disease, the person often becomes less physically active and more withdrawn. Language abilities are severely affected, and communication becomes difficult. She may no longer recognize her husband or children or even her own face in the mirror.

Physical symptoms such as muscle rigidity are also common, and the person is no longer able to dress or feed herself. Swallowing becomes difficult, and incontinence is common. Toward the end the sufferer often loses weight and becomes weak and bedridden.

When death finally comes, it is not due to Alzheimer's disease itself but is caused by other factors such as pneumonia or kidney infection.

? Who is most likely to get Alzheimer's disease?

No one knows the exact cause of Alzheimer's disease, but researchers have identified certain people who are at especially high risk.

Your risk for Alzheimer's increases with age, doubling every five years after age 65. By the time you reach 85, you have a one-in-three chance of getting the disease.

Your risk also increases if someone in your family had Alzheimer's disease, especially before age 65. This suggests the disease has a major genetic component.

In recent years scientists have isolated three genes that may be associated with the development of Alzheimer's. They think mutations in these genes contribute to the abnormal buildup of beta amyloid protein found in the brains of people with the disease.

A recent theory – still unproven – has linked the development of Alzheimer's with a history of severe head injury, particularly in people who carry the mutated genes. Some researchers believe the disease may occur when some type of injury to the brain – for example, a head injury or small stroke – prompts the body to produce beta amyloid protein in an attempt to heal the injury. If you happen to carry the defective genes, your body overproduces the protein, leading to an abnormal buildup that results in Alzheimer's disease.

Another popular theory about the cause of Alzheimer's disease involves the ingestion of aluminum, an abundant element found in soil, water, plants and animal tissues. It is also added to a variety of processed foods and non-prescription drugs such as antacids, and many people cook food in aluminum pots and pans.

Several years ago scientists reported finding high levels of aluminum in the brain cells of people who died from Alzheimer's disease. But many other researchers say this doesn't establish clear cause and effect, and they consider the aluminum theory unlikely.

? How is Alzheimer's disease diagnosed?

A definite diagnosis of Alzheimer's disease can only be made after death. An autopsy, which includes a post-mortem study of the brain, reveals the presence of abnormal plaques and tangles, and clumps of beta amyloid protein – the classic pathological signs of Alzheimer's disease.

Recently researchers have found that people with Alzheimer's show elevated levels of a substance called glutamine synthetase in their spinal fluid. This may be related to the buildup of beta amyloid protein in the brain. If the research is verified, this could one day lead to a simpler diagnostic test for the disease.

Until such a test is developed, however, doctors must diagnose Alzheimer's by observing the person and excluding other conditions that could be causing symptoms of memory loss and confusion.

? How are you tested for Alzheimer's disease?

If your doctor thinks you or a loved one may have Alzheimer's disease, here's what you can expect:

◆ Your doctor will take a thorough *history of symptoms*. Because people in the early stages of Alzheimer's tend to deny their problems, he will probably speak to family members, who are usually the first to notice memory loss and behavioral changes.

◆ Your doctor will carry out *a complete physical examination,* including laboratory tests to detect signs of underlying disease – for example, infections, diabetes, anemia and endocrine disease – that could be causing or aggravating symptoms. This process may take several days, and in most cases can be done on an out-patient basis. He may also do a *mental status exam* (see page 204).

At this point your doctor may decide to refer you to a neurologist for further investigation – especially if the test results don't rule out Alzheimer's disease or some other dementing illness.

The next set of tests may include the following:

◆ *An electroencephalogram*: This painless test measures brain waves and may detect other problems causing symptoms of dementia such as a tumor or seizures.

Advice for Alzheimer's caregivers

As Alzheimer's disease progresses, the ill person requires more supervision, and it often becomes extremely difficult for family caregivers to cope.

If you're the spouse of someone with Alzheimer's, you may be over 65 yourself. You must face the physical and emotional demands of caring for your partner, while at the same time you may be experiencing your own physical illness or other limitations. If you're caring for a parent with Alzheimer's, you may feel trapped between your own needs and those of your aging parents.

The issues raised by Alzheimer's and other dementing illness are complex. Is your relative safe at home? Is he competent to drive and to manage personal and financial affairs? Will he have to be placed in an institution?

It's true that institutional care is usually necessary in the final stages of Alzheimer's, when caregiving demands become overwhelming. But certain strategies can make caring for someone with Alzheimer's at home much easier for both patient and caregiver:

◆ Don't neglect your relative's physical and psychological health. People with Alzheimer's disease can and do develop other problems that cause pain and discomfort. Because those with Alzheimer's can't express themselves clearly, the symptoms may be masked by aggressive behaviors such as shouting or pleading. Also be alert to signs of depression, which often develops in people with Alzheimer's and which can make problem behaviors much worse. Once the depression is treated with antidepressant medication, the situation usually improves. Report any major or sudden change in physical appearance, mood, and eating and sleeping habits to your relative's doctor.

◆ *Brain scans*: Traditional X-rays aren't very useful in investigating dementia, but three relatively new techniques – Computerized Axial Tomography (CAT) scan, Single Positron Emission Computerized Tomography (SPECT) and Magnetic Resonance Imaging (MRI) – can give your doctor a useful picture of brain structures and function. These tests, which are painless and non-invasive, can help your doctor rule out other problems such as a tumor or stroke. They can also show areas of shrinkage or deterioration in people with more advanced Alzheimer's disease or other dementing illness.

◆ *Spinal tap*: This isn't done too often anymore, but your doctor may want to obtain a sample of cerebrospinal fluid to rule out diseases like syphilis that can cause symptoms of dementing illness. The procedure involves inserting a needle into the spinal canal to withdraw fluid. The fluid is then examined in a laboratory.

◆ *Neuropsychological tests*: These have been developed to identify signs of cognitive impairment. For example, you might be asked by the tester, usually a psychologist, to recite the details of a story after hearing it

◆ Try to spread the caregiving responsibilities among family members and close friends. Too often one person takes on the bulk of these tasks and can feel overwhelmed and resentful, especially when other relatives could pitch in. Once a diagnosis of Alzheimer's disease has been made, it's important to have one or more family meetings to make a plan and discuss sharing responsibilities. Don't assume that others won't help. For example, teenage grandchildren can be asked to take on certain household chores or to spend time with an ailing grandparent while you go out for an hour or take a nap.

◆ You can't do everything yourself. Take advantage of community support services. They can provide friendly visiting, homemaker services and nursing care, supervised adult day care and overnight respite care so you can take a vacation or attend to your own personal, social and health needs (see page 261). Your family doctor or a social worker can put you in touch with the appropriate agencies.

◆ Look for a caregivers' support group in your community, where you can meet with other people who are in the same situation. You can share ideas and strategies and ask questions, and you won't feel quite so alone. Alzheimer's Society chapters exist in most communities and are a valuable resource.

◆ If you think the stress is affecting your own health, particularly if you feel depressed, exhausted or physically ill, it may be time to increase the amount of outside help you're getting or to consider placing your relative in an institution where he will receive the best possible care. This is a difficult decision, but there are ways to make the choice and the transition easier (see page 259).

once. Or you may be shown pairs of words – related words such as "shoe" and "foot," and unrelated pairs such as "cat" and "flower" – and be asked to recall them later.

You may be asked to do simple subtraction tests that reveal impairments in mental function. For example, the tester will ask you to "subtract 7 from 100 and continue subtracting 7 as long as you can."

You may also be asked to identify various parts of a familiar object such as a watch. The tester will point to the wristband, the face and the hands and ask you to name them.

You may be asked to draw the face of a clock set at 11:10. Even in the early stages of dementia, people have trouble placing the minute hand on the number 2 and often place it on the 10 instead.

? How is Alzheimer's disease treated?

At the present time no treatment exists that can stop or reverse the progression of Alzheimer's disease. Various drugs have been tested in the hope that they might delay deterioration or improve mental function in people with Alzheimer's, but the results have been disappointing so far.

One drug, tetrahydroaminoacridine (Tacrine or Cognex), has been approved for use in the United States. However, the benefits have been modest and may be outweighed by the risks of liver damage, a side effect of the drug. Another drug being studied is selegiline (Deprenyl or Eldepryl), which is useful in the treatment of Parkinson's disease. Other drugs being tested include vasodilators, which improve blood flow to the brain; drugs that speed up nerve growth; and drugs that replace vital neurotransmitters, which may be depleted in people with Alzheimer's disease.

But even though no drug treatment exists, many advances have been made in the management of Alzheimer's disease. One aspect of treatment involves helping caregivers understand how someone with Alzheimer's disease sees his or her world. In this way, caregivers can minimize problems and help the person compensate for lost abilities. The goal of these strategies is to keep the sick person as active and independent as possible, to delay institutionalization and to minimize stress on caregivers.

What are some ways to manage problem behaviors?

One of the most upsetting aspects of caring for someone with Alzheimer's disease is managing difficult behaviors such as anger, agitation, withdrawal and wandering. The best way to minimize these behaviors is to recognize and eliminate certain triggers that can cause or aggravate them. Here are some tips to keep in mind:

◆ Try to maintain familiar surroundings and a regular schedule of meals and other activities. These provide a sense of security and prevent your relative from feeling frustrated or anxious.

◆ Your relative may have difficulty understanding symbolic language, so use concrete expressions. For example, it's better to say "Peter is coming to visit after lunch" than to say "We're going to have company later."

If you're going out to a restaurant, look for one that features a buffet selection. Choosing from foods that can be seen and smelled is much easier for someone with Alzheimer's disease than ordering from a menu.

◆ People with Alzheimer's often have trouble making choices, so avoid presenting your relative with unnecessary decisions. Instead of asking "Do you want to wear your blue sweater today?" say "Put on your blue sweater."

◆ Speak clearly and calmly. If you argue or try to use logic, your relative won't understand the words but may respond unfavorably to the negative emotions in your face and voice.

◆ It's known that early memories are usually well preserved, even in people with fairly advanced Alzheimer's disease, and this can be useful for caregivers. If your relative doesn't want to try something new (new experiences tend to be upsetting), try to connect the experience to something familiar. For example, your relative may not want to go to the optometrist to have his vision tested for new eyeglasses. Encourage him this way: "You know when we go for your new glasses we have to pass the swimming pool where we used to take the children. Do you remember the little gazebo on the lawn? We could see if it's still there."

- If your relative seems especially anxious, he probably needs extra reassurance with a gentle touch or smile.

- Fatigue is a common cause of upsetting behaviors. Limit activity schedules and encourage frequent rests.

- If your relative seems withdrawn and apathetic, you may be tempted to provide interesting diversions, thinking this will be helpful, when in fact, he may no longer be able to cope with such stimulation. Sometimes caregivers expect too much of a loved one, simply because they don't want to accept the inevitable. Make sure you have a realistic understanding of his current capacities.

- The environment should not be too stimulating. Bright lights, loud music and too many people can make someone with Alzheimer's anxious or even aggressive.

- If wandering is a problem, install door locks that are difficult to open. Try hanging a picture or mirror on the inside of your front door. This may encourage your relative to think it's a wall rather than an exit. Someone who tends to wander or has trouble navigating should wear an identification bracelet. Ask your local police department if they have a program that registers the names, photos and identifying details of potential wanderers.

- If your relative wants to continue driving a car, this may be unsafe (see page 88). Discuss this matter with your doctor, who may be able to suggest ways to discourage driving – for example, removing the person's car keys and driver's license. In many jurisdictions, doctors aware of such a situation are obligated to notify authorities, who will cancel the driver's license.

Some other causes of dementia in older adults

While Alzheimer's disease is the most common cause of dementia in older adults, it's by no means the only cause. Doctors divide dementing illnesses into two major groups.

Dementias caused by brain disease are caused by illnesses that directly affect the brain – for example, Alzheimer's disease, strokes (once called "multi-infarct dementia" and now known as vascular dementia), Parkinson's disease, Huntington's disease, Pick's disease and a group of rare viral illnesses, including Creutzfeldt-Jacob disease.

Dementias caused by general medical or other problems are caused by diseases in other parts of the body that can affect cognitive functioning. Some common diseases causing secondary dementia are depression (see page 210), Acquired Immune Deficiency Syndrome (AIDS) and Wilson's disease (a disorder in how the body metabolizes copper). Dementia-like symptoms can also occur as a side effect of certain drugs or combinations of drugs, and, once recognized, these are usually reversible.

Even doctors find it difficult to distinguish among these dementing illnesses, so if you or someone you love is showing symptoms, it's vital to seek medical help as early as possible.

A note about delirium

Sometimes an older person who shows signs of what appears to be dementia (such as memory loss and disorientation) is really suffering from another disorder known as delirium.

Unlike dementia, the symptoms of delirium usually develop suddenly over a period of a few hours or days. (Like depression, delirium can also develop in someone with a dementing illness.)

Symptoms of delirium often fluctuate – they appear, disappear, then reappear. They include sleep disturbances, mental confusion, hallucinations, agitation and emotional extremes such as intense anxiety or euphoria (exaggerated happiness).

Delirium in older adults is often triggered by acute infections that feature fever – for example, pneumonia, urinary tract infections and abscesses. Other known triggers are a head injury (signs of delirium appear immediately or a few weeks later), thyroid imbalances, kidney or liver disease, and intoxication from medications and drugs such as alcohol and barbiturates. When the underlying cause is removed, the delirium usually disappears.

Parkinson's disease

Parkinson's disease (PD) is the second most common neurological disorder affecting older adults (the first is stroke). The disease, which usually strikes between ages 50 and 65, affects about 1 percent of people over age 60 and 2 percent of those over age 70.

Like Alzheimer's disease, Parkinson's disease is progressive and there is no cure, but the outlook today is much brighter than it was a decade ago.

? **What causes Parkinson's disease?**

PD is caused by the loss of cells in an area of the brain called the "substantia nigra." These cells produce an important brain chemical called "dopamine" that helps keep levels of another chemical, acetylcholine, in balance. When 60 to 80 percent of the dopamine-producing cells have died off, symptoms of PD start to appear. Researchers still don't know why these cells begin to die.

? **What are the symptoms of PD?**

The symptoms of PD often begin so gradually that they are ignored by sufferers and their doctors, or else explained as "tiredness" or "just part of growing older." Although symptoms can differ widely among individuals, here are some common warning signs:

◆ *Early signs*: These include fatigue, aches and pains that range from vague to severe and tend to disappear after resting; tremors in hands or legs; slowed movements (feeling as though you are walking through water); loss of natural arm-swinging movements when walking; poor balance; muscle stiffness; trouble turning over in bed at night; tripping because the feet aren't being lifted off the ground normally; difficulty writing (feeling as though each letter must be painstakingly drawn); tremor in the limbs, especially when at rest; trouble with fine motor tasks such as buttoning clothes and fastening jewelry; mumbling and problems with pronunciation of words.

◆ *Later signs*: These include increased tremor of hands, feet or parts of the face; loss of balance and movement, often leading to falls; short, shuffling steps; the inability to stop walking and start again, especially backwards or sideways.

◆ *Other possible symptoms*: These include

mask-like facial expression; swallowing problems that can lead to excess saliva and drooling; forced closure of the eyelids.

? How is PD diagnosed?

A diagnosis of PD is usually made by a neurologist who observes symptoms and rules out other causes. For example, you can develop what doctors call "parkinsonian symptoms" without actually having Parkinson's disease.

Certain types of tremor are not related to PD. *Exaggerated "normal" tremor* may be caused by drugs such as amphetamines, antidepressants, some asthma preparations, alcohol (especially during withdrawal) and even large amounts of coffee. *Essential (or familial) tremor* is often present over the person's lifetime and worsens with aging. This hereditary tremor, which usually affects the hands and head but not the legs and feet, usually appears when the person reaches out for something (unlike the tremor of PD). However, in about 10 percent of people with PD, the tremors resemble essential tremors, which can make diagnosis difficult.

Other diseases and conditions that can mimic PD include head injury; hydrocephalus (pressure from water in the brain); progressive supranuclear palsy; certain viruses that affect the brain; a condition that closely resembles PD called "striatal nigral degeneration"; and Shy-Drager syndrome, a type of PD accompanied by extremely low blood pressure upon standing (orthostatic hypotension).

A diagnosis of PD is often devastating for sufferers and their families, but you should know that each person with the disease follows a different course. In some the disease progresses quickly, regardless of treatment, while others continue to enjoy a good quality of life for many years.

? How is PD treated?

Treatment for PD often begins with the drug selegiline (Deprenyl). Some studies suggest that if this drug is given early in the disease, it can delay the onset of disabling symptoms for one to two years. Anticholinergic drugs such as trihexyphenidyl (Artane) and benz-tropine (Cogentin) can also reduce tremors in the early stages, although they are not well tolerated by older people who experience unpleasant side effects.

The mainstay of PD treatment is two medications called Sinemet and Prolopa. These medications combine a drug called levodopa with other drugs. The levodopa resupplies the brain with dopamine, while the other drugs – carbidopa and benserazide – prevent the breakdown of levodopa in the body, allowing it to work more effectively at lower doses. Because these drugs can have side effects such as nausea, low blood pressure and hallucinations, they must be taken under close medical supervision. Improvement of PD symptoms after Sinemet is usually gradual – first rigidity lessens, then movement speeds up, and the person's gait and balance improve.

In recent years researchers have been studying the effect of diet on PD. It's known that protein, found in meat, fish, eggs and dairy products, can inhibit the body's absorption of Sinemet, so patients are often advised to take their medication about an hour before eating. Some doctors and nutritionists recommend that, if you are taking Sinemet and it isn't working, you may need to avoid eating protein-rich foods during the day and take in your daily protein requirement at dinner time. However this should only be done under medical supervision and should be avoided if you are underweight, are recovering from surgery or have diabetes. Some researchers are also looking at whether shifting the ratio of carbohydrates to protein (i.e., seven times as much carbohydrate as protein) can decrease PD symptoms.

If you have PD, exercise and physiotherapy are important. They allow you to maintain your muscle tone and fitness, which helps you to remain mobile. Your doctor may recommend exercises or refer you to a physiotherapist.

People with PD are at increased risk for serious depression – in fact, about half of all sufferers will experience some type of depression, which may be related to chemical changes in the brain. Fortunately, such depressions usually respond to treatment with antidepressant medication. Dementia is also quite common in the later stages of PD, affecting about one-third of all people with the disease.

Depression and other mood disorders

Doctors used to believe that depression was a disease of late life, affecting older people more frequently than younger ones. In fact, recent studies have shown that quite the opposite is true: Depression is slightly more common in people between the ages of 18 and 64 than it is among those over 65.

Even so, depression remains the most common psychiatric disorder among older adults, and it's particularly common among those who are hospitalized for illness or who are living in long-term care facilities. Depression causes untold misery for sufferers and their families alike, and in extreme cases it's so painful and debilitating that people consider and attempt suicide (see page 220).

The most common type of depressive ill-ness is major depression. Other types of depression that affect older adults include bipolar disorder (also known as "manic depression" – see page 217) and dysthymia (see page 219).

Depression can be a special problem in people over age 65 for several reasons:

◆ While younger people who are depressed tend to have classic symptoms of depression – sleep and appetite disturbances, crying, depressed mood – older people often develop physical symptoms that may mask the disorder. These include aches and pains, intestinal complaints, breathing problems and feelings of anxiety.

◆ When asked by a doctor if they feel

depressed, older people are more likely to deny feelings of hopelessness and despair.

◆ Doctors who lack experience with older patients may misdiagnose and mistreat depression, or they may believe it's a normal response to the pressures and losses of old age rather than an illness that can be treated.

◆ It's often easier for older people who no longer work or care for families to conceal their depression than it is for younger people, who must still show up at the office or take their children to school.

◆ Because of the stigma associated with depression and other mental illnesses, older people may be reluctant to seek help. They tend to turn their distress into physical symptoms and then seek medical attention for unexplained headaches, back pain and intestinal problems.

Depression

When doctors talk about the disease of depression, they aren't talking about occasional feelings of sadness or "the blues" that all of us experience from time to time. Depression is a serious condition that can have a variety of persistent physical, emotional and cognitive effects.

Physical effects

◆ *Appetite changes*: Your interest in eating dwindles and you lose weight and energy. In some cases depression may cause you to overeat and you gain weight quickly.

◆ *Sleep disturbances*: You wake up in the middle of the night or early in the morning and can't fall back to sleep. Oversleeping is another problem – you may sleep 12 to 14 hours at night but still not get out of bed the next morning or else return to bed very quickly.

◆ *Changes in energy*: You may feel slowed down, as though you were carrying a heavy weight around with you. Even the simplest tasks – getting dressed, making breakfast – seem like enormous obstacles. Some depressed people feel abnormally restless and are unable to sit still or relax their bodies.

◆ *Sexual problems*: If you enjoyed sexual activity before, you now feel a lack of interest and desire.

Emotional effects

◆ *Loss of pleasure*: You no longer enjoy what used to give you pleasure – hobbies, conversations with friends, a visit from someone you love.

◆ *Increased anxiety*: You feel nervous much of the time and may spend many hours worrying about your health or other problems in your life.

◆ *Sadness*: You feel despondent and often feel like crying. There may also be feelings of worthlessness and guilt.

Cognitive effects

◆ *Changes in concentration*: You seem unable to focus on what you're doing and have difficulty making even small decisions.

◆ *Impaired judgment*: You have trouble making accurate assessments and tend to exaggerate your own faults, blaming yourself for your illness. This loss of judgment may cause you to "catastrophize," turning minor events into major upsets.

What causes depression?

Although the exact cause of depression is unclear, there's good evidence that depressed people have abnormal levels of certain brain chemicals called "neurotransmitters." These chemicals, which transmit signals between brain cells, play a vital role in how you feel, think and behave. However, doctors still don't know if abnormal brain chemistry actually causes depression, or if this chemistry is merely the result of depressive illness.

It's unlikely that depression stems from a single cause. Most experts now think that certain factors such as heredity or childhood influences predispose you to the illness, while an event or combination of events – for example, stress caused by loss or change – actually triggers the symptoms. Here are some factors that have been implicated in depression.

Family history

If a close relative (a grandparent, parent or sibling) has suffered from depression, you are at increased risk. Although this suggests a genetic component to the illness, it's also possible that depression runs in families for other reasons – for example, children who are raised by a depressed parent may fail to learn healthy ways of coping with stress, and this can leave them vulnerable to depression. But this doesn't explain why depression is more likely to affect someone whose aunt, uncle or a distant grandparent suffered from it than someone who has no family history of depression.

Early loss

Researchers have noted a striking pattern of childhood loss among people who suffer from depression – for example, the early loss of a parent because of death, divorce or serious illness. This may cause deep-rooted emotional problems that leave them open to depression later in life, especially when they experience other losses.

Physical illness

Depression often accompanies physical illness, although researchers aren't sure why. It's possible that the stress of illness triggers depression, but in some cases – particularly with depression after stroke – biochemical changes in the brain may occur that cause depression.

Certain diseases and conditions that seem to trigger depression are more common in older adults – for example, cancer, chronic pain, stroke, Alzheimer's and Parkinson's diseases, thyroid failure and vitamin B_{12} deficiency. One study found that about half of all people who suffered a heart attack became clinically depressed, and more than 70 percent of them remained that way for at least a year.

Medication

Certain drugs that older people take to treat other illnesses are known to cause mood changes as a side effect (see page 214). If you think your depressed mood may be related to a medication, tell your doctor. She may decide to switch you to a different class of drug.

How do you know if you're depressed?

Every one of us feels unhappy, bitter or disappointed from time to time. While such emotions shouldn't be ignored, they don't necessarily mean that you're suffering from depression.

It's also easy to confuse certain age-related changes with depression – for example, if you're sleeping fewer hours than you used to, this may simply be a normal part of growing older and not a warning sign of depression.

You should seek medical advice if:

◆ you develop new signs and symptoms (see page 211) that trouble you most of the day, nearly every day, for a period of two weeks or longer;

◆ you experience significant weight loss not due to dieting, or significant weight gain: i.e., more than 5 percent of your total body weight in a month (if you normally weigh 150 pounds, this means a gain or loss of eight pounds within a month);

◆ you experience memory loss, confused thinking or difficulty concentrating (see page 196);

◆ you experience persistent depressed feelings and physical symptoms after being diagnosed with a serious or chronic illness, or following bereavement (see page 229);

◆ you have recurrent thoughts of death (not just fear of dying), thoughts of suicide without a specific plan, or a specific plan for committing suicide.

❓ How is depression diagnosed?

The good news about depression is that for most people, treatment can significantly relieve and even cure your symptoms. But before treatment can start, it's absolutely vital that the problem is properly recognized.

Sometimes people go to their doctor complaining that they feel depressed. In many cases, however, depression is diagnosed after you've sought help for a problem such as insomnia, digestive upset, headache or nervousness.

Your doctor may sometimes want to rule out underlying disease that might be causing these symptoms, so you may be asked to undergo a physical examination, including laboratory analysis of blood and urine. She will review your current medications, question you about your general mood and observe you for clues that may suggest depression – slowed speech and gestures, restless motions such as handwringing or pacing, stooped posture, irritability, a sad or empty expression, tearfulness or an unkempt appearance.

❓ How is depression treated?

Older people who suffer from depression tend to experience more rapid physical and mental deterioration than a younger person with the same illness. That's why depression in an older adult requires prompt and vigorous treatment, usually in the form of medication, psychotherapy, or a combination of medication and psychotherapy.

In some cases your family doctor or a geriatric specialist may be able to treat you for depression. But if your depression is incapacitating, if it doesn't respond to treatment, if it reoccurs or is accompanied by suicidal thoughts, you will probably be referred to a psychiatrist. The best specialist is a geriatric psychiatrist – if one is available in your

◆ *Benzodiazepines*, a class of tranquilizers, can cause symptoms of depression with chronic use.

◆ *Propranolol and other beta blockers* used to treat heart disease can cause depression.

◆ *Cimetidine, ranitidine* and other drugs used to treat ulcers can cause depression, especially in higher doses and in people with kidney disease.

◆ *Non-steroidal anti-inflammatory drugs (ibuprofen, indomethacin)* used to treat arthritis symptoms can cause depression.

◆ *Levodopa* used to treat symptoms of Parkinson's disease may cause mood changes.

◆ *Antihypertensive drugs* used to control high blood pressure can cause depression. One such medication, *reserpine*, is known to have depressive effects, especially at doses of 0.5 milligram or more daily, and most physicians no longer use it for this reason.

◆ *Sedative drugs such as barbiturates* may also cause depression.

community – or a psychiatrist with experience in treating older adults.

Medication

◆ *Antidepressant drugs:* This group of drugs has proved extremely effective in treating depression. While there are many kinds of antidepressant drugs, they all work in basically the same way, causing subtle changes in the brain's neurochemistry that seem to relieve symptoms.

Finding the best antidepressant for you can be a challenge. Don't be surprised if you have to try more than one drug before you find one that works well for you.

Many doctors continue to rely on well-established drugs known as tricyclic antidepressants. These drugs are often very effective in relieving depression, but they usually take some time – two to six weeks – to become fully effective. They may also have unpleasant side effects such as constipation,

dry mouth, blurred vision, urinary retention and drowsiness, and they may be less safe for people with heart disease than some of the newer drugs. Even though these side effects diminish or disappear after a few weeks, many older people find them especially difficult to tolerate and they may stop taking the medication altogether.

Your doctor may recommend an older tricyclic antidepressant such as imipramine (Tofranil) and doxepin (Sinequan). Although these can work well, a newer group of tricyclics – for example, nortriptyline (Aventyl) and desipramine (Norpramin) – seem to be better tolerated, especially by older people.

In recent years a new generation of antidepressant drugs known as SSRIs (selective serotonin reuptake inhibitors) has been developed. These drugs include fluoxetine (Prozac), sertraline (Zoloft), paroxetine (Paxil) and fluoxamine (Luvox). They also take between two and six weeks to show some benefits, and while they are usually (but not

When someone you know is depressed

It can be devastating to watch someone you love – a spouse, companion or aging parent – suffer from depression. Here are some things you can do to help.

◆ Insist that the person be seen by a doctor so the depression can be diagnosed and treated. If he refuses, understand that this is just part of the disease, and keep trying. Your doctor may be willing to make a house call or recommend a psychiatric outreach service that assesses people in their own homes.

◆ Treat the person as normally as you can, and encourage him to be as physically active as possible.

◆ Try not to add to the person's feelings of guilt by blaming him for his symptoms or getting angry because he won't "snap out of it." You need to realize that he can no more "snap out" of his illness than he could snap out of heart disease or diabetes. Avoid making useless statements such as "You have nothing to be depressed about," or "Try to think positively."

◆ If the person is supposed to take medication or attend therapy, make sure that he is following the doctor's orders. When medication or other therapy isn't working, don't count on him to raise the issue with his doctor. You may have to speak to the doctor yourself.

◆ Be alert for danger signs that could mean the person is at increased risk for suicide (see page 220), and if you notice them, tell his doctor right away.

◆ Finally, take care of yourself by eating properly, getting enough exercise and taking part in enjoyable activities with friends and family. Studies have shown that people who live with a depressed person are themselves more prone to depressed moods.

---

always) as effective as the older drugs, they tend to have fewer or at least more tolerable side effects. This makes them ideal for many older people. If you take one of these drugs, you may experience some nausea, headaches or agitation, but such side effects may disappear. Even so, they should always be reported to your doctor.

Finding the right dosage is extremely important. If the dose is too low, the drug won't be effective; if it's too high, you may experience unpleasant side effects. Recent studies have shown that older people can obtain relief with lower doses of antidepressant medication, so your doctor may adopt a "start low, go slow" approach.

Because antidepressants start to work only when they reach what doctors call a "therapeutic level" in your body, it's vital that you give these drugs enough time to work. This can be difficult if you're experiencing side effects, but most doctors recommend that you try each medication for at least four weeks before giving up and switching to a different drug.

Most people have to remain on antidepressant medication for many months, even after they begin to feel better. How long you continue to take the drug depends on your general health, the severity of the depression and whether your depressions tend to recur. You should never stop taking antidepressants suddenly, since this can cause problems. Instead, your doctor will advise you to taper the dosage down gradually. If your symptoms recur, you may have to take antidepressant drugs indefinitely.

◆ *Other drugs:* Many older people who suffer from depression are bothered by physical and emotional symptoms of anxiety that can be upsetting and debilitating. Until your antidepressant medication begins to work, your doctor may prescribe a mild tranquilizer to help you relax.

Psychotherapy

While medication is extremely important in the successful treatment of depression, supportive psychotherapy may also be helpful.

It's not uncommon for older people who are depressed to resist the idea of psychotherapy. You may not "believe in" psychotherapy as a way to resolve your problems. You may feel uncomfortable about discussing such personal, private matters with a stranger. Or, if you're extremely depressed, you may simply find it difficult to summon up enough energy to see a therapist.

But psychotherapy, which involves regular sessions of talking and listening to a therapist over a period of months, is extremely useful in treating depression for a number of reasons.

It can help you identify negative patterns that may be contributing to or aggravating your depression. For example, you may tend to put down your own accomplishments while at the same time you exaggerate how happy and successful other people are. You will be encouraged to understand these patterns in relation to your life experiences, including your childhood and your relationship with your family. This can relieve guilt and also help you start thinking more realistically and positively.

Psychotherapy can help you resolve current conflicts and issues that may be contributing to your depression. For example, you may be having family or financial problems, or perhaps you're experiencing stress due to retirement, chronic illness or the death of a spouse.

Finally, psychotherapy can help you deal with the negative emotional consequences of depressive illness. If you've been depressed, it's not uncommon to feel a sense of guilt and worthlessness. You may feel that you've let other people down by becoming ill, and you may worry that your life will never be the same. Just talking about these feelings with a supportive, knowledgeable therapist can be a great relief.

Psychotherapy can take many forms and occur in a variety of settings (see page 194). In some cases, a spouse or other family members may be encouraged to attend with you.

It's important that you find a therapist with whom you feel comfortable, or else therapy won't be effective. Your therapist should be someone who is experienced in treating older people and who is sensitive to issues that are more likely to arise later in life.

Just as you may have to try more than one antidepressant drug before finding the one that works for you, you may also have to try more than one type of therapy or therapist. You must also be patient when it comes to psychotherapy. The process of self-discovery and change is usually slow.

Many depressed people notice that psychotherapy "begins to work" at around the same time as their antidepressant medication starts to kick in. As you start to feel better physically and emotionally, you will find yourself taking a more active role in your psychotherapy.

Electroconvulsive therapy

If your depression is severe, and if drug treatment and psychotherapy don't seem to be working, your doctor may suggest electroconvulsive therapy (ECT). The treatment, which involves delivering a brief electrical current to the brain, is seen as a life-saving therapy for those whose depressions are so severe that they stop eating or contemplate suicide.

Unfortunately, many people are intimidated by the idea of ECT, once popularly known as "shock therapy." This is partly due to the gruesome images portrayed in movies, and partly because in the past, ECT was sometimes used inappropriately – for example, on people with personality disorders rather than depression.

If you have to undergo ECT, you should know exactly what will happen. The procedure is done in hospital or at a special clinic, sometimes on an out-patient basis, and usually involves a total of six to twelve sessions, two or three times per week.

You will be given a muscle relaxant and a short-acting anesthetic prior to treatment. While you're unconscious, a quick, painless burst of electricity is delivered via electrodes attached to your head. You may feel somewhat groggy afterward, so you should always have someone accompany you. You may experience a brief period of mental confusion or memory loss after several treatments, but this is usually temporary. Some people who have undergone ECT have reported more profound and long-lasting memory loss. However, doctors say it's not clear whether this is related to the treatment or the underlying depression itself.

Manic depression

If you experience depressive symptoms and feel sad all the time, you're probably suffering from what doctors call a "unipolar" disorder. But some older people develop another type of depression called "bipolar" disorder or manic depression, in which their low moods alternate with episodes of mania or exaggerated elation. Although the disorder tends to show up earlier in life, it can also develop for the first time after age 65.

Here are the warning signs of mania. (Mania can also occur on its own, unaccompanied by periods of depressed mood.)

◆ Unlike other types of depression, manic episodes tend to develop suddenly, within a period of days or weeks.

◆ The person seems to be in an unusually cheerful or "high" mood all the time, although there may also be periods of suspicion or irritability that can lead to violent outbursts.

◆ There's often extreme physical and mental restlessness – the person seems to be rushing around constantly from place to

Depression or dementia?

An older person who experiences memory loss and confusion may worry that these symptoms signal the start of Alzheimer's disease or some other dementing illness. But these problems can be a sign of depression.

In such cases a correct diagnosis is absolutely vital, especially because, unlike most dementias, depression can be successfully treated. (However, you should also be aware that depression and dementia can and do occur at the same time in some older people.)

Here are some ways you and your doctor can tell the difference between depression and dementia:

Depression
◆ progresses unevenly over weeks and months;
◆ person complains of memory loss;
◆ often worse in the morning, gets better as day goes on;
◆ person is aware of problem and may exaggerate it;
◆ person may turn to alcohol or other drugs for relief.

Dementia
◆ progresses steadily over months or years;
◆ person may try to hide memory loss from others;
◆ gets worse later in the day or when the person is tired;
◆ person is unaware of problem or tries to minimize it;
◆ person rarely abuses drugs.

place, project to project, thought to thought.

◆ Speech is unusually loud and rapid, and it's difficult for someone else to stop or interrupt the flow of conversation.

◆ The person spends much less time sleeping or resting.

◆ There's often a lack of judgment, which can lead to involvement in high-risk activities such as gambling, shopping sprees, new business ventures or investments, and sexual promiscuity.

◆ The person may show signs of grandiosity or inflated self-esteem, imagining himself to be someone famous. Sometimes this can progress to actual hallucinations or delusions.

Manic episodes can be extremely debilitating for the sufferer and upsetting for family members who must cope with their relative's frantic activity. In extreme cases the person must be hospitalized to protect himself and others.

If you or someone you know seems to be suffering from manic depression or mania alone, it's important to get treatment right away.

Your doctor will want to rule out delirium (see page 207) and eliminate the presence of an underlying physical illness such as a thyroid disorder. She will also examine whether the behavior might be a side effect of certain medications – for example, some tranquilizers, ulcer drugs, antidepressants, anti-Parkinson drugs and amphetamines can cause manic symptoms, as can alcohol and cocaine.

Treatment for manic depression involves medication in the form of lithium salts, which can stabilize moods in about half of all sufferers. Because lithium usually takes about two weeks to become effective, you may also be given a short course of antipsychotic medications such as haloperidol, or other drugs such as carbamazepine and valproic acid, which can stabilize your moods.

Since lithium can be toxic in excess, you will probably need to have regular blood tests. Common side effects include thirst, frequent urination, nausea, diarrhea and weight gain.

Here's some advice to remember should you or someone you know be diagnosed with manic depression:

◆ Most researchers now believe that manic depression is a hereditary disease involving an imbalance in brain chemistry. This means that the symptoms aren't under your control, and you shouldn't blame yourself for your behavior.

◆ It's absolutely vital that you continue taking your lithium, since you can easily suffer a relapse. If side effects are a problem, let your doctor know.

Dysthymia

A diagnosis of dysthymia may be made if you experience a chronically depressed or low mood most of the time for at least two years, and if you also suffer from two or more of the following symptoms:

◆ poor appetite or overeating;

◆ inability to sleep or oversleeping;

◆ low energy or fatigue;

◆ low self-esteem;

◆ poor concentration or trouble making decisions;

◆ feelings of hopelessness.

This mood disorder tends to show up early in life, but it's not uncommon for it to begin in the later years. Many older people who experience major depression may also suffer from underlying dysthymia.

People with dysthymia often appear resigned to their situation, saying "That's just how I am" or "I've always been this way." Older adults who suffer from this disorder may not mention the problem to their doctors unless asked. Like other types of depressive illness, dysthymia seems to run in families, and it's also more common in people with a family history of major depression. Dysthymia may respond to treatment with antidepressant medication and/or psychotherapy.

Adjustment disorder

This mood disorder is less serious than major depression, but it can cause upsetting symptoms, including crying, worrying, and physical complaints such as headache, upset stomach, and unexplained aches and pains.

Adjustment disorder normally develops within three months of some stressful event – for example, the loss of a spouse, retirement or moving to a new environment like a nursing home. People who suffer from a serious or prolonged physical illness are also vulnerable to adjustment disorder, perhaps because they feel disconnected from their usual world and feel a loss of control and competence.

If you or someone you know seems to be suffering from this disorder, see your doctor. He will check for any underlying illness or other problem that could be causing the symptoms. While antidepressant medication

Suicide and older adults

If you're over 65 and suffering from a major depression, you are at increased risk for suicide. According to one U.S. study, 85 percent of older people who committed suicide were known to be suffering from a depressive illness.

Besides depression, another well-established risk factor for suicide is old age. Statistics show that the suicide rate among older people – especially those over age 75 – is much higher than it is for younger people:

◆ In North America, the average rate of suicide among people age 25 to 64 is about 15 per 100,000.

◆ The average rate of suicide among people age 75 to 84 is about 26 per 100,000.

◆ The average rate of suicide among people over age 85 is about 20 per 100,000.

Here are some other facts about suicide you should know:

◆ Older people who try to kill themselves are much more determined to die than younger ones and are less likely to fail or be stopped in their attempt.

◆ Older men are much more likely to attempt or commit suicide than older women, particularly in the first six months after the death of their wives.

In most cultures, men have been raised to be assertive and in control, and they often find it hard to deal with retirement and the loss of physical health and power. In addition, because they tend to develop fewer social supports than women, many older men become extremely dependent on their wives for personal care (cooking, cleaning, shopping) and social and emotional well-being (keeping in touch with friends and family). When an older man loses his wife through death, serious illness or divorce, he can become extremely depressed and may see suicide as the only way out.

◆ Alcoholism is common among people

isn't usually necessary, you may be referred for psychotherapy, which can help you deal with your unhappy feelings.

Seasonal affective disorder

In recent years doctors have identified a group of people whose depressive symptoms seem to be related to changes in their exposure to certain kinds of light, particularly ultraviolet light. They become extremely lethargic and depressed, often gaining excessive amounts of weight, in the winter months when days are shortest. When spring and summer arrive, their symptoms ease up or disappear altogether.

This pattern of depression is called "seasonal affective disorder" (also known, rather appropriately, as SAD). Researchers think that SAD may be related to a deficiency of melatonin, a hormone secreted by the pineal gland in the brain. Melatonin secretion increases with exposure to sunlight.

The actual prevalence of SAD in older people isn't known, but some researchers suspect it may be more common than any-who attempt or commit suicide, especially older men who may turn to alcohol in an effort to ease the painful symptoms of depression.

The link between alcoholism and suicide may be related to the fact that drinking lowers inhibition, causing people to act out their impulses in a violent way. But it may also be due to the fact that alcoholism erodes family and other social supports, leaving alcoholics more vulnerable to despair and depression.

Here are some danger signs of suicide. The more signs, the higher the risk:

◆ current major depression;

◆ a major loss such as the death of a spouse;

◆ a history of major losses;

◆ a recent suicide attempt or a history of suicide attempts;

◆ a major mental, physical or neurological illness;

◆ a crisis in the family such as divorce;

◆ expressing feelings such as "I'm a burden to everyone" or "There's no hope";

◆ communicating suicidal intent either directly – "I'm going to kill myself" – or indirectly – "You'd all be better off if I was dead";

◆ actions such as giving away valued possessions, storing up medication or buying a gun;

◆ alcoholism or increased drinking;

◆ living alone with few friends (this includes the social isolation of a married couple).

Note: If you or someone you know appears to be suicidal, you should get help immediately. Call your family doctor or psychiatrist, or bring the person to the emergency department of the nearest hospital.

one thinks, especially among housebound older adults who rarely see the sun because of illness, isolation or disability.

If you think that you or someone you know is suffering from SAD, tell your doctor, who will probably want to rule out any other problems first. Many people with SAD can be helped by supervised, daily exposure to full-spectrum light, usually delivered by a lamp or a special device worn on the forehead.

Anxiety and anxiety disorders

Feeling anxious from time to time is part of being human and alive. While there's no evidence that older people are any more anxious than those who are younger, anxiety seems to be a fairly common experience later in life. Studies show that about 20 percent of those over the age of 65 report being troubled by the physical and emotional symptoms of anxiety.

? Are there different types of anxiety?

In recent years doctors have learned to distinguish between several basic types of anxiety.

Normal anxiety

Feeling anxious from time to time is a normal part of living. You might even say that we are designed to feel anxious in order to protect ourselves from danger. When you perceive a threat, your nervous system becomes activated in a "fight or flight" response: Your muscles become tense and ready for action, and in order to supply them with more blood and oxygen, your heart pumps more quickly and your breathing quickens. This response occurs even when there's no immediate danger – for example, when you're worried about your health or the well-being of your children. When the worry is resolved, the anxious sensations usually disappear.

Anxiety as a symptom

Anxiety and physical illness often go together. The most reasonable explanation for this is that being sick causes you to worry. Is your illness life-threatening? Will it cause pain? Will treatment work? Will you regain your health and independence? Can you afford health care costs?

Although doctors don't know why, it appears that certain health problems themselves – not just the worries they trigger – are associated with anxiety. These include depression, especially among older adults (see page 210), Alzheimer's and Parkinson's diseases, and some types of cancer. Older people with hearing loss also tend to be more anxious, especially in social situations.

It's easy to blame certain symptoms on anxiety when they're actually caused by illness. For example, weakness, dizziness, sweating, shortness of breath and feelings of dread can be provoked by a silent, atypical heart attack, pulmonary embolism or a small stroke. Trembling, rapid heartbeat and restlessness may be caused by hypoglycemia (low blood sugar), hyperthyroidism (overfunctioning of the thyroid) or a rare tumor of the adrenal gland known as pheochromocytoma.

Anxiety can also occur as a side effect of certain drugs. In fact, there are hundreds of prescription and over-the-counter medications that list anxiety or agitation as a possible side effect. These include calcium channel blockers such as verapamil, which is used to treat angina, and ephedrine and pseudoephedrine, which are often found in over-the-counter cold remedies. A drug called "theophylline," sometimes used to treat asthma and chronic bronchitis, can also produce anxiety symptoms, and because of this, few geriatricians recommend using this drug in older people.

Another common source of anxious symptoms is caffeine, found in coffee, tea, cola drinks, chocolate and some non-prescription medications. Studies show that as little as 200 milligrams of caffeine (one cup of coffee contains about 150 milligrams) can cause rapid heartbeat, shakiness and sweating in some people.

Anxiety symptoms are also common during withdrawal from drugs such as alcohol and sedatives.

Anxiety disorder

There's a major difference between the normal, explainable types of anxiety and intense, often crippling anxieties that aren't so easy to explain or understand. Doctors call these "anxiety disorders."

It's estimated that 10 percent of North Americans will experience one of these disorders at some point in their lives. In the past doctors believed that these disorders were directly related to deep-seated psychological problems. Now researchers are finding that genetics and subtle imbalances in brain chemistry may play a significant role.

Common symptoms of anxiety

◆ *Physical symptoms*: trembling, twitching or feeling shaky, muscle tension, aches or soreness, pain or discomfort in the chest, shortness of breath, palpitations, sweating, cold or clammy hands, dry mouth, dizziness or lightheadedness, nausea, diarrhea or stomach complaints, flushes or chills, frequent urination, a lump in the throat;

◆ *Emotional symptoms*: feeling edgy or nervous, easily fatigued, abnormally focused on surroundings or physical sensations, easily startled or upset, trouble concentrating, irritability.

Anxiety and depression

The link between anxiety and depression is well-known. About 80 percent of people who have been diagnosed with major depression suffer from high levels of anxiety, and about 35 percent of those with anxiety disorders will develop depression. While most psychiatrists still believe that anxiety and depression are separate illnesses, the diseases often overlap, especially in older adults.

 Are some people at greater risk for anxiety and anxiety disorders?

While older people frequently report anxiety as a symptom, they are less likely to suffer from anxiety disorders than people under age 65.

Certain negative experiences associated with aging may make you more vulnerable to anxiety. These include the loss of loved ones, the fear of increased dependency due to health problems, changes in economic or social status, loneliness and fear of isolation, and finally, the fear of dying.

Most people find they can recover from the effects of change and loss if they have enough time. But these stresses tend to pile up in the later years, and it's easy for you to become overwhelmed. Some experts think that the so-called "young old" – people in their 60s and 70s – are most vulnerable to anxiety because they are still adjusting to the realities of older age. Those in their 80s and 90s may actually be less prone to anxiety because longer exposure to loss and stress has given them a measure of resistance.

Women are more likely to experience certain anxiety disorders than men, but the reasons for this aren't clear. It may be that women, particularly older women who are widowed or divorced, are more likely to be exposed to poverty and powerlessness, which makes them vulnerable to anxiety. Another explanation may be that, in general, women are more likely than men to admit that they have a problem and to seek medical help. Some researchers believe that men also experience anxiety but are more likely to mask their symptoms with alcohol.

Your risk for anxiety later in life seems to be greater if you are poor and if you live in a situation that makes you feel completely dependent on others.

? What should you do if you suffer from anxiety?

If you're feeling normal anxiety over a personal problem or situation, here are some suggestions:

◆ Don't keep your worries bottled up inside. Often just sharing your fears with someone you trust can bring relief.

◆ If you seem to worry a lot, you may have a tendency to exaggerate the seriousness of certain situations. Try to be more realistic. You may also feel anxious because you assume too much responsibility or try to control those around you. You may find that letting go a bit can be an enormous relief.

◆ Many people worry when faced with an important decision. If you have to make such a choice, try to be organized about it. Consider the pros and cons, and if possible, give yourself a deadline so you don't worry endlessly.

◆ Keep as physically active as possible –

exercise is a natural tranquilizer.

Sometimes these strategies don't work. The worst thing you can do is to suffer in silence. Call your family doctor if:

◆ you continue to feel anxious, if periods of anxiety seem to recur, and if the symptoms are interfering with your life and relationships;

◆ a personal loss or stress has caused severe, ongoing anxiety symptoms;

◆ you don't feel anxious but are bothered by headaches, stomach upsets, skin rashes and sleeping problems;

◆ you experience symptoms of depression (see page 211).

? How is anxiety treated?

Your doctor will examine you first to make sure that your symptoms aren't due to some underlying illness or a side effect of medication. She may question you about what's happening in your life and see if there's some obvious explanation for your distress. It's important to answer her questions honestly so that she can help you.

If your doctor thinks it's necessary, she may prescribe a mild tranquilizer to see if this helps. If she believes you might be suffering from an anxiety disorder, she may refer you to a psychiatrist or other specialist. Anxiety disorders are usually treated with a combination of medication, psychotherapy and/or behavior therapy and relaxation training.

? What are anxiety disorders?

The following disorders are classified by doctors as anxiety disor-

A word about tranquilizers

It's estimated that up to half of all people over age 65 use tranquilizers at some point to relieve tension or as part of treatment for a medical illness. Although short-term use of these drugs, commonly known as benzodiazepines, can be extremely helpful, you should be aware of potential problems.

Tranquilizers can become habit-forming when taken over a long period of time. It's easy to become dependent on them.

As you grow older, your body becomes less efficient at metabolizing certain drugs and you may suffer from diseases or take other drugs that make you more sensitive to benzodiazepines. Both can lead to a toxic buildup of the medication in your system. Symptoms of tranquilizer toxicity include memory loss and problems concentrating. If you take tranquilizers at night, impaired physical function the following day can cause falls or other injuries.

If your doctor prescribes a tranquilizer, it should be a drug that tends to remain in your body for a relatively short amount of time. Short-acting tranquilizers include oxazepam and lorazepam.

Always follow your doctor's orders when it comes to taking tranquilizers. Never take more than the recommended dose or seek prescriptions for tranquilizers from more than one doctor. You should also ask certain questions. For example: How long will the drug remain in your system? Will you feel sedated or sleepy the next day? How long does the doctor think you'll need to take this medication?

If your tranquilizers don't seem to be helping you, if you find that you want to take more, or if you think you might have a problem with tranquilizers, speak to your family doctor.

---

ders. Although they usually manifest themselves early in life, they can begin at any age, and untreated, they can be extremely upsetting and debilitating.

If you or someone you know suffers from one of these disorders, it's important to seek medical help, even if you're convinced that nothing will work. Although many of these conditions tend to recur, with the right treatment most people will enjoy a remission or a lessening of their symptoms.

Simple phobia

A phobia is defined as a persistent fear of a particular object or situation – for example, fear of snakes, dogs, heights or flying. This is the most common type of anxiety disorder, as well as the most common psychiatric disorder in older women and the second most common psychiatric disorder in older men.

Most of us have a normal fear of objects or situations that we perceive as dangerous. Phobias, however, are usually triggered by an unpleasant experience that causes you to dread the object or situation involved.

If exposure to the stimulus causes extreme fear and unpleasant physical sensations and if the fear is in any way disabling, it's likely that you're suffering from a phobia.

Very few people seek treatment for simple phobias because the source of the phobia can usually be avoided. But if a phobia interferes with your normal routines or relationships, you should get help. Most phobias can be cured by exposure therapy – gradually confronting the dreaded situation or object – and relaxation techniques such as deep breathing.

Generalized anxiety disorder (GAD)

This disorder, characterized by ongoing excessive or unrealistic anxiety, is often difficult to distinguish from everyday anxiety. The most common symptoms are trembling, restlessness, fatigue, shortness of breath, rapid heart rate, sweating, dizziness, trouble swallowing, stomach upset, insomnia and irritability. A diagnosis of GAD is usually made if you experience several of these symptoms on most days for at least six months.

GAD is usually treated with a combination of psychotherapy and medication.

Panic disorder

You have this disorder if you suffer from recurring panic attacks – episodes of severe anxiety or fear accompanied by symptoms such as palpitations, shortness of breath, chest pain or tightness, sweating, tingling in hands or feet, fear of losing control and fear of dying. Many (but not all) people with recurrent panic attacks begin to avoid leaving home or going to public places – a condition called "agoraphobia."

Doctors believe that panic disorder is caused by a combination of biological and psychological factors. Researchers have found that people with panic disorder are significantly more sensitive than normal people to a certain brain protein called "cholecystokinin." It's also likely that there's some link between panic disorder and excessive anxiety about separating from important people, places or things early in life.

Panic disorder is usually treated by a combination of psychotherapy, which can help you identify panic "triggers," and medication, including antidepressant drugs and tranquilizers.

Social phobia

This is a persistent fear of social situations. Its symptoms may include a fear of public speaking, fear of eating in front of other people and being unable to urinate in a public lavatory. People with social phobia often go to great lengths to avoid being placed in dreaded social situations, and they may become extremely isolated.

Some people are born with a shy or insecure temperament that may predispose them to social phobia. An embarrassing incident, particularly in childhood, may trigger it. Sufferers often have a distorted perception of themselves and others, believing that other people are better than they are.

Social phobia is usually treated by psychotherapy, which may help you discover the emotional roots of your extreme shyness and social avoidance. Some doctors also recommend medication to control symptoms.

Obsessive-compulsive disorder (OCD)

This disorder involves recurrent compulsions (repetitive actions) or obsessions (repetitive thoughts) that are severe enough to cause distress or interfere with your normal activities and relationships. Common compulsions include hand-washing, counting, checking and touching; common obsessions include fear of contamination and thoughts of violence toward a loved one.

Doctors used to think this crippling disorder was a psychological condition caused by strict upbringing and early obsessions with cleanliness. Now they think it's linked to an imbalance in brain chemistry, in particular a deficiency in serotonin.

OCD is treated with a combination of psychotherapy and behavior therapy that helps you understand and resist compulsions. Serotonin-activating drugs such as fluvoxamine, fluoxetine and clomipramine can also help suppress symptoms.

Post-traumatic stress disorder (PTSD)

This disorder occurs in people who have been victims of war or who have experienced or witnessed a trauma such as a car accident, a physical assault or a natural disaster. Symptoms include anxiety, anger, insomnia, difficulty concentrating, flashbacks of the trauma, a sense of unreality, and withdrawal from family and friends.

Psychotherapy can help you control the intrusive memories of the traumatic event, and antidepressant drugs can relieve unpleasant physical symptoms.

How do you know if you have an anxiety disorder?

Anxiety disorders tend to show up fairly early in life, usually when you're in your teens or 20s, so if you suffer from one of these problems, you probably know about it by now.

Unfortunately, many people who suffer from crippling anxiety don't seek or get help. Either they hide the problems and endure their symptoms for many years, or else they haven't been properly diagnosed and treated. In the past it was common for people with anxiety disorders to be misdiagnosed, and they often underwent extensive tests for heart disease or other medical problems. Many more were sent to psychiatrists in the belief that their crippling anxiety was caused solely by psychological factors.

Over the past decade or so, doctors have learned a great deal about anxiety disorders. They have a better understanding of what causes them, they are more skilled at diagnosing them and they can offer more in the way of treatment. So even if you or someone you know has suffered from crippling anxiety for many years, it's not too late to seek help.

Other problems affecting mental health

Psychotic illness

Psychosis is one of the most severe forms of illness affecting the mind. While psychotic symptoms and disorders are far less common among older adults than depression or anxiety, they still account for a considerable amount of suffering in later life.

People with psychotic illness often appear to have completely lost touch with reality, and when their symptoms are severe, they are unable to function normally and may require hospitalization.

The main feature of psychotic illness is delusions – false and sometimes bizarre beliefs. These beliefs are real in the sufferer's mind and cause him to misinterpret ordinary perceptions or experiences. Often the person suffers visual or aural hallucinations that seem extremely real. He may believe he is being tormented, followed, tricked, spied on or ridiculed, and this makes him suspicious and agitated.

People who are psychotic may also become extremely withdrawn and apathetic. This may be mistaken for laziness or uncooperativeness. When their symptoms are severe, they may find it nearly impossible to function normally in the world.

Older people are most likely to experience psychotic symptoms in the course of a depression or dementing illness, as the result of physical illness such as Huntington's disease or after certain types of brain injury. Alcohol or drug intoxication is another common source of delusions or hallucinations in older adults (see page 231).

Sometimes older people become extremely afraid that they're having hallucinations when they aren't. The following experiences are common among healthy people and *do not* qualify as psychotic hallucinations:

◆ hearing or seeing things just as you awaken or fall asleep;

◆ hearing someone call your name occasionally when there's no one there (this is especially common in the weeks and months following the death of a spouse or loved one);

◆ a musical humming inside your head that clearly isn't coming from the outside.

The most common type of psychotic illness affecting people of all ages is *schizophrenia*, which is estimated to affect about 1 percent of the population. Although there are cases of schizophrenia beginning fairly late in life, most people tend to develop symptoms when they are young – the average age of onset for men is sometime in late adolescence or the early 20s, while for women the disease usually shows up between ages 25 and 30.

There are several types of schizophrenia, but symptoms usually include delusions, hallucinations and obvious disorders in speech, thinking and perception. In many cases these symptoms alternate with periods of extreme apathy and withdrawal.

Doctors still don't know what causes schizophrenia. In the past it was falsely blamed on poor parenting or other psychological factors. Now researchers believe that biochemical factors are involved, most likely an imbalance in the brain chemical dopamine. That's why certain anti-psychotic drugs that suppress dopamine can often control psychotic symptoms and help many people with schizophrenia live relatively normal lives.

Schizophrenia is an extremely difficult illness for those who suffer from it and for their families. Older adults who have had schizophrenia for many years may face additional problems when their spouses become ill or die.

Unfortunately, very little research has been done into how aging affects schizophrenia. There's some evidence that older adults suffer less from the active symptoms – such as delusions and hallucinations – and more from symptoms such as apathy and social withdrawal. Studies have also shown that as they age, people with schizophrenia tend to require lower dosages of anti-psychotic medication to control their symptoms.

If someone you know seems to be developing psychotic symptoms, either spontaneously or in the course of another illness, it's vital to report this to your doctor.

Hypochondria

The popular image of the hypochondriac is a Woody Allen–type character who goes from doctor to doctor, anxiously takes his temperature every hour and imagines any headache to be a brain tumor.

Most of us suffer mild episodes of hypochondriasis (commonly known as hypochondria) from time to time. But when hypochondria becomes chronic and severe, it's no laughing matter. Hypochondria is a psychological condition that doctors categorize as a somatoform disorder – the presence of physical symptoms suggest illness, but no illness can be diagnosed.

If you suffer from hypochondria, you are constantly preoccupied with sickness. You believe you have a serious illness, based on your own interpretation of certain symptoms and sensations, and go from doctor to doctor in search of a diagnosis and a cure. These fears and beliefs persist, even when no illness has been diagnosed and despite many reassurances from numerous doctors.

People with hypochondria know their own medical histories in great detail, and often say that previous physicians who found nothing wrong with them were insensitive or incompetent.

It's tempting to label anyone who does this a hypochondriac – unfortunately, many people with real illnesses have been dismissed as hypochondriacs until their diseases were finally recognized. However, hypochondria clearly exists as a mental disorder, and the preoccupation with imagined illness can become so severe that it impairs relationships and interferes with the person's ability to function normally.

The incidence of true hypochondria in the general population isn't known, but doctors estimate that between 4 and 9 percent of people they see in general practice suffer from some degree of hypochondria. The problem usually begins after age 30 and tends to persist into older age.

Many people who suffer from clinical depression or anxiety become abnormally vigilant about their bodies, focusing on every little change, and it's not uncommon for them to develop hypochondria. The good news is that when these disorders are successfully treated, the hypochondria tends to disappear.

Abnormal grief

When you experience the death of a loved one, it's normal to feel grief. This may include feelings of sadness and loss, as well as physical symptoms of stress such as insomnia and fatigue. While these feelings vary widely from person to person, they tend to follow a normal course (see page 241).

But sometimes grieving is intense and/or long-lasting enough to be considered abnormal or even pathological. Such grieving can take a tremendous toll on your emotional and physical health and should be recognized when it occurs so you can get help.

Delayed grief

While a slight delay in grieving is normal, an absence of grieving for weeks and months is unusual. All too often people who delay grieving are praised by others ("She's so strong that she didn't even cry at the funeral," or "Isn't he amazing to be able to carry on so well?"). By delaying grief, you may be denying the fact that your loved one has died.

Prolonged grief

Sometimes people become "stuck" in the first or second stages of grieving and can't seem to move forward toward resolution. You may feel excessive guilt about the person's death, blaming yourself in some way, or you may turn your anger onto others, such as doctors or other family members. It's not unusual for someone in this state to develop a major depression and experience a decline in physical health.

Detachment and isolation

You feel numb and cut off from the world, and insist that people leave you alone. You generally refuse to take part in any social activities, saying that you "have no feelings" and are better off this way. If friends and family take you at your word, they may stop calling. You may begin to feel angry and resentful at being left alone, and you can also start to feel suspicious of other people.

Grief following an unnatural death

If you have lost someone to suicide, accidental death or homicide, you may experience some added symptoms. These may be normal or abnormal, depending on how intense they are and how long they last.

If your loved one committed suicide, you may feel excessive guilt over failing to prevent the act. You may also feel angry at the person who killed himself and embarrassed about others finding out about the suicide.

If the death was traumatic, you may notice that you are easily startled and upset, and you may experience intrusive thoughts and images of the person's death, even if you didn't witness it. If the death was the result of violence, you may feel victimized and extremely anxious about your own safety.

Taking on the person's symptoms

You may begin to believe that you are suffering from the same disease that killed your loved one. You may actually develop symptoms that the dead person suffered, even though nothing is actually wrong with you.

If you think you or someone you know is experiencing an abnormal reaction to grief, seek help right away. Your family doctor may be able to help you manage some of the physical symptoms with the short-term use of medication, but abnormal grief usually requires working out your feelings through individual or group psychotherapy.

Alcohol abuse

Recent studies have suggested that when taken in small amounts – for example, a glass of wine with dinner or an occasional shot of whiskey – alcohol may be physically and psychologically beneficial for some older people.

But it's important to establish the difference between sensible drinking and problem drinking. In general, you shouldn't drink more than two drinks a day, and some experts say you shouldn't drink every day. *Note: One drink equals a regular beer (12 oz. or 340 ml. 5 percent alcohol) OR one glass of wine (5 oz. or 145 ml. 12 percent alcohol) OR one shot of liquor (1.5 oz. or 45 ml. 40 percent alcohol).*

There are several reasons why people should curtail their drinking as they age:

◆ You become more sensitive to the effects of alcohol, especially alcohol-induced cognitive impairment such as memory loss and poor concentration.

◆ You are more prone to illnesses such as high blood pressure, heart disease and diabetes later in life. Because these ailments can be aggravated by drinking, your doctor has probably told you not to drink.

◆ You are more likely to be taking medication to control illnesses and have been warned not to mix these drugs with alcohol.

But many experts believe that the true extent of alcohol abuse among older adults may not be known for the following reasons:

◆ Older drinkers tend to be middle class and don't conform to the popular image of the alcoholic.

◆ Older adults tend to be more isolated from those who typically recognize and report problem drinking in younger people – for example, co-workers and employers.

◆ Doctors may believe that older people "don't do that" and miss symptoms of alcohol abuse.

◆ The older person's family may excuse excessive drinking ("What else does he have to do at his age?") and actually supply him with brandy or wine. As well, relatives may be so embarrassed about an older family member who abuses alcohol that they deny or hide the situation.

If you suffer from alcohol-related problems now, it's likely that you started drinking when you were younger. But about 30 percent of older drinkers start abusing alcohol after age 60. These late-onset drinkers tend to explain their drinking as a reaction to retirement, the death of a spouse or other stresses of older age. Some may turn to alcohol in an effort to relieve symptoms from chronic pain, insomnia, depression and anxiety that occur later in life.

However, it's not clear why some older people who are under stress begin to abuse alcohol, while many others who face similar or even more severe stress never develop a problem. In fact, researchers still aren't clear what causes alcoholism at any age.

Some studies have suggested that alcoholism tends to run in families – either because of a genetic factor or because drinkers saw alcohol consumed at home and learned that this was an acceptable way to handle stress. In recent years some experts have put forward the idea that alcoholism is a disease that shouldn't be blamed on the victim. Others disagree, saying that this view discounts any notion of individual personal control.

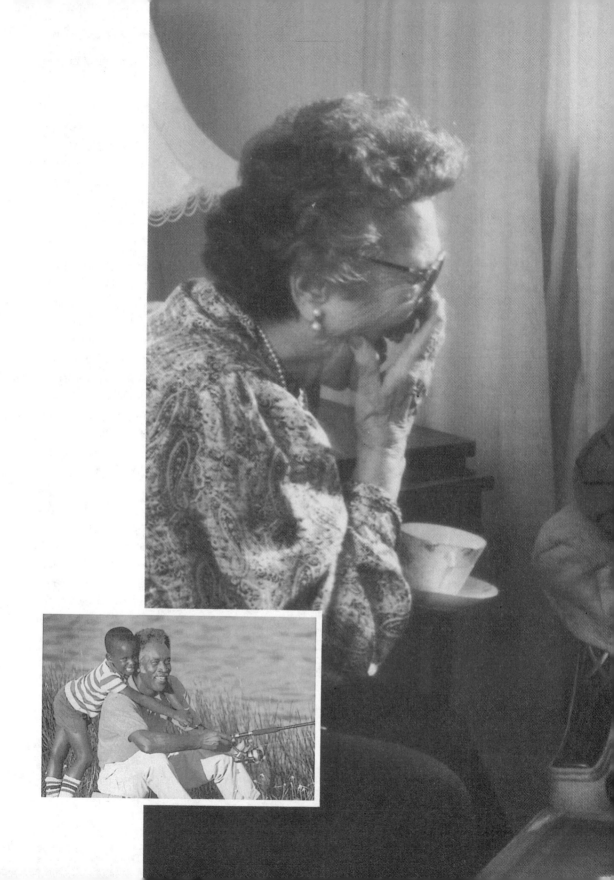

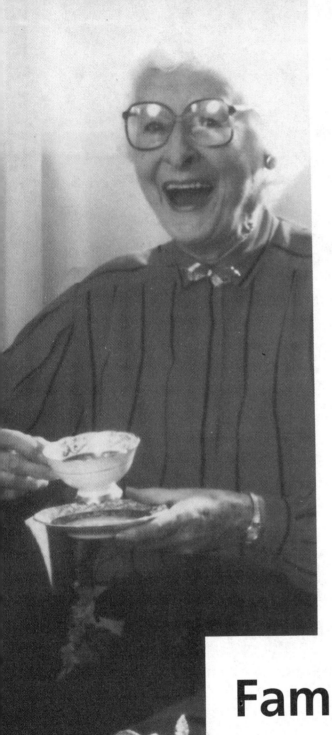

7

*A group of closely
related persons
living under one roof:
It is a convention,
often a necessity,
sometimes a pleasure,
sometimes the reverse.*

ROSE MACAULAY

Family Matters

IT'S IMPOSSIBLE TO DISCUSS YOUR health and well-being without exploring an extremely important subject: growing older in the context of your family.

Each of us comes from what experts call a "family of origin" – your grandparents, parents and siblings. These are the people who have had the most profound effect on you, whether by their example, their influence or their absence. They have shaped you, in good ways and bad, and their presence endures in your life regardless of death, illness, distance or estrangement.

In addition to our families of origin, most of us go on to choose partners and have children of our own, who may then go on to give us grandchildren and great-grandchildren. In effect, we establish a new family of origin, and the cycle continues as joys and sorrows are passed down through the generations along with the family silver.

Keep in mind that families are like snowflakes – no two are alike. It's impossible to describe the complexity of relationships and feelings that exist in just *one* family, let alone to present a blueprint for all families.

Even so, it may be useful for you to read about some of the issues which tend to arise later in life and which can have an impact on your health and well-being. Knowing that such experiences are common may help you feel less alone when they happen in your own family. If you can understand how and why certain problems develop, you may be able to prevent them or, at the very least, cope with them more effectively.

First, take a moment to think about your family and your own place in it. Most people don't take the time to do this, unless there's a crisis, and that may not be the best time to reflect on these issues.

Here are some creative ideas to help get you started. You can certainly try some of these suggestions on your own, but it's a good idea to involve other family members.

♦ Draw your family tree. You'll need a fairly large sheet of paper to make room for different generations and branches. Circles are used to represent the women in your family, squares are used to represent the men.

Put yourself in the middle of the tree, then start drawing lines to link you to your various family members. Lines drawn upward connect you to your parents, grandparents, aunts and uncles. Don't forget to make room for their spouses and children. Lines drawn horizontally connect you to your own spouse (or spouses, if you've remarried). Moving downward, the next set of lines connects you to your adult children, their partners (if they have them) and your grandchildren.

Once you have drawn your tree, sit down with a family member or close friend and tell them what you know and feel about these people in your family. What happened to them? How well did you know them? What stories did you hear about them? How did they relate to other people in the family? Were these relationships positive or difficult?

As you work on your family tree, certain patterns will begin to emerge. Pay attention to events such as illness, the unexpected loss of a family member, relocation from another city or country, family quarrels leading to estrangement and wartime experiences. These can give you important insights into your family and yourself: For example, there's evidence that older people who suffer from depression have experienced some profound loss in early life – for example, death or serious illness of a parent during their own childhood.

◆ Go back through your family photos. If necessary, reorganize them in a new album or albums and invite family members and friends to go through them with you.

◆ Make a greater effort to connect with family members who live far away. Perhaps you've lost touch with nieces and nephews, or you may have become estranged from a brother or sister. Getting past these issues can be emotionally challenging, especially if many years have gone by, but there's great potential for emotional peace and satisfaction in resolving these problems.

◆ Compose your autobiography or life story, beginning with your earliest childhood memories. You can write it or dictate it into a tape recorder, or your spouse, an adult child or teenaged grandchild can interview you on audio or videotape. This can be an extremely fulfilling experience for you and makes a wonderful legacy for your children and grandchildren.

When you look through your albums or boxes of family photographs, you may feel amazed that so many years have passed and marvel at all the changes you've seen and experienced. It's often difficult to see these changes in ourselves. Many older people, including those in their 80s and 90s, say that in some ways they still think of themselves as being much younger than their chronological age.

In the same way, we don't always recognize the changes that have occurred in our family members. Even though your son is now a grown man with a family of his own, in some ways you may still see him as a young boy. This can cause problems for you both if you continue to treat him as a child by overprotecting him or trying to control his life.

Families grow in many ways and many directions. As you grow older, certain events are more likely to occur, and these may have a profound impact on you as an individual and on your family relationships.

Coping with illness

Illness in your family can occur at any age. By the time you've reached 65, you may have already experienced what you consider to be your fair share. However, because many serious and chronic diseases tend to occur with aging, you and your spouse or companion should be prepared to face some illness later in life.

When an older person becomes sick, it's usually the spouse or other partner who takes on the role of caregiver. Adult children and other family members may provide help, but they don't become the main caregivers, unless you're alone or your partner can't care for you because of his or her own illness or disability.

Caring for a sick person is a difficult job at any age, but it can be a special strain for older caregivers, both physically and emotionally.

Besides offering moral support and encouragement, you may have to help your partner manage daily activities such as eating, bathing, toileting and dressing. You may have to keep track of medication and doctor's appointments, and also take care of day-to-day tasks such as cooking, cleaning, laundry, shopping and banking. If your partner suffers from cognitive losses due to Alzheimer's disease, care becomes more complicated and there are added concerns about safety.

How you cope with illness as a couple depends on many factors. If the illness is acute rather than chronic, you may find it easier because there's hope for recovery and you can both work toward that goal. Chronic and degenerative illnesses are usually more difficult to face. Not only do they place ongoing physical and emotional demands on both of you, but the demands persist over time and may become greater as the illness progresses.

While coping with serious physical illness is stressful, many people say that conditions such as Alzheimer's disease are even more difficult for caregivers. As well as facing the illness itself, you must watch someone you've known and loved for many years undergo dramatic changes. The person continues to be physically present, but in the later stages of the disease you are left feeling terribly alone.

A serious illness tests the nature of your relationship. Commitment in a long-term relationship varies a great deal. At one end of the spectrum are those who think: "I'll stay with you as long as my needs are met." At the other end are those who feel: "I'll stay with you through sickness and in health till death do us part." Most couples fall somewhere in between these two extremes.

If your relationship has been good, it's likely that your commitment to each other has deepened over the years, and this can make illness easier to face. But if you've experienced unhappiness or abuse, this can erode your commitment and make the situation more complicated.

Here are some of the normal emotional responses that can occur when you or your partner develops a serious or chronic illness.

When you are sick

◆ You dislike feeling dependent on the other person, especially if you were very independent before.

◆ You feel guilty watching your partner struggle to cope with the demands created by your illness.

◆ You may become critical of your partner's efforts if he or she has to take over tasks that you once handled.

◆ You feel upset and angry about being sick, and because your partner is present more than anyone else, you tend to take your anger out on him or her rather than on your adult children or your doctor.

When your partner is sick

◆ You feel upset at seeing your partner in pain or coping with a disabling illness.

◆ You feel overwhelmed by the physical and emotional demands of caring for your partner, particularly if you have to deal with intimate tasks such as bathing and toileting.

◆ You feel unprepared to take over certain tasks that used to be handled by your partner – for example, cooking, cleaning, gardening, home maintenance or dealing with finances.

◆ You feel worried about the future and the possibility that your partner will die or have to be placed in an institution, leaving you alone.

How to face illness together

A serious or chronic illness can disturb the balance of your relationship, especially if you don't make an effort to understand what is happening. Even in this difficult situation, you can still maintain some control.

Be honest with yourself and your partner. This means talking about problems when they come up rather than burying them and letting resentment creep into your relationship.

Know your limits and don't be afraid to ask for help.

If you're the caregiver, you may feel guilty about asking others for assistance, believing that you should be able to do it all. But by doing too much, you're placing your own health in jeopardy, which may cause your partner to suffer later on. So it's vital that you ask for help from family members or professional caregivers (see page 259).

It's also important to avoid the trap of "overcaring" or becoming a martyr to your partner's needs. Such exaggerated devotion is usually a two-edged sword: On the one hand, you feel needed and you enjoy receiving emotional "pats on the back" from others who say how wonderful you are to spend so much time and energy helping your partner. On the other hand, you may be unaware of the tremendous physical, emotional and social toll that such caregiving is taking on you. In some ways – however unintentional – by overcaring, you may also be encouraging your partner to remain in a dependent state.

If you're the one who's sick, you need to take responsibility for what's happening to you and your partner. If you think that your spouse is having trouble coping, you might suggest that it's time to ask for help. This can be a wonderfully loving thing to do for your partner – it relieves the well person of guilt and shows that you still care about his or her well-being.

Be generous when your partner takes over one of "your" household tasks. It's only human for us to want to feel irreplaceable and special, but being openly critical only undermines your partner's efforts and leads to resentment and hurt feelings. Try to accept that your partner may not cook, fold the laundry or vacuum the house exactly the way you did.

It's not unusual for illness to have an impact on the sexual part of your relationship, if it still exists (see pages 182 and 186). This can be a particular problem if you're giving intimate care to your partner – taking him to the bathroom, cutting his toenails, helping him dress. Such familiarity can easily stifle sexual feelings.

If your relationship is strong enough, it can be helpful to talk about these feelings – you may find a way to resolve them over time. If not, you can still enjoy holding hands, caressing your partner's face and giving a shoulder rub. This is especially important if you are the one who's sick – a caress or a back rub at the end of a long day is one thing you can still do for your partner.

Caring for your aging parent

It's possible that one or both of your own parents are still alive, and you may be caring for them. If they are still living in their own home, you may be providing hands-on care and help with tasks such as cooking, shopping and banking. If they live in a retirement residence or nursing home, you probably spend time visiting and may help out with tasks such as laundry, making financial arrangements and dealing with staff.

If you're over 65, your parent is probably 85 or older and may be suffering from a cognitive illness such as Alzheimer's disease. This adds another layer of difficulty for you as a child and caregiver.

The strain of dealing with your own aging parents is often compounded by other troubling events and circumstances in your life such as your own health problems or the needs of your partner.

Some people take great joy and comfort in having a parent who has lived to a very old age. Such a parent can be a wonderfully positive role model for their own aging. But it can be hard to watch your parent struggle with illness and dependency, and this can trigger upsetting thoughts and feelings about your own aging and mortality.

If you find yourself struggling to balance your own problems and needs with those of your parent, you probably need help. Asking for help is often difficult, but in this case it is absolutely vital for your own health and well-being and also for the health and well-being of your parent (see page 259).

Coping with divorce and remarriage

If you're over 65 now, you grew up in an era when marriages seldom ended in divorce. Later-life divorces are more common today, and an older person who leaves – or is left by – a spouse faces certain unique problems:

◆ After living with someone else for so many years, it can be extremely difficult to adjust to being alone.

◆ Older women are more likely to suffer economic hardship after a divorce than older men. This seems to be true for women in general, but younger divorced women have more opportunities for employment and remarriage.

◆ While some adult children actually encourage the breakup of an unhappy marriage, others react negatively. Even if they're mature adults with grown children of their own, your adult children may feel hurt and angry when you tell them you're getting a divorce.

◆ If you're over 65, you're more likely to be facing the breakup of your adult child's marriage than your own. This is often an emotionally wrenching experience for older parents, and you may have a variety of concerns (see page 251).

◆ Remarriage after divorce is less common among older people than remarriage after the death of a spouse – mainly because divorce is less common than widowhood among people of your age.

Although later-life remarriage can be a wonderful experience, it also presents certain challenges to you and your family (see page 249).

◆ Although divorce is difficult and painful, it can also be an opportunity for happiness and growth. But when you divorce later in life, it may be harder for you to see these possibilities. You have fewer years left, and less time to find another life partner, if that's what you want.

When your partner dies

Even though such a loss may be predictable and even expected, for most older people the death of a partner is the most profound event that occurs in later life. How you cope with it depends on many factors.

It's common sense that if your relationship was happy, the loss may be especially hard to bear. But even if your life together was unhappy, your partner's death can trigger many difficult emotions, including anger, guilt and regret.

The timing of your partner's death may affect how you cope with loss. Some experts believe that a sudden or unexpected death is harder on the surviving partner than death after a long or terminal illness. Being forewarned, they say, allows you to "rehearse" the event emotionally, to express unsaid feelings to your partner and to make practical decisions about such matters as the funeral and finances.

But being forewarned may have its disadvantages, too. A long or difficult "death watch" can take a tremendous emotional and physical toll on an older person. When her partner finally dies, she may be so numb from the ordeal that her adjustment is delayed.

Previous experiences of grief and loss can also affect how you cope with the death of a partner. If you haven't faced much loss so far, your partner's death may be extremely traumatic. If you have already survived the deaths of parents, other relatives and friends, you may be somewhat better prepared. Many older people find, however, that nothing can fully prepare them for the loss of someone with whom they have shared 40, 50 or 60 years. And when such a loss follows on the heels of so many others – a common experience later in life – you may find it especially hard to endure.

How people react to the death of a partner varies widely. In one survey, nearly 70 percent of older adults said the death of their spouse had affected them greatly. They mentioned the loneliness of living without a

The stages of normal bereavement

Many factors affect how you grieve after a major loss. Men and women may show their emotions differently, individual families tend to have different "styles" of grieving and there are many cultural variations in how grief is expressed.

Experts who study the bereavement process have identified three stages of normal grieving. This process lasts, on average, a total of two years. While some people are able to work through these stages in a fairly short period of time – as little as six months – others experience pain for many years until they eventually resolve their grief.

First stage

This usually begins with the death itself, although if the dying process has been slow and drawn out, grieving can actually begin before the person dies. This stage usually lasts from four to six weeks but varies widely.

◆ You feel shock and disbelief, which are accompanied by feelings of numbness, emptiness and confusion. These emotions are more pronounced if the death was sudden, unexpected or unnatural.

◆ You may be preoccupied with the actual details of the person's death.

◆ You experience distressing physical symptoms such as tightness in the throat and chest, shortness of breath, insomnia and loss of appetite.

◆ You are more likely to feel anxious rather than depressed, and your mood fluctuates greatly. Weepiness, guilt and irritability are common.

◆ You may experience a worsening of your own health problems and seek medical help for your symptoms.

Second stage

This stage usually lasts about a year.

◆ The numbness begins to wear off and you may feel more depressed.

◆ Friends and family become less available, and this loss of support may cause crying, insomnia, decreased energy and fatigue, and withdrawal from your usual routine and interests.

◆ You feel a strong sense that your loved one is near you, and it's not uncommon to hear the person's voice or even see him sitting in his usual place.

◆ You may feel a greater sense of unreality about being alone and may also experience feelings of denial.

◆ You spend time thinking about your relationship with your loved one. If there is unresolved guilt or anger, you try to work these feelings out.

◆ You have periods of feeling better, but certain events – birthdays, wedding anniversaries, special holidays and events that were planned but never happened – can make you feel much worse again.

Third stage

This stage usually lasts another year.

◆ You make new social contacts and begin to take part in activities and interests that didn't involve your loved one.

◆ You may still feel depressed and empty from time to time, but periods of crying are less frequent, and physical symptoms such as insomnia, decreased appetite and fatigue disappear.

◆ You are able to recall your loved one with pleasure and welcome the chance to talk about her with others.

Advice for the newly widowed or divorced person

◆ In the weeks and months after the death of your partner or the end of your marriage, you may be tempted to give up your house or move to another community to be closer to other family members. But your emotions may be clouding your judgment. Avoid making any drastic changes in your life for at least six months to a year.

◆ Don't ignore your physical health – eat properly, get some physical activity every day and avoid using alcohol or tranquilizers to help you cope. Some studies have found that older people, especially men, are more likely than younger people to get sick and even die in the first six months after the death of a spouse.

◆ Expect to see some changes in how other people treat you. Your adult children may suddenly become more anxious about your safety and well-being. Friends of your own age may treat you differently because you're no longer part of a couple – for example, they may exclude you from dinner parties and events that you once attended with your partner. Widowers are more likely than widows to receive certain types of support – friends and relatives assume men can't look after themselves, so they rush in to help with food and invitations.

◆ You shouldn't spend too much time alone in your house or apartment. If you don't feel like being with anyone, it's still a good idea to get out every day for a walk or a drive. If you're fortunate enough to have supportive friends and family, don't turn them away. If you're alone, consider joining a support group in your community where you can meet and talk with older women and men in your situation.

partner and said they missed their spouse as an individual.

But while grief is the most common reaction, it isn't universal. Nearly 17 percent of older people surveyed said the death of their spouse had affected them relatively little. This might have been because the relationship wasn't especially happy or because they felt that other life events such as the death of a child, a war, or changes in their own health had an even greater impact.

Women are more likely to experience the death of a partner than men. That's because females outlive males, and because traditionally women tended to marry men who were several years older than themselves.

Although many older women are emotionally devastated by the death of a beloved partner, studies show that they fare somewhat better than men in a similar situation. Women are more likely to have developed a support system of family and friends and are often closer to their adult children and grandchildren. Women who have watched as female relatives and friends coped with widowhood may also prepare themselves emotionally by "rehearsing" the loss of their partner.

Grief after loss

When your partner dies, you will probably go through a period of grieving. Feelings of grief can also occur after some other type of bereavement, such as the death of an elderly parent, a cherished sibling or friend, or an adult child.

Older people are also more likely to experience extreme grief following the death of a beloved pet. Studies have found that people who are mourning the death of a companion animal experience the same emotions and stages of grief as those who are mourning a human being.

There's no "right" way to grieve after losing someone you love. Some people adjust to their loss within weeks or months while others may go on grieving for years. Sometimes grief becomes so profound or prolonged that it requires professional help (see page 229).

When you have no immediate family

If you've never married or if you have no children, you may face special challenges later in life.

Many people imagine that never-married or childless people are abnormally lonely or unhappy, especially later in life. In fact, you may well experience some loneliness and find that you have fewer resources in times of trouble.

But you only need observe the lives of your friends and relatives to realize that being married and having children isn't a sure-fire guarantee against loneliness later in life. Spouses become ill and die, children move away, parents become estranged from each other and their children.

Many older people who never married or didn't have children compensate for the lack of an immediate family by cultivating a loving extended family of siblings, nieces, nephews and devoted friends who provide support. However, if you can't rely on this support in times of illness or crisis, you may need to ask for other kinds of help from community services and professional caregivers (see page 261).

Some experts believe there may actually be certain advantages to reaching older age without having married. You avoid the emotional suffering and the struggle to reorganize your life that accompanies widowhood or divorce. Also, by living alone for many years, you have probably developed qualities of independence and self-reliance that will help you cope with old age.

Being a grandparent

The experience of grandparenting varies from generation to generation and from culture to culture. In previous generations, grandparents were more likely to live under the same roof as their grandchildren than they are today, and this may have allowed them to play a more active role in their grandchildren's lives. This kind of intergenerational togetherness is still practiced by some families, especially if living with older parents is the cultural norm.

How you feel about being a grandmother or grandfather depends on many factors. Were your experiences with your own grandparents happy ones? Did you appreciate the role that your own parents played in the lives of your children? Do you have a good relationship with your adult children and their partners?

There are many kinds of grandparents, and one kind isn't necessarily "better" than another. Here are three basic grandparenting styles:

♦ Your contact with your grandchildren is limited. You may see them on special occasions or send them a gift or card on their birthdays.

♦ You have a friendly, involved relationship with your grandchildren and see them often at your home or theirs.

♦ You are actively involved in raising your grandchildren. You may be caring for them during the day to help their parents, or you may actually have custody of them and be raising them yourself.

Your grandparenting style may change over the years. For example, you may feel more attached and devoted to your grandchildren when they're young. Grandmothers enjoy having the opportunity to nurture a baby again, and grandfathers often discover they have more time and patience for a grandchild than they did for their own children.

Other grandparents are less interested in changing diapers and reading stories when their grandchildren are young, but form strong attachments to older grandchildren.

Some common later-life situations

The following questions aren't based on actual case histories, but they do illustrate certain situations and problems that occur later in life.

The joys and opportunities of grandparenting

Being a grandparent offers many potential rewards for you and your family. The rewards are obvious:

◆ You have the opportunity to enjoy your grandchildren without bearing total responsibility for them. Every grandparent knows the pure pleasure of handing a cranky toddler back to his or her parents!

◆ You have a "second chance" at loving and influencing a child, and because you have more experience now, you may avoid certain mistakes you made with your own children.

◆ Your grandchildren's presence, their experiences and questions, help keep you connected to the future. They are often rapt and willing listeners to stories, especially stories about your youth and their own parents' childhood. (Chances are your own children have heard these stories a thousand times by now and are less-than-willing listeners!)

There are also potential rewards for your family:

◆ The presence of grandparents can provide a stable structure for grandchildren, providing them with a sense of security apart from their parents.

This may be especially important for adolescent grandchildren who are rebelling against parental rules but who still want some kind of safe haven in the family. According to one survey, 80 percent of high school students said they discussed personal issues with their grandparents, and more than 70 percent reported that they still spent time with their grandparents.

◆ Grandparents can offer important emotional and practical support for grandchildren whose parents may be experiencing marital or financial problems.

◆ When it comes to teaching your grandchildren about life, you have a unique advantage: You've lived a much longer life than anyone else in the family and have learned how to cope with misfortune and how to adapt to change. You can share some of the strength and wisdom you've gained with grandchildren.

◆ Your continued presence in the lives of your grandchildren proves that, contrary to what society often teaches them, older adults are valuable people. This awareness and appreciation will pay off in many ways as they grow older themselves.

If you've faced any of these dilemmas, you may have already solved them on your own. Perhaps you obtained helpful advice and support from friends who had gone through similar experiences, or you may have received professional help.

The answers presented here are based on expert advice from social workers and other counselors who work with older people and their families. Such advice is general and certainly doesn't apply to every family. However, it may give you ideas and insights that will help you find your own solutions.

Losing contact with your family

My husband and I are in our mid-70s and live in a small town. Our three children have all moved away and are living in cities several hundred miles from our home. We try to visit them a few times a year, but it's difficult, and when we get there, our children seem so busy with their jobs and families. I often feel as though we're losing touch with them and becoming strangers, especially to our seven grandchildren, who hardly know us. Sometimes I think we should sell our house and move closer to one of them. What should we do?

It's not unusual today for family members to live in different cities and even countries. Although some families don't have a problem with this and even prefer it, when you're older it may be especially hard to live far from your children and their families for all sorts of practical and emotional reasons:

◆ You miss spending time with your children and grandchildren. This may make you feel that you're no longer important to them and that you don't have a place in their lives.

◆ Traveling is expensive and may be particularly stressful if you have health problems.

◆ When you do visit each other, the time you spend together may not be satisfying. For example, you and your family members may not want to "spoil" the visit by bringing up problems or sensitive issues. Or the opposite situation develops: You need to discuss everything in a limited amount of time, and the built-up tensions explode into arguments or confrontations.

◆ When you do need help during an illness or some other crisis, it's much more difficult for your children to provide assistance and support. (This works two ways: You may not be able to give them immediate help and support when they require it.)

Many older people feel so cut off from family members that they consider relocating to be closer to their adult children. This is a complicated decision that shouldn't be made without a great deal of open, honest discussion. Here are some questions to consider:

◆ Do you and your children feel equally positive about such a move?

◆ Do you and your partner agree about the desirability of moving?

◆ Will you be able to make a positive adjustment to an unfamiliar environment?

◆ Do you have a realistic idea about how much time your children and their families will be able to spend with you?

◆ Are you prepared to establish friends and

activities in your new home so that you don't become totally dependent on your children for company?

Before moving to another community to be closer to your son or daughter, consider relocating on a trial basis if you can afford to maintain two residences for a few months. If all goes well, then you can make the move with a clear mind. If you find the situation isn't to your liking, you still have the option to remain in your own community.

In the meantime, you can make a greater effort to keep in touch with your children and grandchildren and hope that this encourages them to do the same.

Long-distance telephoning is a good idea, but you should establish a regular calling time – for example, once a week on Sunday. This gives you something to look forward to, and you'll know that your children and grandchildren won't be out when you call. Such calls should be made at a mutually convenient time. Don't hesitate to make an unscheduled call occasionally, though, either to discuss a problem or just to say "I'm thinking about you."

If you don't already have one, get a phone extension so you and your partner can speak to family members together – that way you won't be repeating what each person says.

To save money on long-distance phone calls, try recording personalized messages or stories on audiotapes and sending them to your grandchildren. Be creative. If your grandchildren are still young, make up a story on tape and then ask them to continue it – you can keep sending the tape back and forth until the story is finished.

Letters are always a good way to stay in touch, but keep them short. Save jokes, riddles, interesting clippings and photographs for your grandchildren and tuck them into the envelope.

When an adult son or daughter asks you to move in

My wonderful wife passed away last year, and I'm still living in our apartment. I'm 76 and in pretty good health, except for some high blood pressure and diabetes. A few months ago I fell down at home and broke a bone in my wrist, so it's been hard to cook. My daughter comes to help me out with the laundry and cleaning, but lately she's been talking about me moving in with her. On the one hand, I don't want to hurt her feelings and make things harder for her, but on the other, I'm not sure I want to live with her and her family. What should I do?

In the past it was common for older people to move in with their children – for companionship, to save money, to help with household tasks and to look after grandchildren while parents were working.

But this is no longer the cultural norm in most Western societies, where older people seem to value their independence. In fact, *most older adults don't see moving in with adult children as an ideal option*. A recent survey asked women and men where they would choose to live if they couldn't manage on their own, and most said they would rather live in a seniors' facility than move in with an adult child!

There may, however, be emotional and practical benefits to such a move. You have a chance to rebuild or deepen your emotional ties with your child and grandchildren. You can help each other on a day-to-day basis, and there may be financial advantages for you both in sharing a home and other expenses.

This is a sensitive issue for older people who come from a cultural background where it's normal for an older person to move in with an adult child, usually a daughter, when he or she can no longer manage alone. Sometimes this works out well, but there can be problems: For example, your adult child may have become assimilated into the new country's culture and doesn't feel the same way you do or perhaps your child's partner has a completely different set of expectations about whether parents should live with their children. In such a situation, it's important to remember that no one is "right" or "wrong" – you simply have different feelings. Talking to a family therapist about these issues may be extremely helpful.

Before making such a complex decision, you should ask yourself the following questions:

♦ Are there alternatives to moving in with your adult child that you haven't considered? You and your children may not be aware of the services in your community that can allow you to remain in your own home or apartment, if that's what you would prefer (see page 261). For example, an older person who can't shop or cook because of a physical problem or disability may be able to manage quite well at home by having meals delivered daily from services such as Meals-on-Wheels.

♦ Is the location of your child's home convenient for you? It's important that you still have access to places and people, otherwise you risk feeling trapped in your new situation.

♦ Will you be spending most of your day alone? If loneliness is a problem now, you may think moving in with family will solve it. But this may not be so. It's likely that your child and his or her partner will be away working all day and your grandchildren will be away at school or with friends. If you expect to be alone much of the day, you'll still need to find activities and interests to keep you busy (see page 52).

♦ Is there enough room for you to live comfortably with your adult child and her family? If the house or apartment is small, if bedrooms are close together, or if you have to share a bathroom with other family members, this may create strain. Many families who do decide to live together find that living quarters that allow you to live separately but close by – for example, in a so-called in-law apartment – work best.

♦ Will the move cause members of your family to feel displaced or invaded? For example, if a teenaged grandchild has to give up a bedroom to make room for you, this can lead to feelings of resentment and probably isn't a good idea.

♦ Will you be able to adapt to moving in together? Consider whether your child's lifestyle suits you and vice versa. For instance, will your son-in-law's smoking bother you? Does your daughter keep a much neater – or messier – home than you're used to? Do they have pets who might bother you?

♦ Do you have a good relationship with your son-in-law or daughter-in-law? Remember: You won't just be moving in with your adult child, but also with his or her partner.

◆ Will you be expected to contribute to household expenses? Many families find it difficult to discuss money, but this can become a problem if you haven't talked it over beforehand and come to some mutual agreement about who pays for what.

If you do decide to move in with an adult child, here are some tips to ease the transition:

◆ Cooperate with your family in establishing and maintaining private time for all of you. For example, if you live in a downstairs apartment, you may agree to join your family for dinner two nights a week on an ongoing basis. If you live in the main part of the house, you may agree to be together for the first hour after dinner with your family, and then spend the rest of the evening on your own. Grandchildren should be involved and included in setting up such arrangements.

◆ Respect one another's privacy. A good rule to follow is that each person in the household has control over his or her room. This means your daughter shouldn't be "tidying up" your space and possessions, and you shouldn't venture into her personal areas for whatever reason. When it comes to mutual areas such as the kitchen, try to agree on your rights and responsibilities.

◆ Remember that your child is an adult who deserves respect and should treat you with respect. It's easy for parents and children who live under the same roof to fall back into old, familiar roles – for example, your 50-year-old daughter may be especially sensitive to your criticisms, which have the power to make her feel like a rebellious 16-year-old again.

◆ Try to keep silent and avoid taking sides during arguments between spouses and problems between parents and children. Every family has disagreements, and you may feel uncomfortable finding yourself in the middle of these situations rather than being a casual observer. It's a good idea to discuss such problems before they occur and to set up some ground rules. If the situation becomes very tense, you may choose to remove yourself by going to your own room – although this may cause you to feel upset and lonely if it happens too often.

◆ Finally, if you find that living with an adult child isn't working out for whatever reason, don't be afraid to leave. Talk to other family members or a social worker who can help you explore more desirable options. Even if your health is poor or you have financial problems, solutions can be found. If you feel you're being abused in any way, it's even more important that you find another living situation (see page 262).

When your family doesn't want you to remarry

I'm 72 and my husband died a few years ago. I'm in reasonably good health, I have enough money to live comfortably and I love to travel – although I don't enjoy traveling alone. I recently went on a cruise where I met a terrific man. He's a few years older than me, divorced with three grown sons. Lately he's been talking about us getting married. I might decide to say yes, but my own children are against it. They say he just wants my money and someone to look after him. How can I get married if my family is so negative about it?

Where do older people live?

◆ Forty-three percent have lived in their present home for more than 20 years.

◆ Five percent live in retirement communities.

◆ Nearly 30 percent live alone (32 percent of women, 22 percent of men).

◆ Thirty-three percent of men and half of all women over age 65 who are widowed, divorced or separated live with adult children or other family members.

◆ Fewer than 5 percent of those over age 65 live in nursing homes, although 25 percent can expect to be in a nursing home at some point in their later years.

Source: Wendy Lustbader and Nancy R. Hooyman, Taking Care of Aging Family Members *(New York: The Free Press, 1994)*

Many older women find themselves alone later in life, either through divorce or because they've been widowed. Because women tend to outlive men, they also outnumber them later in life, which means that widowed or divorced men have a better chance of finding a new spouse than widowed or divorced women.

Some women who have been widowed or divorced never even consider the idea of remarriage. If you had a happy marriage, you may still feel loyal to your partner's memory; if the marriage was unhappy, you may be reluctant to try again with someone else.

But there are many good reasons to remarry later in life – the comfort of intimate companionship, the opportunity to share your daily joys and problems, the presence of someone to lean on in times of stress and access to two incomes rather than one.

If you do find someone who seems compatible and decide to marry or live together, don't be surprised if an adult child or children raise some initial objections or oppose the idea completely:

◆ Your children may feel upset about the idea that someone else is going to "replace" their other parent.

◆ Like many younger people, they may accept certain stereotypes of aging and believe it's silly to think about marriage "at your age."

◆ They may be uncomfortable picturing you in an intimate relationship with someone other than their father (or mother) or in any intimate relationship whatsover. Children – of all ages – often have a hard time thinking about their parents' romantic or sexual needs.

◆ They may be worried about losing your attention and affection to a new spouse or to children and grandchildren that your partner may bring into the family.

◆ They may be upset to think that when you die, they could lose their inheritance – either in the form of money or cherished family possessions – to your new partner and his or her family.

◆ They may be genuinely concerned that you're making a poor choice.

If your children raise serious objections to your remarriage, listen to their concerns courteously and with an open mind. Try to hear the feelings that may lie behind their opposition, and if possible, reassure them that they will still have your love and support. If their concerns center on your finances or their inheritance, consider talking to a lawyer about the pros and cons of signing a marriage contract with your new spouse.

If your family continues to oppose the idea of remarriage, you have to decide whether remarriage is worth the risk of damaging your relationship with your children. But don't forget: It's quite possible that the opposition will fade once you've remarried and your children see that you're happy. It's also possible that relationships in the family will continue to be strained for some time.

You have as much right to be happy now as you did when you were younger. Don't let anyone convince you that you're "too old" to get married again if that's what you really want to do.

When your adult child goes through a divorce

Our daughter is going through a very bitter divorce. I feel depressed about it and am very worried about what will happen if my son-in-law gets custody of their children. My husband is extremely angry at our daughter and says she should never have asked for the divorce. Now we're arguing about this between ourselves. What can I do?

If you're a loving parent, it's difficult to watch your children suffer at any age. But when an adult child goes through a divorce, there may be added pressures and concerns:

◆ If you have grandchildren, you may be concerned about the negative emotional effects a divorce will have on them.

◆ You may also worry about losing touch with your grandchildren if the other parent gets sole custody. This parent may move away or remarry, and in some cases, may actively discourage contact between you and your grandchildren.

◆ You may feel guilty because, as a parent, you somehow didn't do enough to help your adult child avoid divorce. If you're divorced yourself, you may believe that this played some role in the failure of your son's or daughter's marriage.

◆ If divorce is creating financial problems for your adult child, you may be called upon or feel the need to offer assistance. In many cases where parents have sole custody of children but can't afford babysitting or daycare, grandparents may help out with childcare.

You have every right to be concerned about your grandchildren, and you may also have reasons to be afraid of losing contact with them. Some research has found that this is a greater problem when sons divorce, since mothers are still more likely to be given sole custody of children than fathers.

If you feel you're being denied access to your grandchildren, speak to a lawyer. In many jurisdictions, grandparents can pursue visitation rights after a divorce if it's found to be in the best interests of the children.

An adult child's divorce is bound to create stress in the family, and it may become an issue between you and your own partner.

Here are several ways to cope with this situation:

◆ Don't blame yourself for what's happening in the life of an adult child. Even if you could have helped the situation in some way, your advice might well have been rejected. If you did express doubts about the marriage before, this isn't the best time to say "I told you so."

◆ Offer whatever help and support you can. This might be in the form of giving financial assistance (if you can afford it), helping with your grandchildren, or simply providing a loving, non-judgmental ear.

◆ Don't add to feelings of bitterness by verbally attacking or putting down the other parent in front of your child or grandchildren.

◆ How you or your own spouse feels about an adult child's decision to divorce is a separate issue. Parents don't always know the intimate details of their children's private lives, and there may have been some very good reasons why the marriage ended.

When an adult child asks to move back home

Our youngest son is 30 and married with a new baby. He just lost his job and has asked if he and his family can move in with us for a few months, just until he finds a new job. He lived with us until he got married two years ago. We have a large home and I feel we should help, but my husband isn't sure this is the best idea. What should we do?

Adult children facing unemployment, divorce, health problems or drug dependency often turn to their parents for help, and many parents offer that help gladly. Such assistance can take many forms – you may be able to help out financially, or provide care for your grandchildren.

Once you agree to have an adult child move back home, it can be difficult to ask him to leave. That's why it's important to ask yourself certain questions before agreeing to such a request:

◆ Is this the best thing for you? Consider whether you have enough space, and whether your home is properly equipped to meet the needs of extra adults and young children. Decide whether you're ready to give up much of your own privacy.

◆ Is this the best thing for your adult child? While moving home may meet his needs in the short-term, will it encourage him to become dependent on you and prevent him from getting his life back in order? This may be a special problem if a child has been unusually dependent in the past.

◆ Does your spouse agree to having a son or daughter move home, even temporarily? If one of you is opposed, this is bound to cause problems later on.

Here are some suggestions to consider if your adult child does move back home:

◆ Set some mutually agreeable limits. For example, your son and his family can move in with you for three months or until he gets a new job. After that, you expect him to make other arrangements. If you don't set limits, the situation can drag on beyond everyone's endurance, resulting in resentment and arguments.

◆ Discuss what you expect from your child. This includes whether or not he will contribute to rent and living expenses, who will be taking care of extra cooking, housework and laundry, and what's expected in terms of "house rules" (Who disciplines the children? Can he and his wife smoke?).

◆ If the situation doesn't work out or persists beyond the terms of your agreement, discuss the next step. You may agree to having your child and his family remain with you for another few months, or you may decide they need to move out.

◆ You may decide that you want to help, but living together isn't the best idea. In that case, you could offer an adult child financial help in the form of a gift or loan to help him support himself and his family until he gets back on his feet.

When you are abused by a family member

My wife and I are in our 80s and still living in our own home. We have no children, but our nephew has always been very devoted to us, and we depend on him a great deal. A few years ago we gave him authority to manage some of our investments, and I just found out that a large part of the money is missing. When I asked him about it, he got very angry and said some terrible things. For a minute I even thought he was going to hit me. We are extremely upset about this. What should we do?

Although most older people enjoy positive relationships with their families, a minority will experience some type of neglect or abuse. Some experts estimate that at least 4 percent of older adults living in the community are neglected or abused.

While abuse by strangers and professional caregivers does happen, research has shown that most abusers are related to their victims. A recent study found that in 27 percent of elder abuse, the perpetrator was a son, in 24 percent of cases it was a husband and in 11 percent of cases the daughter was the abuser.

Abuse of older family members rarely happens without some other problem being present – for example, past episodes of conflict or violence, financial problems or alcohol and drug abuse.

◆ *Financial abuse:* This is the most common type of so-called elder abuse. It occurs when someone handles your money or property without your knowledge or consent. For example, an adult child or other relative may convince you to let them make investments for you that they turn to their own advantage. Or there may be outright theft or fraud involving property or pension checks.

◆ *Physical abuse:* This ranges from neglect to actual violence. Neglect means failure to provide the necessities of life to a dependent parent or other relative. Violence may include pushing, hitting, slapping or throwing objects that can result in bruises, cuts or even broken bones.

◆ *Psychological abuse:* This often accompanies other types of mistreatment. It may include cruel or belittling remarks and threats of physical harm or abandonment.

Some studies have found that two groups of older people may be especially vulnerable to abuse: those who are economically dependent on an adult child or other caregiver and those who are cognitively impaired due to illness such as Alzheimer's disease or stroke.

Many older people are reluctant to admit

that someone is mistreating or taking advantage of them:

◆ You may feel ashamed and embarrassed that this is happening to you and don't want anyone else to know about it. This is especially true if you're being abused by your own child.

◆ If your self-esteem is already low, you may feel that you deserve to be treated poorly. If you were mistreated in the past, by either a spouse or a parent, you may simply be accustomed to abuse.

Who provides care to older parents?

◆ Nearly 80 percent of caregivers are women.

◆ Daughters outnumber sons 3 to 1 as primary caregivers.

◆ One-third of caregivers are over age 65.

◆ Women today can expect to spend 18 years of their lives helping an aging parent.

◆ Most family caregivers provide about four hours of care each day, seven days a week.

◆ Fewer than 10 percent of caregivers say they use paid services.

Source: Wendy Lustbader and Nancy R. Hooyman, Taking Care of Aging Family Members (New York: The Free Press, 1994)

◆ If you're financially and/or emotionally dependent on the abuser, you may hesitate to complain or fight back because you fear being abandoned or losing their "love."

◆ You may worry that by revealing the abuse, you'll be forced to press charges against the person who is hurting you.

If you think someone is abusing you financially and don't want to confront that person directly, speak to someone else – another family member, a trusted friend or a lawyer. You need to find out what's happening and get control of the situation.

If you're being abused physically or psychologically by someone in your family, you need to break the cycle and get outside help. Unfortunately, very few people are willing to disclose this type of situation to a complete stranger. If there's no other relative you can talk to, call your family doctor or your clergyman. They may put you in touch with a social worker at a family service agency or seniors' center in your community that can help.

When your adult children don't share caregiving equally

I'm 74 years old, and my husband is in a nursing home with Alzheimer's disease. My arthritis has gotten worse recently, and I'm finding it hard to manage the laundry and shopping. My daughter has been wonderful to me, and my daughter-in-law tries to call, but she's looking after her own father, who is quite ill. My son is very busy at work and doesn't have time to see me, except on the weekends. My daughter just started a part-time job, and I'm afraid to tell her that

I need more help. What should I do?

When you need help at home, it's natural for your adult children – if you have them – to help out. In many families this assistance is offered lovingly and generously, but it's not unusual for one person to take on the bulk of caregiving responsibilities.

In a family with sons and daughters, daughters are more likely to take on the role of helping older parents when they need it. This is partly because women have been raised to nurture others, while many men don't feel comfortable in this role. Some families continue to make the incorrect assumption that women who don't work outside the home have more time to help a parent with shopping, laundry or doctor's appointments than men.

Geography is another factor that determines caregiving. For example, if your daughter lives in another city and you have a son living nearby, he's more likely to help out. But if he's married, he may rely on his wife to get involved.

It's likely that one of your adult children is seen as the so-called family leader. This role usually develops over many years and is often taken on by the eldest child or the child who has guided the family in previous crises. A sibling who also happens to be a nurse, social worker, doctor or other health care professional is often expected to take the lead when a parent is ill or needs help.

Some parents have only one adult child to rely on. It's easy to become very attached and dependent on an only son or daughter, especially if you have no other supports. But you should be aware that such adult children, who have families of their own and in-laws, can become physically and emotionally overwhelmed by a parent's needs.

What can you do if you or one of your children feels that too much is being expected of one member?

♦ If you sense that your daughter is becoming overwhelmed, ask her about it. This may give her "permission" to ask other members of the family to increase their participation.

♦ Call a family meeting to discuss the situation. This can involve you, your partner (if possible) and your adult children. You may decide to involve your children's partners and older grandchildren too.

♦ If your son isn't helping out, ask yourself if you've somehow let him "off the hook." Many older parents expect less from their sons because they accept that men are "too busy" or that their work is "too important" to be interrupted. They may ignore the fact that a daughter or daughter-in-law is often just as busy.

♦ When it comes to helping older parents, families must be flexible. Sometimes a situation that worked well in the past must change, either because a parent needs more help, or because an adult child faces added work or family responsibilities.

♦ If you require more help than your children can give, you should consider getting outside help – for example, a paid caregiver or help from a community service such as Meals-on-Wheels. Or it may be time to consider moving from your home or apartment into some kind of assisted living situation (see page 262).

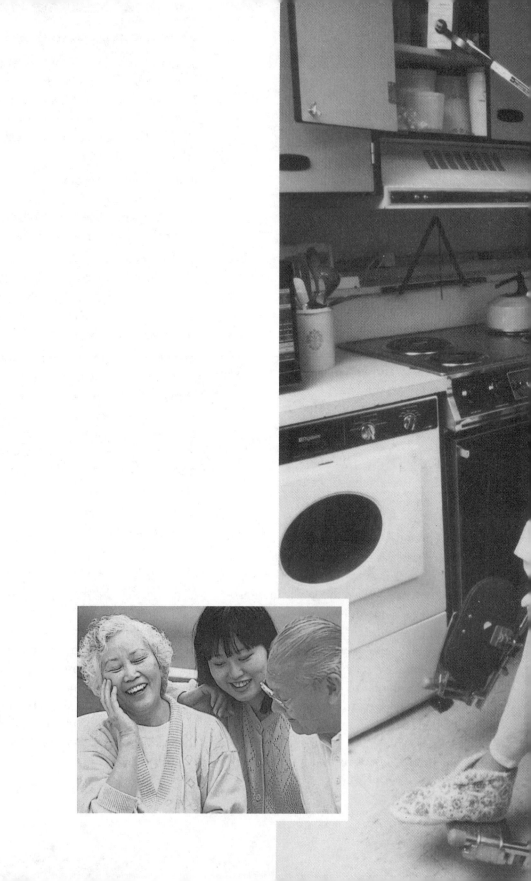

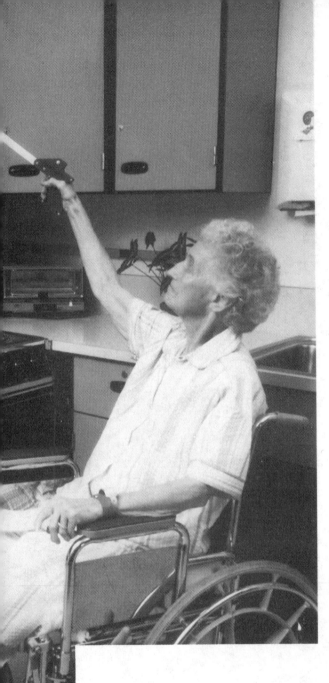

8

Old age is not a
disease – it is strength
and survivorship,
triumph over all kinds of
vicissitudes and
disappointments, trials
and illnesses.

MAGGIE KUHN

When You Need Help

ALL OF US NEED HELP SOMETIME during our lives, but as we grow older it can become more difficult to admit to this need. Over your lifetime you have probably offered help and support to other people – friends, family, strangers – on countless occasions. If you're like most people, chances are you feel more comfortable giving help than receiving it. But asking for and accepting help is a normal part of life.

If your health is good and you have a support system of relatives and friends, you can remain quite independent well into older age. Life is unpredictable, though, and your situation could change. That's why it's vital that you and your family know what kinds of help are available.

Many older people are reluctant to ask for help because they fear it means a loss of independence. In fact, *asking for and accepting help allows you to maintain your independence for a longer period of time*. By making proper use of in-home and caregiver support services available to older people and their families, you may prevent or delay moving to a nursing home.

When to ask for outside help

As you get older, it's possible that certain experiences and situations will challenge your ability to remain independent. These include illness, loss of physical or mental strength, the death of a spouse, isolation from family and financial vulnerability.

You or your partner, if you have one, may reach the sensible decision that help is necessary. You may decide to reach out to your adult children for assistance with shopping, meal preparation, banking, home maintenance or transportation to appointments.

Or you may decide that it's time to obtain professional help in the form of community services such as a visiting nurse, meal assistance or a homemaker or live-in companion (see page 261).

Unfortunately many older people are unaware that they need help. Others recognize the problem but stubbornly resist until they experience a close call or a minor disaster such as a fall or a kitchen fire.

More often than not, it's a family member – usually an adult child – who suggests that outside help may be necessary. Some older people feel upset or hurt by such a suggestion and want to reject it. But it's important to consider why the suggestion is being made.

Your children may be genuinely worried about your well-being and want to make sure that you are safe and happy. This is a special concern if you aren't in good health or if you've recently become widowed and are living alone for the first time in many years.

If your children have been helping you, they may feel that they can no longer provide all the assistance you need.

Your children may feel that, by accepting some outside help, they will be able to spend more time actually talking and visiting with you instead of running around on errands or doing housework.

Why some older people resist help

There are many reasons why an older person might refuse to seek or accept outside help:

◆ You may genuinely feel that you don't need assistance and that family members are suggesting it in order to relieve their own feelings of anxiety or guilt.

◆ You were raised to believe that asking for help, especially from someone outside your family, is a sign of weakness.

◆ You may believe you're doing just fine on your own and don't realize how dependent you have become on a son or daughter. It's easy to categorize what your adult child does for you as a "favor" or something done out of love – which it probably is. But just how "independent" would you be without this help?

◆ You may worry that if you agree to outside help, your family will stop coming to see you. Although it's true that they may not come as frequently as they do now, you may find that when you see them, your time together is more enjoyable.

◆ You may not like the idea of "strangers" coming into your home. Perhaps you don't want to give up your privacy, or you may be concerned that they will damage or steal something that belongs to you.

◆ If your family thinks you're spending too much time alone during the day, they might suggest that you become involved in a community program for older adults. Some older people resist such involvement because they don't identify themselves as "joiners." The idea of associating with other older women and men, especially those who appear infirm, can be threatening because it forces you to confront the reality of your own aging – or at least your fears of aging.

Admitting that you need some help is just the first step. Next you must decide what type of help will best meet your needs and then find out how to access it in your community.

Finding the right kind of help

This can be a bewildering experience, especially if you're alone or coping with illness. You may not be familiar with what type of help is available in your community. You may not be sure if you're eligible to receive certain community-based services. Or, you may feel uncomfortable about the idea of accepting free, government-funded services, or fret about the added expenses if you aren't eligible for free services or covered by insurance for the added expense.

How do you go about finding help for yourself or someone in your family? Many communities operate senior information and referral hotlines, which can be a valuable source of information and can also save you time and energy. The hotline will tell you what types of services are available in your area and supply you with phone numbers and contacts. The phone number may be listed in the front of your telephone directory, or you can ask the telephone operator to find it for you.

Other sources of information might include a local seniors' center or hospital, your family physician, a local family support agency or the public health department.

A guide to community support services

Community support services exist to meet the special needs of older people who are still living in their own homes or who have moved in with an adult child.

If you're the one who needs assistance, these services can help you preserve or even improve the quality of your life and allow you to remain as independent as possible. They can make your life easier on a day-to-day basis and ease the pressure on your partner or other family caregivers.

If you're looking after a spouse or parent, these services can preserve your own physical and emotional health, which is vital to you and also to the person you are caring for.

Services in your home

◆ *Homemaker services* provide in-home help with chores such as meal preparation, housecleaning, laundry and even shopping. Many home health care agencies offer these services on a sliding scale based on your ability to pay.

◆ *Meal home delivery programs* prepare and deliver hot, nutritious meals to you as often as you need them. This is helpful for older adults who can no longer shop or cook for themselves and who might become malnourished. Besides providing meals, many older people enjoy the regular contact with the volunteers who make the deliveries.

◆ *Home health care services* provide education and assistance with health care procedures and treatments when you're ill or recovering from surgery. For example, if you have diabetes, a specially trained nurse can visit you at home and teach you and your caregiver how to monitor your blood glucose levels and how to deliver insulin injections. Or she might show you how to care for a colostomy. Other home health care services such as hearing tests, foot care and physiotherapy may also be available.

Services away from home

◆ *Day programs* offer structured activities and companionship for older people who are living alone or with family members who are away during the day.

These programs provide a variety of activities, including outings, guest speakers, music, art and discussion groups. In some communities day programs are available for older people whose first language is not English. The programs, which may include transportation and one or two hot meals each day, are usually staffed, by social workers, recreation and program staff and volunteers. You can choose to attend as often as you'd like, and fees may be partly or completely subsidized, depending on your ability to pay.

Some day programs are designed for people with mild to moderate cognitive impairment due to Alzheimer's disease or another type of dementing illness. They provide a secure environment for cognitively impaired people, offer activities geared to their abilities and give information and advice to family members.

◆ *Respite care* is designed to provide a break for those who are caring for a partner or parent in the community. Even if you're making use of community-based services, you still need some time away from your caregiving responsibilities. If you're caring for someone who can't be left alone due to cognitive impairment, respite care may be extremely helpful and may help delay the need to place your relative in institutional care.

Respite care may be provided in various settings, including your own home, a nursing home or hospital. It may involve medical supervision, physiotherapy and recreational activities geared to the needs of your relative. This allows caregivers to rest, to take a much-needed vacation or to attend to their own health care needs, which are often ignored. Respite services can also help when a personal illness or family crisis takes you away from your caregiving responsibilities.

A guide to alternative living situations for older people

Even if you locate and take advantage of

community-based support services, you may find it difficult to continue living on your own or with an adult child.

This may lead you or your family to conclude that it's time for a nursing home. But this may not be necessary. Here are some other options to consider.

◆ *Subsidized apartments*, available in many communities, are built especially for older people who are reasonably independent but require some assistance. Rent is often geared to income, which is important for older adults who are living on a fixed income.

These buildings are often designed to meet the needs of older individuals and couples, including those with physical disabilities. For example, wheelchair access, wider-than-average corridors and doorways, accessible kitchen cupboards, doorbells with flashing lights for the hearing-impaired and grab bars in the bathroom may be standard features. Meals and housekeeping are not included, although you can make these arrangements on your own. The buildings may also offer extra security, including an emergency button in each apartment and a manager on duty 24 hours a day.

Subsidized apartments are often located close to shopping areas and seniors' centers, and may provide daily or weekly van service to nearby malls.

◆ *Retirement homes* are similar to subsidized apartments but provide extra services such as meals in a central dining room, recreational activities and weekly housekeeping help, which are figured into the rent. You may also receive certain personal care services and assistance with medications for an additional fee.

◆ *Group homes* offer a type of communal living that meets the needs of older people who are widowed and don't want to live alone, but who may not want to live in an apartment and can't afford a retirement home.

These are usually converted family homes, run by licensed operators or agencies. They provide private or shared bedrooms and bathrooms, and common kitchen, laundry and recreational areas. A house manager and other staff members live on the premises to provide supervision and security. There may be access to a garden, and pets may be allowed.

◆ *Assisted living apartments* offer all the services of a retirement home but also provide daily help with personal care, including on-site nursing care.

How to find and keep a good professional caregiver

Some older people who are too disabled to live alone but who don't want to leave their home or apartment may decide to hire a professional caregiver. Such care is expensive, so you must be able to afford it, either on your own or with help from your adult children.

If you decide that you want the person to live with you, your home or apartment must be large enough to provide private accommodation for the caregiver, and you must be able to provide extras such as a television, telephone, dishes and linen.

A paid helper can provide a variety of services based on your needs. He or she may help with daily care such as bathing, dressing and meals, accompany you on outings or to appointments, and provide companionship

Is the home-sharing option right for you?

What if you don't want to give up the familiarity of your home but can no longer afford or manage to stay there? Some older people in this situation find a solution in a home-sharing arrangement.

There are several ways to approach home-sharing:

◆ You might decide to ask a relative – an unattached adult child or a young adult niece or grandchild – to move in with you. They get free or reduced rent in exchange for keeping you company in the evening and helping you with household tasks, shopping and driving.

◆ If no family member is available, you could ask someone else to move in with you under a similar arrangement. This could be another older adult or a student who is willing to exchange help and companionship for reduced or free rent. You may be able to find such a person through an accommodation registry in your community or by advertising for a housemate in a local newspaper.

Before moving ahead into a home-sharing arrangement – whether the sharer is a family member or a stranger – consider the following questions:

◆ Are you confident about finding the right kind of person to share your home?

◆ Do you have realistic expectations about what this person can and can't provide for you? For example, if you want regular company, it's unlikely that a young relative or student will be prepared to eat every meal and spend every evening with you.

◆ Are you willing to give up your privacy and make compromises?

◆ Are you prepared to set up a system of rules that will be mutually agreeable? These rules would cover areas of potential conflict such as privacy, noise, pets, smoking, having guests spend the night, sharing of expenses and household tasks.

◆ Will the benefits of home-sharing actually outweigh the disadvantages?

If you advertise for a housemate, ask those who respond to supply you with personal and landlord references and then check these references thoroughly. Consider asking the person for a deposit to be kept against any damage to your home. The terms of the sharing agreement – for example, whether rent or expenses will be paid and how much notice each party must give before terminating the arrangement – should be put in writing and signed in the presence of a witness. If you have any doubts about the person or the arrangement, ask for a trial period and put this provision in writing.

by talking, reading to you or playing cards. In the best situation, mutual trust and affection can develop, and the caregiver can become a friend to you and your family.

Hiring a paid helper is a major decision. You want to find the best possible person – someone who is reliable and trustworthy, who is capable of meeting your needs, both physically and emotionally, and who respects you as a person, regardless of age or disability. It's also important that you be compatible, because you'll be spending lots of time together. If you enjoy chatting, don't hire someone who seems particularly shy or quiet; if you're naturally reserved, you may not want someone who is too loud or boisterous.

You can find a paid caregiver in several ways: by advertising for one in the newspaper under "Domestic help wanted"; by answering ads from people seeking employment, usually under "Domestic employment wanted"; or by hiring an agency to supply you with the best person.

While hiring through an agency is more expensive than doing it yourself, there may be certain advantages. Many agencies ask caregivers for references and carry out a security check on their backgrounds. Some agencies are bonded, meaning they may be liable should you be able to prove that the person they recommended has stolen from you or damaged your property. However, agencies vary widely in quality and honesty. The best way to choose one is through a personal recommendation from someone who has used and is satisfied with their services. You can also call the Better Business Bureau in your community (listed in the white pages of your telephone directory) and ask what they know about the agencies on your list.

If you're hiring a caregiver to look after your partner or a parent – even through an agency – you should go about it carefully.

It may be a good idea to exclude your relative from the initial interview. This allows you to give the applicant information and ask certain questions that you might not want to share in your relative's presence.

You can also use this interview to narrow down the choices before introducing applicants to your relative.

Once you have a short list of candidates, arrange for each one to meet your relative at home. Encourage the older person to be actively involved in the interview if he or she is mentally capable of doing so.

Observe how each applicant acts with your relative. Is her approach respectful? Does she seem warm and caring? Does she ask questions about your relative's life and listen to the answers?

Always ask for references and check them thoroughly. If you can't track down an applicant's references, this is usually a warning sign that he or she may be dishonest.

You should always have a signed contract, spelling out the terms of employment – salary to be paid, salary to be deducted for social security, hours and days off and notice of termination (see page 266). To find out what your legal obligations as an employer are, call the social security office in your community. It's listed under "federal government" in your telephone directory.

Once you've hired a professional caregiver, you should do everything you can to make the arrangement work.

It's a good idea to have a trial period of a few weeks. This gives your relative and the caregiver the opportunity to get to know each other and decide if the arrangement is suitable. If not, you can feel free to back out.

It's important that you and your family state clearly what you expect from the caregiver and stick to the deal. If you make a habit of asking for more help – extra chores, longer hours – the person will become resentful and probably start looking for other work.

Sample agreement with a salaried live-in caregiver

1. Room and Board

Employer will provide three meals a day and a private room.

2. Salary

Employer will pay $_____ gross monthly. $_____ will be deducted for Social Security, leaving a net pay of $_____ per month.

3. Time Off

Employer will provide two 24-hour periods off per week, on _____ and _____. Live-in will give at least one week's notice if these days need to be changed.

4. Extra Work Days

If substitutes fail to arrive on live-in's days off, employer will pay live-in $_____per day.

5. Duties of Live-In Helper

_____

_____

_____

_____

6. Termination of the Agreement

Either party can terminate this agreement with two weeks' notice. If a hospitalization occurs, normal pay will continue for _____ days. Thereafter, if live-in does not seek other employment, $_____ will accrue each day, payable in a lump sum once the hospitalization ends.

Employer_____   Date:_____
(signature)

Live-in_____   Date:_____
(signature)

Source: Wendy Lustbader and Nancy R. Hooyman, Taking Care of Aging Family Members *(New York: The Free Press, 1994)*

Even though it may be hard to do so in the face of illness or disability, you and your family should make every effort to treat a paid caregiver with friendliness and respect. Expressing your personal appreciation on a regular basis is often just as important to an employee as the salary she is being paid.

Always have a back-up plan ready in case of a crisis – for example, if the caregiver becomes ill, has family problems or leaves on short notice. You might want to write these into the agreement and also have the signature of a witness.

When a nursing home becomes necessary

Many older people and their families eventually must face the fact that some type of nursing home or chronic care is necessary.

In many cases this difficult decision is reached after a gradual process of decline caused by chronic, debilitating illness. In other cases, the main caregiver – usually a spouse – dies or falls ill and can no longer care for a dependent partner. Or a sudden illness requiring hospitalization occurs and it seems unlikely that the person will be able to manage at home after being discharged.

The decision to enter a nursing home is extremely complex, and the reasons for making it vary greatly from person to person and family to family.

Here are some warning signs that it may be time to consider a nursing home for yourself or someone in your family:

◆ Incontinence is an ongoing problem. The person must be changed and bathed frequently, and soiled bedding must be laundered. These factors place an extreme burden on the caregiver. (It's vital that all proper steps to diagnose, treat and manage an incontinence problem have been taken; see page 158.)

◆ Cognitive impairment caused by Alzheimer's disease or some other illness is severe enough that the person can no longer be left alone safely and must be supervised at all times.

◆ The person is becoming too heavy for caregivers to manage safely at home – for example, there may be problems with transferring the person in and out of bed or chairs, onto the toilet or in and out of the bathtub.

◆ The main caregiver – usually a spouse – is losing sleep and becoming physically and emotionally exhausted by the person's needs. Other help may not be available or affordable.

◆ The main caregiver experiences illness or injury or faces stress from other directions –

A nursing home checklist

Before choosing a nursing home for yourself or someone in your family, it's important to do some research. You should be prepared to visit the home on more than one occasion, and it's a good idea to make one of those visits during the evening or on a weekend when staffing levels tend to be lowest.

Besides looking over the facilities and speaking to staff, talk to some residents and their family members and ask them to tell you about the home.

Location

People who receive the best care in nursing homes are those whose family members visit them often. That's why the location of the home should be convenient for your visitors – for example, it should be located near your child's home or office and accessible to public transportation if your partner doesn't drive.

Certification

Check to see that the home has a current license to operate (this should be posted in a prominent place) and that it is certified to participate in government assistance programs if you expect to receive benefits.

General atmosphere

The home itself should appear clean and well maintained, with good natural lighting. Proper ventilation is important to minimize unpleasant odors. Do the residents generally look clean and content? Notice whether they are up and dressed and if they've been encouraged to wear their own clothes. Do staff members seem to be cheerful and willing to answer questions?

Resident rooms

Whether a room is private or semi-private, it should have at least one window and open into a corridor. Check to ensure that steps have been taken to allow for privacy – for example, there should be a drape or screen around the bed in a semi-private room. Is the layout of the room practical? There should be ample storage space, a bedside table,

for instance, another illness or death in the family or financial problems.

Facing your feelings

Some older people make the decision to enter a nursing home with good grace. Perhaps you recognize that there's a genuine need for such care, or you may wish to spare the health of your partner and protect your family from worry. But most people have some difficulty accepting the idea, and others are violently opposed:

◆ You may feel upset and betrayed, especially if your family raises the subject of nursing-home care abruptly. If you feel that you have no control, you may resist simply out of anger.

◆ You may feel as if your family is abandoning you and worry that you won't see them anymore.

◆ You fear that entering a nursing home means your life is over. You feel anxious about how you will be treated there, and you grieve over the expected loss of independence and privacy.

◆ Like many people, you may have a nega-

adequate light for reading or sewing, an easy chair and chairs for guests. Look around to see whether residents have been allowed to decorate their own rooms with personal possessions such as bedspreads, knickknacks and photos.

Common areas

There should be some common areas where residents can go to get away from their rooms – for example, a lounge where they can chat, read, watch television or sit with guests. A separate dining room, where residents can take meals together, is a good feature. There should also be some outdoor areas where people can go for some fresh air and sunshine.

Safety

The home should be fully wheelchair accessible. There should be a call button beside the bed and in the bathroom and grabbars beside the tub and toilet. The home should be equipped with smoke detectors and automatic sprinklers, and exits should be clearly marked. Find out whether the home has a no-smoking policy.

Professional services

There should be a physician on staff or on call at all times, and registered nurses on duty 24 hours a day. A good nursing home will offer other services and programs – for example, a pharmacy, dental care, social workers, some type of physical and/or occupational therapy, recreational and cultural activities, pet visiting and access to religious services.

Food services

Ask to see a sample menu and meal schedule. There should be three meals offered daily at reasonable hours, as well as nutritious snacks. Is assistance available to those who need help with meals? Check to see if the kitchen can supply meals for people on restricted diets and ask how much choice is available. If you really want to check the quality of the food, ask if you can taste it.

tive impression of nursing homes. Perhaps you visited a relative or friend in one that was less than adequate, and can't forget the sights, sounds and smells.

Here are some emotional reactions and situations that can occur:

◆ You're willing to assume certain risks in order to remain at home. However, your adult children aren't willing to have you assume those risks, because this creates feelings of anxiety and guilt for them. Whose feelings should prevail?

◆ When your family raises the issue, you may try to bargain them out of it – for example, you may promise not to call them so often, or to stay in bed all day in order to avoid falling.

◆ The situation may become complicated when family members disagree about the need for nursing-home care. One adult child may press for the decision, while another says it's premature. Sometimes this kind of disagreement is based on long-standing alliances or conflicts between parents and children. Or it could simply be based on different perceptions

What you should know about nursing-home care

Nursing homes provide five basic types of service:

◆ *Medical care:* Most nursing homes have physicians on staff and/or on call to deliver basic medical care. If you wish to remain in the care of your own personal doctor, and he is willing, some homes will allow it.

◆ *Nursing care:* This includes the services of registered nurses (RNs) or licensed practical nurses who administer medicines, injections and treatments that are ordered by a doctor.

◆ *Personal care:* This includes help with bathing, eating, dressing and grooming, which is usually provided by health care aides.

◆ *Therapeutic services:* These may include social, recreational and spiritual activities and programs.

◆ *Residential services:* This includes room and board, meals, housekeeping, supervision and protection.

– for instance, a daughter who lives nearby and helps you on a day-to-day basis may have a clearer understanding of your current needs than a son who lives out of town and only speaks to you on the phone.

◆ You and your family may differ about what should happen when a parent becomes frail and dependent. Perhaps you spent years looking after your own parent at home and now you expect the same from your adult children. You must be prepared to accept that they are unable or unwilling to meet those expectations.

How to make a difficult decision easier

Many families have difficulty communicating about emotionally charged issues. But such communication is absolutely vital now.

If you're the one who is in need of nursing-home care, it's important that you feel able to express your fears. Once your family understands the source of your anxiety, they may be able to relieve it.

If a partner or parent is in need of nursing-home care, listen to his fears and try to respond constructively. He may simply want reassurance that he won't be abandoned, that you will continue to visit him and that you will do your best to handle any problems that arise.

Such reassurance may be difficult to convey to a partner or parent who is suffering from cognitive impairment due to illness. This can place an extra burden of guilt and sorrow on family members.

If a serious family conflict exists over the nursing-home decision, it may be useful to speak to a professional social worker or family therapist. All nursing homes and many community agencies employ social workers who may be able to help.

Most people tend to focus on the negative consequences of moving to a nursing home. Instead, try to explore the positive aspects and potential benefits to you or your family member.

For example, families who are relieved of the physical and emotional strain of caregiving may begin to enjoy better relationships.

You may look forward to improvements in your health and well-being because of better nutrition, more frequent bathing, attentive nursing care, and access to certain types of therapy and recreational activities.

If you lived alone or with minimal help, you may be relieved to have the company and assistance of other people and be freed from anxiety about your safety. There may also be an opportunity for greater social contact with other residents and family members, volunteers and staff. If you had few social contacts before, this may give you renewed pleasure in life and even improve your memory and alertness.

As acute care hospitals cut back on length-of-stay in order to save health costs, many families are faced with the pressure to discharge an older person directly into a nursing home. In some cases this can't be avoided. However, some people find it extremely difficult to accept the idea of moving directly into a nursing home. They may be afraid, but they may also genuinely feel that they would be able to cope at home.

In this situation, you may want to arrange a "trial period" at home. It's possible that, contrary to everyone's expectations, you are able to manage quite well. Faced with the option of a nursing home, you may be more willing to accept help such as Meals-on-Wheels or a visiting homemaker. However, the trial period may help some older adults recognize the full extent of their limitations. While this can be stressful for family members, who must watch their relative struggle, the experience may make it easier for an older person who has vehemently rejected the idea of a nursing home to finally accept that there's no other choice.

Should you have a living will?

By the time you've reached age 65, you may have already made out a will. This is a formal legal document, usually prepared and held by your lawyer, that determines the disposition of your property after you die. While it's absolutely vital that you have a will, its terms only come into effect after your death. It doesn't address certain complex situations that tend to occur toward the end of life.

We live in an era where high-tech medical care can save lives that would not have been saved even a decade ago. Doctors now have the ability to prolong life – sometimes beyond the point where we may feel it's worth living. In the face of such realities, many people today are less concerned about the fact of dying than they are about the manner in which they will end their lives:

◆ You may wonder what will happen if illness or injury prevents you from expressing your wishes to your doctors and relatives.

◆ You may have strong feelings about what type of treatments you would and would not want in certain situations.

◆ You may wish to spare your partner or

your adult children from the anguish of making certain decisions on your behalf when they don't really know your wishes.

All about advance directives

In recent years there's been a growing interest in the use of advance directives, particularly so-called living wills, which are designed to give people a greater say in various life-and-death decisions.

A living will is a legal document. It allows you to set down certain wishes in advance, giving you some control over your medical treatment in case you become unable to speak for yourself. For example, you might develop an illness such as Alzheimer's disease that affects your ability to make choices or to communicate your desires to others. Or you might lapse into a coma following an illness or injury and be unable to speak for yourself.

Some people choose to prepare living wills while they are still relatively healthy. Others are prompted to make the move after watching a friend or relative suffer a lingering death.

A living will gives you the opportunity to state in advance whether you would accept or reject life-sustaining treatment and care such as tube feeding, the use of artificial breathing machines known as ventilators, blood transfusions, kidney dialysis, certain kinds of emergency surgery and resuscitation after heart attack or stroke.

In some jurisdictions, living wills are not considered legally binding on doctors or family members. If you are considering a living will for yourself or someone you care about, speak to a lawyer who can advise you how to proceed. It's also a good idea to discuss your concerns with your doctor. Even though your own physician may not be directly involved in your care later on, she may be able to advise you.

Here are some points to consider:

◆ A living will is no substitute for discussing your wishes with your doctor and members of your family. If you haven't prepared such a will, they may use these discussions as a guideline to determine your care later on. If you do have a living will, it's important that they know about it. If other people are convinced that the document is an accurate expression of your wishes, they are less likely to challenge the provisions you have made.

◆ When making a living will, be certain that the wording is clear. Stating that you would prefer "no extraordinary measures" isn't enough – you must be specific. Perhaps you wish to decline the use of measures such as resuscitation unless there's a reasonable chance that such treatment will restore you to active independent life instead of just prolonging the dying process. (Even so, doctors and family members may still have trouble deciding what a "reasonable chance" is.)

◆ When making provisions, be sure that you understand the medical implications of what you are requesting. If you aren't a doctor, you may not have a thorough enough understanding of certain conditions and treatments. For example, someone who has cancer may state that he doesn't want surgery or radiation if the situation is hopeless. But sometimes such treatment can reduce the size of a tumor and actually make you more comfortable in your final days.

- You should review your living will regularly – once a year if you are still reasonably healthy, more often if your health is poor or is deteriorating. It's not unusual for people's wishes to change over time, and you can certainly make amendments.

- If you do decide to draw up a living will, many experts now advise you to designate a proxy, someone who can interpret the will later on and make decisions in case of unforeseen circumstances. Such a person should be someone whom you trust and who understands your values and wishes.

- You can ask a lawyer to design a living will, or you can use a form that is available from organizations such as Dying with Dignity in Canada and Concern for Dying in the U.S. Some experts say that while a legal document is best, writing your wishes on a piece of paper and signing it is better than doing nothing at all. The paper should be kept with you at all times and a copy given to a trusted relative.

- Instead of a living will, some jurisdictions allow for another arrangement known as a health care power-of-attorney. This is a legal document that appoints another person – for example, your partner or an adult child – to make health care decisions on your behalf should you become unable to do so. Unlike a living will, a health care power-of-attorney may allow this person to make a variety of decisions on your behalf, not just decisions regarding end-of-life care. For example, your partner could refuse or request a particular treatment on your behalf. Your lawyer can advise you about the possible advantages of a health care power-of-attorney.

When competency becomes an issue

Imagine how you would feel if you lost the ability to perform certain tasks and make everyday decisions about your life. Such a situation would be devastating. You would lose your sense of independence, other people might begin to see and treat you in a different way and your self-esteem would be threatened.

Now imagine that you have lost this ability but aren't fully aware of it, or perhaps you don't want to accept that a problem exists. In this situation, you might continue to make decisions or act in a way that places you or someone else in a potentially harmful situation. For example, some older people who should not be driving because of health problems continue to do so, even though they are putting themselves and others at risk (see page 88).

Certain illnesses of later life – particularly those known to affect the brain and behavior – can alter your ability to make decisions and perform certain tasks. But remember: Just because someone has such an illness doesn't mean they are or will become incompetent!

Sometimes another person, usually a close relative or friend, will notice these changes and decide to challenge your competency to manage your own financial affairs or to choose where you should live. Their intentions may be completely honorable. They may feel they have an obligation to act in order to protect you from doing harm to yourself or to others. Unfortunately, sometimes such actions are undertaken for less selfless reasons – perhaps to gain financial control over an older person's estate.

However, even if the intentions behind such a challenge are honorable, any situation involving an allegation of incompetency is bound to be difficult.

What is incompetency?

Incompetency can occur at any age. It's defined as the inability to make decisions and perform specific tasks in an adequate manner. An incompetent person is no longer legally able to make certain decisions and act on them.

There are many kinds and degrees of incompetency. Sometimes a person becomes temporarily incompetent during an acute illness – for instance, delirium due to an infection, or an episode of mania (see page 217). If the problem is correctly diagnosed and treated, it's possible that competency will be restored.

In extreme cases, a person may become totally incompetent because of a serious illness or injury and is unable to manage his life. Such a person requires extensive care and supervision, including the appointment of a legal guardian who will make important health care and financial decisions.

But incompetency that arises later in life often tends to be much less dramatic. For example, someone in the early stages of Alzheimer's disease may still be competent enough to decide how and where she wants to live. However, she may have memory problems that make it difficult for her to do her banking – she may write several checks to pay the same bill, or she may make out checks in the wrong amount.

The best way to determine whether someone is competent is through an assessment process. Before a person is subjected to an actual competency assessment, family and friends should explore the situation on a less formal basis. You may have reasons to question an older person's competence in one or several areas, but that may not be enough to justify a formal assessment.

An informal assessment can take place during a family meeting, or you may wish to include the person's doctor in your discussion. Here are some questions that should be considered.

◆ What is the person's problem or problems? Are there real risks if the person continues to live in his present situation?

◆ Has everything been done to help solve these problems – for example, medical care to treat underlying illness, adding safety features to the person's home or apartment and taking full advantage of community services and in-home care?

◆ Will a formal competency assessment help solve the problem?

◆ Whose interests would be served by a formal assessment – those of the person at risk or those of family members?

Because there are still no generally accepted standards regarding formal competency assessment, procedures can vary dramatically from place to place. If you decide that a formal assessment is necessary, you should seek out the advice of a geriatrician or psychiatrist. They may be able to refer you to a competency clinic in or near your community. Here's what will happen.

First, the person should be informed as gently and respectfully as possible that an assessment is going to be done. This should probably come from someone familiar – a family member or trusted physician, rather than a strange doctor.

There is one way to introduce the subject: "We would like you to go for a competency assessment because we're worried about you. You sometimes seem to be confused or upset about things, and we would like to see if you are making decisions that are in your best interest – we're sure that you want to also. We want to help you, but we can't unless we know what kind of help you need."

The actual assessment will be carried out by several health care professionals, usually under the supervision of a psychiatrist, psychologist or geriatrician. The assessment will probably take place in several stages and include the following: psychological testing to identify problems with memory and comprehension; observation of the person in his own environment to see how well he carries out specific tasks; discussions with the person and his family to help identify the problems.

A competency assessment may find that, contrary to the opinions expressed by family or friends, the person is still competent. However, if she is found to be incompetent, legal steps may be taken allowing a family member or a court-appointed guardian to make certain decisions on her behalf.

Facing the end of life

We have now come to the last section of the final chapter, and it discusses a subject most of us prefer to avoid. Denying death is natural, and it may even serve a healthy purpose when you're young, but this denial often becomes harder to maintain when you grow older, especially if you are sick and have watched loved ones pass away.

Of course it's impossible to fully explore the subject of death and dying in such a short space. Many excellent books have been written on the topic. But it would be wrong to end this book without examining certain important issues regarding death and dying today.

Just a few generations ago, most deaths occurred at home, usually in the presence of family members. In fact, if you are now in your 70s or 80s, you may vividly recall the experience of having an older relative – perhaps a grandparent – die at home.

However, in recent years, death and dying have been removed from this natural environment, and today approximately 80 percent of the population die in hospitals or nursing homes. For many of us, this has led to an increased fear of death – either our own or that of a loved one – and, in particular, to increased anxiety about the dying process.

You may be afraid that you'll die in the impersonal surroundings of an institution, surrounded by strangers and hooked up to machines that sustain your life beyond the point where you feel it's worth living. You may also worry that dying will be accompanied by severe or uncontrollable pain. Such fears play a major role in the decision to commit suicide or to ask for help in ending one's life.

Although each of us will die, most of us don't know when death will come. Some of us, however, will develop an illness that progresses to the point where the doctors say we are unlikely to recover. If you or someone you know is facing a terminal illness, you should be aware of certain choices that may be available and that can make the process easier to bear.

The palliative care option

Finding out that you probably won't recover from an illness is likely to bring on feelings of hopelessness and despair. You may believe that your life is over at that very moment and that "nothing more can be done" for you. But just because a cure seems unlikely, that doesn't mean nothing more can be done. In fact, a great deal can be done.

You can still have goals, and the most important one now is to live as independently and comfortably as possible for as long as you can.

Many communities now offer some type of palliative care service, also known as hospice care, to people facing terminal illness. Such programs may be self-contained or they may be affiliated with local hospitals.

Palliative care is delivered at home and/or in the hospital by a specialized team of caregivers who are trained to recognize and meet the special needs of dying people and their families. The palliative care team includes specially trained nurses, doctors, pharmacists, social workers, therapists, chaplains, homemakers, volunteers, and – last but certainly not least – the person's family and friends.

Your family doctor should be able to refer you to a palliative care service in your community. In general, these services begin working with people and their families when the medical prognosis suggests that death will occur within three to six months. (A growing number of doctors hesitate to make such predictions, simply because they have seen so many people outlive them.) Some programs are more flexible and focus on the person's actual symptoms and needs, rather than how many months or weeks may be left.

If you or someone in your family is facing a terminal illness, your doctor may raise the subject of palliative care. Sometimes relatives may discuss the idea with the doctor before raising the issue with the person who is ill.

This is often a difficult step for people and their families to take, because it forces them to admit that the sick person is probably going to die. You must weigh the situation carefully: Does it do more harm to raise the palliative care option and rob the sick person of his desire to deny death? Or will that person suffer more by remaining at home or in hospital where care is probably inadequate?

It's easy to become overwhelmed and feel out of control when someone you love is dying. If you understand the process and know what to expect, this can make the situation a bit easier to bear.

Experts who study death and dying have identified several stages of terminal illness. The process generally begins with disbelief and denial, and progresses through other emotions, including anger, bargaining, depression and acceptance. But there are no absolutes: Some people may remain in the first stage of denial until they are very close to death. It's also very common for people to move back and forth between these emotions, depending on the progress of their disease.

Try to remember that your doctors and nurses are only human – they have their own personal fears about death. Because they have been trained to see death as a failure, some doctors are uncomfortable answering questions from seriously or terminally ill patients and their families. If you have a good relationship with your family doctor, he may be the best one to answer your questions and help you deal with your fears.

Finally, depression is extremely common among people facing terminal illness. Some experts believe that, especially in the later stages of illness, such depression may actually serve a purpose: This withdrawal into oneself allows the person to separate from others and also to contemplate both the meaning and the ending of life. However, in the earlier stages of illness, a deep or prolonged depression may jeopardize whatever quality of life remains. In this situation antidepressant medication may be useful in easing the depression.

What to expect from care services

With the support of a palliative care or hospice program, you can remain at home comfortably for much longer than you could without such support. If it's your wish, you can also die at home.

Here's what usually happens:

◆ Once you've decided to seek palliative care for yourself or a family member, your doctor or local hospital can put you in touch with palliative care services in your own community.

◆ If you have a large family or rely mainly on friends, one person will be asked to serve as the "primary caregiver." The palliative care team will coordinate its efforts through that person.

◆ Your medical care may be directed by your own personal physician or by a doctor attached to the palliative care service. The doctor will devise a treatment plan to manage symptoms and control pain, allowing you to be as comfortable and active as possible.

◆ A home care nurse may visit you on a regular basis to monitor your physical condition and dispense certain medications and treatments. A health care aide or attendant may also be available to assist with daily activities such as bathing, dressing and eating.

◆ A social worker can help you and your family access community services such as Meals-on-Wheels or homemaker support and will also provide counseling and emotional support.

◆ If necessary, you can be transferred from home to a palliative care unit in a hospital. The goal of care in this setting remains essentially the same: to meet your physical, emotional and spiritual needs and allow you to remain comfortable for as long as possible.

What you should know about pain control

Certain diseases which end in death are relatively painless, and in many cases, nature generously bestows a sudden heart attack during sleep or a final period of unconsciousness. But pain and fear of pain are often a major factor in dying.

One of the main goals of palliative care is

to relieve pain. Here is what you should know about pain control:

◆ *Non-drug approaches:* Feelings of anxiety, despair, loneliness and a sense of losing control can all intensify the physical sensations of pain. That's why providing emotional support is an important aspect of pain control. Other non-drug approaches include massage, hypnosis or deep relaxation, electrical nerve stimulation and acupuncture. Cancer pain may be relieved by using chemotherapy and radiation that shrinks pain-causing tumors. Some types of nerve pain respond to the injection of an anesthetic (called a "nerve block").

◆ *Drugs:* Mild to moderate pain may be relieved by a mild analgesic such as acetaminophen, or acetaminophen combined with a narcotic such as codeine. Other drugs not usually considered to be painkillers may also be useful – for example, some anti-depressants and anti-convulsant drugs. Sedatives may be prescribed to help the person sleep.

If pain becomes severe, more potent narcotics such as morphine may become necessary. Unfortunately, many people – even some doctors – have certain misconceptions about narcotics, and they may hesitate to use these painkilling drugs. Or if they do prescribe them, they may not prescribe enough to provide adequate pain relief.

◆ *Myth:* Narcotics are "last ditch" drugs, and once they are used, nothing else is available.

◆ *Fact:* Narcotics can be given regularly, with continuing benefit, for as long they are needed. Most people obtain pain relief on low to moderate doses, and very few will ever need extremely high doses – although most narcotics can be given safely in high doses.

◆ *Myth:* If you take narcotics for pain, you will become addicted.

◆ *Fact:* People who become addicted to narcotics don't usually take these drugs for pain relief. In fact, addiction to drugs like morphine that are given for pain control is extremely rare. It's true that some people may develop a tolerance for narcotics – that is, their bodies become accustomed to the drug and higher doses become necessary in order to obtain the same level of relief. But many other people never develop this tolerance – if they do need increasing doses of medication, in most cases it's due to a worsening of the underlying illness. If a person needs to come off a narcotic drug, this can be done safely under medical supervision.

◆ *Myth:* If you take narcotics you will become sedated and unable to communicate.

◆ *Fact:* It's true that when a narcotic is first given or the dose is increased, you might experience drowsiness or a "spacy" feeling. However, as your body adjusts to the drug, these effects subside – usually within 48 to 72 hours.

The way pain-controlling medication is delivered may be just as important as the drugs that are used. Many hospitals continue to give painkilling drugs "as required," and this can cause problems. *To maintain an effective level of pain control, you should be taking the prescribed drug regularly every four hours around the clock – even if you aren't experiencing pain.* If a dose is missed, the pain will recur. Not only does this "breakthrough pain" cause needless suffering and anxiety, but you will probably need a higher dose of medication to control it.

Caring for a dying person at home

Given the choice, most people say that they would like to die at home in familiar surroundings, preferably in the company of those who love them, perhaps with a beloved cat or dog nearby. Family members and friends may want to honor a person's wish to die at home, and this can certainly be arranged with enough support. However, taking care of a dying person at home is physically and emotionally exhausting, and you should ask yourself certain questions before taking on the challenge:

◆ Are the bathroom facilities adequate?

◆ Is there enough room for the sick person and any necessary equipment?

◆ Can you afford the extra expense of equipment and paid caregivers to relieve you if necessary?

Here's a partial list of equipment needed to care for a dying person at home:

◆ adjustable-height bed;

◆ bedside commodes, bedpans, urinals;

◆ special mattresses and sheepskins to protect skin;

◆ grab rails and/or mechanical lifts in the bathroom;

◆ oxygen and suction equipment;

◆ recreational equipment, including TV, games, a stereo player.

Many people are able to die peacefully and well at home, and their families often speak positively of the experience, saying it was incredibly meaningful and helped them to overcome their feelings of grief and loss.

But sometimes the plan to die at home, however well-intentioned, doesn't work out. The ill person may feel extremely anxious away from the hospital, or she may begin to feel guilty about the demands being made on caregivers. Caregivers themselves may soon discover that they underestimated how emotionally and physically difficult such an arrangement would be.

In these cases, families should not feel guilty about changing their minds and having the person admitted to a palliative care unit in a hospital. They can spend their time and energy working within the system to help their loved one die as peacefully as possible.

Some palliative care programs encourage a system of "patient-controlled analgesia" or PCA. A special apparatus allows people on subcutaneous (delivered continuously by a needle under the skin) pain medication to control the amount of drug they are receiving according to their own needs, within a safe limit. Studies have found that when people have this control, they tend to be less anxious, experience less pain and even use less medication than those who must wait for a nurse to bring them their next dose.

Unfortunately many hospitals still don't employ the latest pain-control techniques for terminally ill patients, and this can lead to unnecessary suffering. If you find that hospital staff hesitate to increase pain medication or give medication on a continual, as-needed basis, ask the doctors why. If you aren't satisfied with their answers, you should consider moving to a more progressive facility.

What happens during the final days?

One reason people fear dying is that they don't know what to expect during the final days and hours.

Although no one can predict when someone will die, certain physical changes may occur that suggest that the body is slowing down and preparing for death. If family members are aware that such changes are normal and even expected, the situation may be less stressful. *It's important to understand that the following changes may or may not occur, and the process itself can last hours, days or even weeks.*

Restlessness

The person may seem agitated, calling out or pulling at bed linens or clothing. This is often due to hallucinations caused by changes in body chemistry. Holding the person's hand, speaking in a calm reassuring voice or playing soft, familiar music may help ease restlessness now.

Forgetfulness and confusion

These may be part of the person's disease or the result of fatigue, pain, changes in body chemistry or a side effect of medication. Such confusion can be upsetting for family members, but they should understand this is a natural part of the dying process.

Difficulty swallowing

Muscle weakness may make swallowing more difficult, and the person may refuse to eat or drink. If they are pushed to take nourishment, people often refuse all sustenance. But when families and caregivers refrain from forcing food, the person may show an interest in taking small sips of water or ice chips.

Sleeping patterns

The person may begin to sleep for much longer periods and have trouble waking. Family members should avoid overstimulation and plan conversations during periods of alertness.

Changes in the skin

Bluish or purple markings may appear on the person's arms or legs, and the skin may feel cool due to poor circulation. Since the person is unaware of feeling cold, there's no need for extra or heavier blankets, which will only make the person feel weighed down and restless. A light mohair blanket can provide warmth without excessive weight.

Changes in breathing

Shortness of breath may occur at this stage, and may be relieved by oxygen or morphine. Sometimes saliva collects at the back of the throat and in the upper airway – because of muscle weakness, the person isn't able to swallow this saliva, and noisy breathing may develop. This may be upsetting to others but probably doesn't bother the person. Irregular and shallow breathing are common in the final hours, and there may be brief periods when respiration stops completely for many moments. These silences are often followed by a huge sigh or gasp as breathing begins once more. Again, these sounds may be upsetting to loved ones, but they are a normal sign that the body is slowing down and death is near.

Acknowledgment of professional reviewers

This book would not have been possible without the contributions of the following staff at Baycrest Centre for Geriatric Care in Toronto, Ontario, who reviewed all or part of the material:

Shayna Alpern, BSc PT, Director of Physiotherapy, Baycrest Centre

Dana Bach, BA, D. Grt., Fitness and Health Promotion, Baycrest Centre

David Conn, MD, MB, BCh, BAO, BA, Psychiatrist-in-Chief and Program Director, Department of Psychiatry, Baycrest Centre; Assistant Professor, Department of Psychiatry, University of Toronto

Morris Freedman, BSc, MD, FRCP (C), Director of Behavioural Neurology Program, staff neurologist, Baycrest Centre; Associate Professor of Medicine, University of Toronto

John Gasner, DDS, Acting Chief of Dentistry, Baycrest Centre

Etta Ginsberg-McEwan, MSW, CSW, formerly Director of Social Work, Baycrest Centre

Michael Gordon, MD, FRCP (C), Vice President of Medical Services and Head of Geriatrics and Internal Medicine at Baycrest Centre; Professor of Medicine, University of Toronto

Moshe Greengarten, MBA, CHE, PhD, Vice President of Public and Community Affairs, Baycrest Centre

Wulf Grobin, MD, staff physician, Fellow in Research and Consultant in Diabetes, Baycrest Centre

Edward Gutman, MD, CCFP, attending physician, Palliative Care Unit, Baycrest Centre

Linda Kremer, PT (reg.), OT (C), Supervisor of Fitness and Health Promotion, Baycrest Centre

Susan Lieff, MD, Consultation Liaison Psychiatrist, Baycrest Centre; Assistant Professor of Psychiatry and Postgraduate Education Coordinator, Division of Geriatric Psychiatry, University of Toronto

Margaret MacAdam, PhD, Senior Vice President, Baycrest Centre

Mortimer Mamelak, BSc, MDCM, staff psychiatrist, coordinator of Sleep Disorders Clinic, Baycrest Centre; Associate Professor of Psychiatry, University of Toronto

Kit Martin, RN, Head Nurse, Palliative Care Unit, Baycrest Centre

Aruna Mitra, BSc, OT, Director of Occupational Therapy, Baycrest Centre

Guy Proulx, PhD, C. Psych., Director of the Department of Psychology, Baycrest Centre

Carol Robertson, BA, BAA, RD, Manager of Clinical/Patient Food and Nutrition Services, Baycrest Centre

Paula A. Rochon, MD, MPH, FRCP (C), staff geriatrician and clinical evaluator/epidemiologist, Baycrest Centre; Assistant Professor, Division of Geriatric Medicine, Assistant Professor, Department of Preventive Medicine and Biostatistics, University of Toronto

Jennifer Schipper, MA, ABC, Director of Public Relations Department, Baycrest Centre

Michel Silberfeld, BSc, MDCM, MSC, FRCP (C), Coordinator of Competency Clinic, Department of Psychiatry, Baycrest Centre; Assistant Professor of Psychiatry, University of Toronto

Allan Steingart, BSc, MD, FRCP, staff psychiatrist, Coordinator of the Psychiatric Day Hospital, Baycrest Centre; Assistant Professor in the Departments of Psychiatry and Preventive Medicine and Biostatistics, University of Toronto

Don Stuss, BA, BPh, MA, PhD, Vice President of Research, Director of Rotman Research Institute of Baycrest Centre; Professor in the Department of Psychology, the Department of Medicine (Neurology), and the Centre for Studies on Aging, University of Toronto

Sorele Urman, BA, BSW, MSW, Director of Coordinated Client Service, Baycrest Centre; Social Work Practice professor, Faculty of Social Work, University of Toronto

The material was also reviewed by the following people from outside Baycrest Centre for Geriatric Care:

Rory Fisher, MD, FRCP (C), FRCP (E), Medical Director of Northern Service, Metropolitan Toronto Regional Geriatric Program; on staff in the Division of Geriatric Medicine, Department of Medicine, Sunnybrook Health Science Centre; Consultant Geriatrician to Toronto Grace Hospital and Riverdale Hospital

Harvey Kaplovitch, MD, CCFP, Family Physician in private practice

Blossom T. Wigdor, CM, PhD, Professor Emeritus, Centre for Studies of Aging, Departments of Psychology and Behavioural Science, University of Toronto

Index

A

Abuse by a family member, 253–254
Accidents, 84
Acetaminophen, 77
Acetylsalicylic acid (ASA), 27, 77, 117, 130, 156
Acquired Immunodeficiency Syndrome (AIDS), 47
Acute pulmonary edema, 152
Adjustment disorder, 219–220
Aerobic exercise, 31–32, 35, 36
Aging, 11, 51, 78. *See also* "Old age"
  negative aspects of, 12
  positive aspects of, 12–13
Agoraphobia, 226
AIDS, 47
Alcohol, 230
  abuse of, 220–221, 230–231
  and sleep, 42
Aluminum, and Alzheimer's disease, 203
Alzheimer's disease, 200, 201–207
  advice for caregivers, 204–205, 206–207
  diagnosis, 203–205
  early warning signs, 202
  management of, 206–207
  stages, 201–202
Analgesics (painkillers), 76, 77
Anemia, 20
Anesthesiologists, 63
Angina, 150–151
Angioplasty, 114, 156
Antacids, 76–77, 110
Antibiotics, 27, 73, 112, 115
Antidepressants, 214–216

Antihistamines, 98
Antihypertensive drugs, 173, 214
Anurex, 109
Anxiety, 100, 222–223, 229
  disorders, 223–227
Apartments
  assisted living, 263
  subsidized, 263
Aphasia, 172–173
Appearance
  attitudes toward, 39, 53
  changes in, 53–54, 55, 56–57
Appetite, loss of, 29
Arrhythmia, 84
Arteries, hardening of the, 113, 150
Arthritis, 48, 126–131
  common types, 126–127
  strategies for living with, 131
  surgery, 129–131
  treatment, 128–129
ASA, 27, 77, 117, 130, 156
Aspirin. *See* ASA
Atherosclerosis, 113, 150
Athlete's foot, 103
Atrial fibrillation (AF), 155, 171

B

Back pain, 93–96. *See also names of specific back disorders*
Back surgery, 96
Balance, sense of, 36, 84, 85, 100
  medications affecting, 44
Baldness, 55
Beano, 25–26
Bed, confinement in, 113–114
Behavior therapy, 194
Benign tumor, 140
Bereavement, stages of normal, 241
Biopsy, 140
Bipolar disorder. *See* Manic depression

Bladder
  displacement, 162
  neck suspension surgery, 163
  retraining, 161
Bleeding
  gastric, 130
  rectal, 98, 109
Bloating, 25
Blood analysis, 68
Blood pressure, taking, 65
Bone(s), 163. *See also* Fractures
  loss, 36, 163, 167
Bone spurs, 93
Boredom, 43, 52, 102
Bowel cancer, 25
Breast(s)
  cancer, 188–189 (men), 133–136 (women)
  enlargement of male, 188
  reduction surgery, 56
  regular clinical exam, 65, 136
  self-examination, 136–137
Brown age spots, 54
Bunions, 103, 104

C

Caffeine, 26, 42, 222
Calcium, 165–166, 167
Calorie requirements, 23, 29
Cancer, 132–143
  pain relief, 278
  prevention strategy, 133
  surgery, 142. *See also names of specific types*
Cardiac arrest, 151
Cardiac arrhythmias, 154–155
Cardiologists, 63
Caregivers, 254
  family, 237, 238, 254, 255, 261, 262, 267
  professional, 263–267
Carotid endarterectomy, 171
CAT (Computerized Axial Tomography) scan, 170, 204

Indigestion, 110–111
Influenza, 97
Ingrown toenails, 103, 104
Injuries due to exercise, 33
Insomnia, 41, 43
Institutional care, 14
Insulin injections, 148
Intergenerational programs, 52
Internists, 63
Intertrigo, 54
Itchiness, 111–112, 146

J

Joint pain, 127
Joint replacement surgery, 130–131

K

Kegel exercises, 161
Ketoprofen, 130
Knee problems, 127, 128

L

Lactose intolerance, 27, 111, 166
Laxatives, 27, 76, 99
Legal guardian, appointment of, 274
Leg pain, 113–114
Leukoplakia, 115
Lightheadedness, 100
Lithium, 218–219
Living arrangements. *See* Apartments; Group homes; Home sharing; Moving in together; Retirement homes
Loneliness, 52, 72, 243, 248
Loss, dealing with, 79, 242
Lubricant jelly, 47
Lumpectomy, 140
Lung cancer, 137–138
Lymph nodes, 140

M

Macular degeneration, 121
"Male pattern" baldness, 55
Malignant tumor, 141
Mammogram, 69, 136, 141

Manic depression, 217–219
Mastectomy, 136, 141
  and sexual activity following, 48
Masturbation, 49
Meal home delivery programs, 21, 262
Medical alert bracelet, 88
Medical checkups, 62, 64–65
Medical tests, 67, 68
Medication(s), 67, 72, 74.
  See also names of specific types of medication
  child-proof caps on, 74
  interactions between, 72, 74, 76, 77
  keeping track of, 74–75
  mistakes, 72–74, 84
  non-prescription, 75–76, 97
  prescription, 75
  rebound effect of, 75
  and sexual response, 48–49
  side effects, 72, 73, 76, 99
  sleeping, 44.
Medicine cabinet, 74, 87
Memory, 50–51, 196–198.
  See also Forgetfulness
Menopause, 167, 179–181
  male, 186
Mental disorders, 193, 195.
  See also names of specific disorders
Mental illness. *See* Mental disorders
Metastasis, 141
Migraine headache, 104, 105, 106
Milk intolerance, 27, 111, 166
Mills, Eleanor, 12
Minerals, 27–28
Minoxidil, 55
Mohs surgery, 140
Morphine, 278
Mouth
  cancer, 115
  dry, 20, 115–116, 223
  lesions in, 115
  pain, 114–115

Moving in together
  adult children with parents, 252–253
  parents with adult children, 247–249
MRI (Magnetic Resonance Imaging) scan, 69, 170, 214

N

Napping, 41, 42, 43
Naproxen, 130
Narcotics, 278
Neck pain, 116–117
Nephrologists, 63
Neurologists, 63, 195
  behavioral, 195
Neuropathy, 145
Neuropsychological tests, 204–205
Nocturnal myoclonus, 45
Non-medical healers, 70–71
Non-steroidal anti-inflammatory drugs (NSAIDs), 77, 117, 130
Nose drops and sprays, 98
Numbness, 104, 116, 146, 169
Nurses, 66–67
Nursing assistants, 67
Nursing homes, 267, 270–271
  checklist, 268–269
  common feelings about, 268–270
  types of services provided by, 270
Nutrition, 19, 20, 21, 22–23, 29

O

Obesity, 35, 133, 147, 152, 161
Obsessive-compulsive disorder (OCD), 226
Occupational therapists, 68, 174, 195
"Old age," perceptions of, 11–12, 13, 45, 46, 48, 78

Stroke, 169–175
  reducing risk of, 35, 171
Suicide, 220–221, 230
Sulfonylurea, 148
Sunlight
  protection from, 54, 139
  and vitamin D, 26–27
Sunscreen, 54, 139
Surgeons, 63
Surgery. *See names of
    specific types*
Swallowing, 20, 68

T

Tamoxifen, 141
Taste, sense of, 20, 28
Teeth
  care of, 57, 66
  loss of, 57
Telecare program, 88
Temperature. *See* Sensitivity
    to heat and cold
Temporal arteritis, 128
Tension headache, 104, 105,
    106
Thrush, 115
Toenails, ingrown, 103, 104
Tranquilizers, 159, 225
Transient ischemic attack
    (TIA), 170, 171

Transurethral prostatectomy
    (TURP), 185
Travel, 52, 80
Tremors, 209
Tumors, 140, 141

U

Ulcers, 111
Ultrasound, 69
Urinalysis, 68
Urologists, 63
Uterus
  dropping of, 162
  removal of, 181–182

V

Vagina, 65
  lubrication of, 47, 180
Varicose veins, 120
Ventricular fibrillation, 155
Vertigo, 100
Vision
  impaired, 120–121
  sudden loss of, 169
Vitamin B_{12}, 26
Vitamin C, 27
Vitamin D, 26–27, 166–167
Vitamin(s), 26
  supplements, 26, 27

W

Walking
  aids, 86
  to improve fitness, 34–35,
    40
  indoor programs, 38
  pain felt while, 113
  three-month program, 37
Warts, 103
Water, importance of in diet,
    26, 54, 99
Weight-bearing exercise, 36,
    167, 168
Weight control, 19, 29, 30,
    35, 133, 152, 168
Weight ranges for older
    adults, 22
Widowers, 184, 220, 240,
    242
Widows, 184, 224, 240, 242
Will, 271
  living, 272–273

Y

Yeast infections, 112

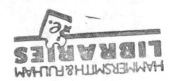